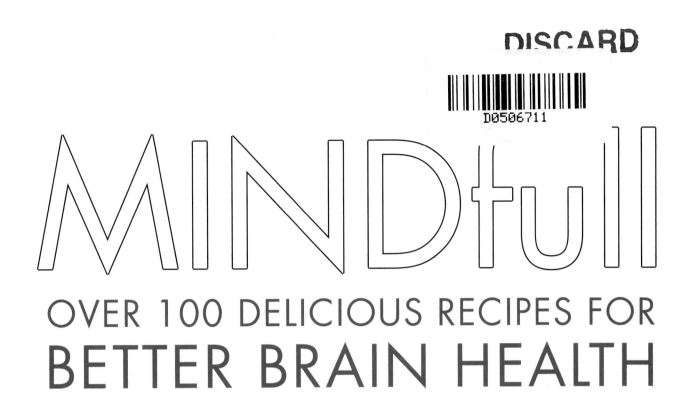

MINDfull

OVER 100 DELICIOUS RECIPES FOR
BETTER BRAIN HEALTH

CAROL GREENWOOD, PhD
DAPHNA RABINOVITCH • JOANNA GRYFE

Collins

Mindfull
Copyright © 2012, 2013 by The Baycrest Centre Foundation

Published by Collins, an imprint of HarperCollins Publishers Ltd

An earlier version of this work was originally published in ebook form only by The Baycrest Centre Foundation in 2012, and was reissued by HarperCollins Publishers Ltd in 2013.

All photographs by David Shuken, except the following: Shutterstock, pp. xvi, 36; iStockphoto, pp. 18, 25, 33, 37, 47, 60, 81, 91, 103, 194, 205, 210, 232, 235, 245, 247, 262

HarperCollins books may be purchased for educational, business, or sales promotional use through our Special Markets Department.

HarperCollins Publishers Ltd
2 Bloor Street East, 20th Floor
Toronto, Ontario, Canada
M4W 1A8

www.harpercollins.ca

Library and Archives Canada Cataloguing in Publication information is available upon request.

ISBN 978-1-44342-408-0

Printed and bound in Canada
TC 9 8 7 6 5 4 3 2 1

MINDfull

Contents

A Message from Baycrest ... vi
Introduction ... vii
Mindfull Living: The Science of Brain Health ... ix
Health Savvy: Using the Nutrition Information in This Book ... xvii

Chapter 1
Breaking the Fast: The First Fuel Zone ... 1

Chapter 2
Morning Brain Boosters: Fuel on the Go ... 39

Chapter 3
Lunch for All: Mid-Day Mindfullness ... 67

Chapter 4
Afternoon Brain Boosters: Slump Ye Not ... 117

Chapter 5
Appetizing Appetizers: Navigating the Witching Hour ... 143

Chapter 6
The Dinner Plate: Colour, Crunch and a Whole Lot of Versatility ... 171

Chapter 7
Delicious Desserts: Sweet Endings, Sweet Dreams ... 237

Acknowledgements ... 268
About the Authors ... 270
References ... 272
Glossary of Cooking Terms ... 276
Index ... 279

A Message from Baycrest

For nearly a century, Baycrest Health Sciences has continually adapted to changing needs to remain at the forefront of seniors' care and brain-health research. Today, we are recognized as the global leader in innovative care delivery and cutting-edge cognitive neuroscience. Affiliated with the University of Toronto, Baycrest is among the world's most respected academic health sciences centres focused on the needs of seniors and our aging population.

We provide care and service to approximately 1200 people a day through a unique continuum of care from wellness programs, residential housing, and outpatient clinics to a 472-bed nursing home and a 300-bed complex continuing care hospital facility with an acute care unit.

Baycrest is leading the charge to reshape the future of aging today. The Rotman Research Institute is home to world-renowned researchers, encompassing a broad spectrum of expertise ranging from behavioural neurology to cognitive psychology to neuro-pharmacology.

At Baycrest, we create, evaluate and transfer new practices, knowledge and products from our health sciences platform and bring them to market to provide a system-wide impact on care delivery, quality of life and health and wellness for an aging population.

Annually, nearly 1000 students, trainees and other practitioners from 24 universities and colleges have a unique opportunity to experience the delivery of high-quality care alongside leading experts on one of the world's most comprehensive campuses of care focused on aging and care of older adults.

Bringing *Mindfull* into your home is one more way that we are changing what it means to age.

To learn more about Baycrest's activities, visit our web site: www.baycrest.org.

Introduction

Lasting memories often revolve around food: the scent of garlic surrounding your grand-mother, the way chocolate stained your mother's hands, your father's famous roast chicken, late-night tubs of ice cream with your friends. So we thought it fitting that food be a driving force in the battle to save the memories and minds of friends, family members and loved ones everywhere.

Fifty percent of Alzheimer's diagnoses are attributed to modifiable risk factors, including diet- and lifestyle-associated disorders like high blood pressure, type 2 diabetes and obesity. This means that our lifestyle choices are as important as our genes in determining our brain health.

While scientists have researched the nutrition of brain health for years, this informa-tion has never been handed over to the home cook. Women of Baycrest, a dynamic group of volunteers focused on brain-health research and healthy aging, decided to create a cookbook that would fill the gap. And that's where we came in.

A leading senior scientist and professor of nutrition and brain health with our Rotman Research Institute—one of the top five ranked cognitive neuroscience institutes in the world—a professional food writer, baker and recipe developer, as well as a curious "foodie" heeded the call to bake, roast, sift, and sauté a delicious translation of the science everyone wants to understand. We are forever indebted to the celebrated cooks, chefs and other food professionals across the country who also generously contributed to this project. The product of this culinary collaboration is *Mindfull*, a cookbook that provides food for your table and even more food for thought.

Our hope is that this book will be a valuable tool for sustaining a brain-healthy diet. From dining room dinners to portable snacks, every page bursts with a fresh approach to cooking designed to take you from morning to night.

From the bottom of our hearts, we thank you for including *Mindfull* in your cookbook collection and, in doing so, supporting Baycrest, a leader in developing and providing innovations in aging brain health. May each morsel and mouthful advance brain-health science and take you one meal closer to sharing more meals with your family and friends for a long, long time.

Here's to many healthy helpings!

Carol, Daphna, Joanna and the Women of Baycrest

Mindfull Living:
The Science of Brain Health

In the last 20 years, a burst of new information has fundamentally changed our thinking about the human brain. No longer is the brain considered a "static" organ that ceases to grow beyond adolescence. Instead, we now know it has a wonderful capacity to refresh, to renew and to repair itself and to create new brain cells and new connections throughout a person's life.

Today, what we refer to as "successful aging" embraces this capacity of the brain to grow and renew—even in the face of the challenges of aging. In fact, we now know that our lifestyle choices can have a huge impact on the degree to which we retain our brain's capacity. The health and lifestyle choices we make as early as age 40 can determine our brain's health and function much later in life. So it is never too early (and never too late!) to adopt a healthy lifestyle to promote successful aging, not just for our bodies but also for our brains.

In the next few pages, you will discover what it means to pursue a brain-healthy lifestyle. Later, you will discover how the food choices you make can play an important role as well. We'll review the current scientific evidence on the best "brain foods," discuss the many myths and misconceptions about the brain and show you what types of changes to make for your own brain-healthy diet.

Rest assured, all the recipes in this book are both easy to prepare and designed to be consistent with the science behind brain health. Think of them as stepping stones on a gradual path towards a diet that increases your ability to strengthen your memory, mental clarity and brain health. All of the information in this cookbook is based on sound science. At the end of the book, we also provide you with helpful links to credible web sites and specific citations if you choose to further your reading in specific areas.

A Healthy Body Leads to a Healthy Brain

In addition to eating a brain-healthy diet, there are many things you can do during the day to boost your cognitive function. This information opens each chapter and is linked to specific times of day or meals. Also emphasized are strategies to help us maintain our body weight. That's because the brain is intimately involved in controlling our feelings of hunger and satiety. As you may know, obesity-related disorders can damage the health of your brain. Maintaining a healthy body weight is an important part of maintaining a healthy brain.

So the first thing we need to focus on when talking about brain health is the overall health of our bodies. Many chronic disorders, including high blood pressure, elevated blood cholesterol and type 2 diabetes, are associated with increased rates of cognitive decline with aging. In some instances, this loss of cognitive function can proceed to actual dementia. We all recognize these as lifestyle disorders that we can control through lifestyle choices, including diet. While adopting a healthy lifestyle may not prevent cognitive decline or dementia, it can help delay the age at which we start to experience symptoms. Here's some advice from the Alzheimer Society of Canada about what you can do to promote healthy brain aging.

Heads Up for a Healthier Brain—Advice from the Alzheimer Society of Canada

Challenge Yourself—Research suggests that mental stimulation enhances brain activity and may help you maintain your cognitive function throughout life. This can take many different forms, such as playing mind-challenging games (e.g., chess, crossword puzzles, Sudoku), learning a new language or musical instrument, and staying engaged in hobbies. While playing computer games may help with challenging you cognitively, many computer games have not been scientifically tested for their ability to improve brain function or to help retain cognitive function over time. So if you select gaming as a means of supporting or enhancing your cognitive function, be certain there is scientific evidence supporting any claim.

Be Socially Active—People who regularly interact with others maintain their brain function better than those who do not. There are many ways to maintain social connectedness: keeping in touch with old friends, volunteering, joining groups, even just saying hello and striking up a conversation with people you meet in public or while shopping.

Be Physically Active—Physical activity not only protects you from developing high blood pressure, elevated blood cholesterol and type 2 diabetes, it also has direct benefits on the brain. Even moderate physical activity helps maintain blood flow to the brain. In addition, research suggests that physical activity may help promote the development of new brain cells and aid in making new connections between existing brain cells. You don't have to run marathons or climb mountains, either. In fact, most experts say just 30 minutes of moderate physical activity a day, such as walking, are enough to make a significant difference in your health. A component of your exercise should be aerobic to maximize its brain-beneficial effects.

Reduce Stress—As you may know, chronic stress can have adverse effects on your blood vessels and can trigger the release of hormones that damage brain cells. While reducing stress is sometimes easier said than done, practicing activities like meditation, yoga, tai chi, deep breathing, massage and physical activity are all examples of ways to relieve stress.

Protect Your Head—With recent media attention, we are all becoming more aware of the terrible danger of concussions and the need to protect our heads. We now know to wear helmets when participating in contact sports or fast-moving sports (e.g., cycling, skiing, skateboarding). And we remember to buckle our seat belt when driving, knowing that hitting the windshield is a common cause of severe head injury that can lead to permanent cognitive loss.

Choose Wisely—Avoid harmful habits such as smoking and excessive alcohol consumption. Also, see your family physician regularly and keep on top of your weight, blood pressure and cholesterol. Be sure to get 7 to 8 hours of sleep whenever possible, as sleep deprivation can have a negative impact on brain function, too.

Healthy Food Choices—The Alzheimer Society of Canada suggests that you consume a diet high in fruits, vegetables, whole grains, fish (and other sources of omega-3 fatty acids) and low in saturated fat, salt and alcohol. They also suggest consuming a wide variety of colourful foods and maintaining your body weight within a healthy range.

Eating Your Way Towards a Healthy Brain

Many scientific studies show a high-quality diet helps protect your brain function as you age. Studies in Canada, Europe and the USA repeatedly demonstrate that a diet high in fruits, vegetables, whole grains, cereals, and fish protects your brain. Conversely, diets high in saturated fat, red meat and highly processed foods are associated with greater rates of cognitive decline and increased risk of developing dementia. A healthy diet filled with fruits, vegetables, whole grains and fish supports your body and brain in so many ways. First, it strengthens your blood vessels, allowing more oxygen and nutrients to reach every cell in your body. Second, it nourishes areas of your brain that are actively involved with speech, learning, and reasoning. Third, it protects your body and brain against inflammation, which has been linked to many diseases. And finally, a nutrient-rich diet promotes the growth of new brain cells and new neural connections.

Delicious Brain-Healthy Nutrients*

Plant-Based Phytochemicals, or Polyphenols

Polyphenols are natural substances found in fruits, vegetables and nuts and range from the anthocyanins in berries, the resveratrol in red wine, the catechins in green tea, the flavonoids in chocolate and the lycopenes in tomatoes to the curcumin in turmeric and piperine in black pepper. All of these compounds were originally felt to exert their brain-protective effects because of their antioxidant and anti-inflammatory properties. Antioxidants help protect tissues, including the brain, from oxidative stress and inflammation and may

---

* Adapted from J. Joseph et al.'s "Nutrition, Brain Aging and Neurodegeneration"; Carol Sorgen's "Eat Smart for a Healthier Brain"; and the Dietitians of Canada web site. (See References section for more information.)

reduce the effects of age-related conditions such as Alzheimer's disease or dementia. More recent research suggests that these compounds may also support brain nerve cell communication and survival.

Where to find them:
Most plants, including nuts, fruits, vegetables, seeds and spices, especially those that are deeply coloured.

Foods that have been studied for these properties and contain high levels of potent phytochemicals include blueberries, strawberries, pomegranates, tomatoes, green tea, chocolate, grapes and red wine, walnuts, turmeric and black pepper.

Vitamin E

Vitamin E functions as an antioxidant and is involved in immune function. Higher levels of this vitamin correspond to less cognitive decline as you get older.

Where to find it:
Nuts, seeds and oils, including sunflower seeds, almonds, walnuts, hazelnuts, Brazil nuts, cashews, peanuts and peanut butter, sesame seeds, and flaxseeds and flaxseed oil.

Omega-3 Fatty Acids

Omega-3 fatty acids are essential for healthy brain function and may help reduce brain inflammation. While fish is the preferred source of omega-3 fatty acids for the brain, those found in other plant foods can also be used by the brain, albeit less efficiently. (For more information on omega-3 fatty acids, see page 157.)

Where to find them:
Fatty fish including salmon, mackerel, sardines, herring and trout; soybeans; flax, soybean or canola oils; omega-3 fortified beverages or eggs.

Monounsaturated Fats

Monounsaturated fats contribute to healthy blood flow throughout your body, including your brain. They also help fight high blood cholesterol and hypertension, which are risk factors in cognitive decline.

Where to find them:
Avocados; olives; olive and canola oils; nuts including hazelnuts, pecans, almonds, cashews, filberts and pistachios.

Fibre

Fibre stabilizes your blood glucose levels and helps lower your blood cholesterol. Your brain depends on glucose for "fuel."

Where to find it:
Lentils and beans; whole grains, such as oatmeal, whole-grain breads, and brown rice.

Folate and Vitamin B$_{12}$

These vitamins help maintain the health of your blood vessels and are required for many biological reactions essential for brain cell communication. Vitamin B$_{12}$ is also needed to maintain the myelin sheath that coats our nerves and allows for faster brain cell communication. While evidence is mounting that these two vitamins can lower your risk of developing dementia, the current evidence remains insufficient to draw firm conclusions.

Where to find them:
Folate is found in dark green vegetables like broccoli and spinach and in legumes such as chickpeas, beans and lentils. In Canada, folic acid is added to all white flour, enriched pasta and cornmeal products.

Vitamin B$_{12}$ is found only in animal foods, including eggs, milk, cheese, milk products, meat, fish, shellfish and poultry and fortified foods, including rice and soy beverages and soy-based meat substitutes (check the Nutrition Facts for levels in these foods).

Spice Up Your Brain for Healthy Aging

In addition to eating brain-healthy foods, certain spices and herbs can also contribute to your intake of brain-protective compounds and help shield your brain from the wear and tear of aging. Some of the more potent spices include turmeric, oregano, vanilla, cinnamon, parsley, basil, sage and pepper. Indian food, for example, contains a potent antioxidant and anti-inflammatory spice called turmeric (curcumin), which is a key ingredient in curry. Because people in India have lower rates of dementia than other countries, scientists are looking at whether curried foods protect the brain from Alzheimer's disease. Many studies conducted in mice report that curcumin protects against inflammation and the cascade of pathologic events contributing to Alzheimer's disease. The relevance of these studies to humans is still awaiting verification, although there is one report of better cognitive performance in elderly Asians who consume curry relative to those who do not.

Scientists are studying other phytochemicals (compounds that occur naturally in plants and are responsible for their colour and taste) in spices (e.g., piperine in black pepper) and foods (e.g., green tea, blueberries, cocoa) that also have antioxidant and anti-inflammatory properties. Similar to results with curcumin, consumption of the isolated phytochemicals or intact food is associated with better cognitive performance and reduced indication of damage to brain areas involved in Alzheimer's disease in animal-based studies.

Clearly, the phytochemicals in both the foods and spices that we eat can play an important role in protecting our brains. In general, we get much more phytochemicals from fruits and vegetables, compared to spices, simply because we eat larger quantities of them. While spices and herbs can contribute to the healthful properties of our diet, we should still be using them primarily for their taste and as a strategy to help increase our fruit, vegetable and grain intakes by enhancing their appeal.

6 Big Myths About Diet and Brain Health

I can wait until I'm older before worrying about brain health.

Recent evidence suggests that our health status in our 50s is a better predictor of risk for cognitive decline in later life. This is particularly true with respect to obesity and other chronic disorders that compromise brain function. As we said before, it is never too early or too late to adopt a brain-healthy lifestyle.

I don't have a history of dementia in my family, so why should I worry?

While a number of genes that increase risk of dementia have been identified, not all individuals who possess these genes develop dementia. Furthermore, many individuals without genetic risk go on to develop dementia, including Alzheimer's disease. Thus, our lifestyle choices, exposure to toxins, occupation, stress level, and socio-economic status play as large a role in our brain health as our genes! These are all areas over which we have some control.

I can focus on a few healthy foods and not worry about the rest of my diet.

We need a large variety of nutrients to support optimal brain function. While some foods may be high in antioxidants, others will be high in other healthful nutrients. Unless you choose foods across all food groups (e.g., meat and meat alternatives, dairy, grains, fruits and vegetables) and across all classes of foods within a food group (e.g., berries, citrus, tree fruits), you run the risk of not meeting all of your nutritional needs. You don't have to give up all your "treats"—but they should be eaten only in moderation.

I don't have time to prepare healthy meals.

Many of the recipes included in this cookbook can be prepared in 30 minutes or less. If you can boil water or cook pre-packaged pasta or microwave frozen foods, you can easily handle these recipes. What's more, home-prepared meals bring more flavour to your plate and help you avoid excessive salt intake. This is important because high levels of salt have been associated with more rapid cognitive decline, especially in those who live a sedentary lifestyle.

You can't prove that certain foods or nutrients improve brain aging.

Well, actually, we can. There are dozens of studies like the ones mentioned above that demonstrate people who consume a healthier diet are more likely to retain their cognitive function with aging. However, these studies simply show associations: those who eat a healthy diet also have better brain function. To provide absolute proof, we need to explore what happens when individuals with a poor diet actually change their eating habits. These types of studies are currently underway, and we are awaiting the results. At present, there is one report of the adverse brain effects of adults at risk for Alzheimer's disease changing their diet to one that is high in saturated fat and high glycemic index carbohydrate foods for four weeks. (See page 32 for more information on the glycemic index.) The results of this study show us that the brain responds quickly to a poor-quality diet. The more important question awaiting an answer is what happens when someone improves their diet.

If a little bit of a vitamin is good, then more is better.

This is absolutely not true. Most of the studies relating to vitamin (or mineral) intake and poor cognitive function include individuals who are vitamin (or mineral) deficient. So, correcting a nutrient deficiency is absolutely a good thing. As we increase our intake of vitamins and minerals, we improve the biologic processes that rely on them, up to a maximal level. Nutrient requirements are established to reflect the level of nutrient intake that supports optimal function. Intake over and above this level is not helpful and can lead to toxicity. In this sense, you can consume too much of a good thing—even vitamins. It is highly unlikely that you would ever achieve toxic levels of a nutrient by eating food alone, but this could occur if you were also taking high doses of nutritional supplements or frequently consuming fortified foods.

Recommendations for a Brain-Healthy Diet

You've probably heard about the health benefits of the "Mediterranean diet." The Mediterranean diet is rich in fruits, vegetables and grains. It relies primarily on olive oil as a source of fat, and fish, chicken, dairy products and beans as sources of protein. While red meat is consumed, it is eaten monthly, rather than weekly or daily.

The Mediterranean diet is a heart-healthy eating plan that also happens to lower your risk of dementia, too. In fact, these findings are even observed in older adults residing in areas far from the Mediterranean, such as New York City. The brain health benefits of the Mediterranean diet have been attributed, in part, to its high reliance on polyphenol-rich foods, including fruits, vegetables and nuts.

While this is clearly one approach to brain-healthy eating, it's not the only one. Many styles of cooking (e.g., Asian, North American and European) can support better brain health provided they are rich in fruits, vegetables and grains and low in fat and highly processed foods. This gives you the opportunity to bring greater variety into your diet and the freedom to explore different tastes and cuisines. That's why the recipes in this cookbook embrace a multi-ethnic perspective and draw upon a vast array of foods, especially fruits, vegetables, grains and fish.

It is also true that no one specific diet is better than all others when you want to change your eating habits to lose weight. While some diets may assist with more rapid weight loss in the first few weeks, the only factor that predicts whether you lose weight and keep it off is your ability to adhere to the diet. That's why the recipes in this cookbook draw on familiar foods that are easy to prepare. General guidelines and not specific formulas are given as there are many ways to adopt healthy eating patterns. This makes changing your diet to a more healthful one that supports not only brain health but also helps you to maintain your body weight easy since it allows you to choose tastes and textures that you enjoy. (For more guidelines on healthy eating patterns, see pages 173–175.)

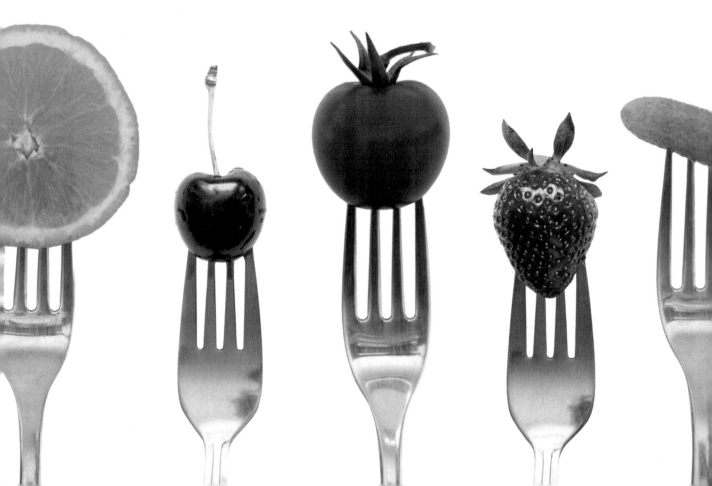

❦ Health Savvy: Using the Nutrition Information in This Book

All of the recipes in this book provide you with important nutrition information. For example, we give you both the weight (in grams or milligrams) of the nutrient and its Percentage Daily Value (%DV) in a single serving. We intentionally focused on nutrients that most individuals need to either reduce (such as fat or sodium) or increase (fibre) to support brain-healthy eating.

The nutrient values for the recipes were calculated using the Food Processor/ESHA software and database and, within that, the Canadian Nutrient File whenever possible.

All calculations were based on: 1) the first ingredient listed when there was a choice; 2) smaller ingredient amounts if there was a range; 3) 1% milk and low-fat yogurt, unless otherwise specified in the recipes; 4) non-optional ingredients; optional ingredients were not included. Nutrient values have been rounded off to the nearest whole number or 0.5 in the case of saturated fat. This information was then used to calculate the %DV based on the same principles employed in the nutrition fact table as outlined by Health Canada.

When it comes to fruits and vegetables, it's simply important that you eat more of them rather than worry about the individual nutrients in each. So we encourage you to do that.

As for Percentage Daily Value, it is a part of the nutrition fact table on packaged foods that we are now all familiar with. The %DV is not meant to be used in absolute terms; rather it can help guide you on whether a specific food, or in this case recipe, has a lot or a little of a particular nutrient and help you compare foods.

The %DV is simply meant to help you make better food choices—not to suggest that these values add up to 100% at the end of the day. We did, however, use the %DV to help guide us, especially for fat and sodium. We wanted to ensure that as we recommend lowering your fat and sodium intakes that we are providing you with recipes that enable you to do so. Wherever possible, we try to keep fat and sodium content below 20%DV, although we were not able to achieve this in all of the recipes, especially those that are meat based.

With meat-based recipes, we tried to keep %DV below 30% for fat. Since these recipes only represent one of several meals and snacks that you may eat daily, you can still keep your daily fat intake low by drawing upon plant-based recipes (e.g., salads, grains, beans) at other meals during the day.

It is important to recognize that while the %DV was developed to help Canadians consume an overall healthy diet, there is currently no information to suggest that the brain's nutrient needs are different from those reflected in an overall healthy diet.

Calories

Caloric, or energy, needs vary greatly among individuals and are dependent on factors such as genetics, body size and body composition. Our level of physical activity also has a profound effect on our daily energy needs. As a general guideline, Health Canada suggests that females aged 51 to 70 should consume between 1650 and 2100 calories per day and males in the same age bracket should consume between 2150 and 2650 calories per day.

These recommendations decrease by about 100 calories per day for people over 70 years of age. This range reflects the impact of physical activity on our daily energy needs. As a general principle, we should adjust our levels of physical activity and daily energy intake to maintain a healthy body weight. It is much healthier to do this by increasing physical activity rather than by decreasing energy (caloric) intake.

Individuals with very low energy intakes (calories) increase their risk of nutrient deficiencies because they are not consuming enough food. According to Health Canada's guidelines, we should aim to engage in 60 minutes of moderate activity, such as walking, each day. This is in addition to the activity of simply going about your day. This amount of activity should not only help prevent weight gain but also enable you to gain the additional health benefits of physical activity.

Protein

The Recommended Dietary Allowance for protein is 0.80 grams of good-quality protein for each kilogram of body weight per day for both men and women.

Most Canadians habitually consume protein well in excess of this level. As a result, your choice of protein should be based more on its overall quality rather than quantity. Be certain to rely on fish, poultry, dairy products, nuts and beans as your best choices for lean, brain-healthy protein.

Carbohydrates

Our specific requirement for glucose—usually consumed in the form of carbohydrate—is actually very low, just 130 grams a day. That's much less than what most people eat each day.

The most important role that dietary carbohydrate serves is as a healthier source of energy compared to fat. Current recommendations are to consume a diet that contains 45 to 65% of calories as carbohydrate and 20 to 35% as fat.

This balance of carbohydrate to fat is a prudent choice for lowering the risk of heart disease, obesity and obesity-associated disorders. Be certain to draw on complex carbohydrates (whole grains and cereals) versus refined carbohydrates (breads, cakes, cookies) as complex carbohydrate sources have been associated with better retention of cognitive function with aging.

Fats and Cholesterol

Fat provides energy, helps in the absorption of fat-soluble compounds including vitamins, contributes to texture and palatability of foods and is an important component of our diet.

Our actual requirements for fat are low and specific to the omega-6 and omega-3 fatty acids found in plant-based oils and fish. Canadians, in general, need to focus on reducing total fat intake, especially saturated and trans fats.

High intakes of saturated fat, found predominantly in meats and higher-fat dairy products, and trans fat, found in shortenings, hard margarines and commercially baked products, can increase blood cholesterol levels and risk of heart disease. By contrast, replacing saturated fat with monounsaturated fat sources, as we have done in this cookbook by using olive and canola oils, helps lower cholesterol. Reducing your intake of fats found in meat will also help you reduce your cholesterol intake, since cholesterol is predominantly found in animal-based foods. In addition to increasing your risk for heart disease, high saturated fat diets are also implicated in accelerated cognitive decline and dementia risk.

Current recommendations are to limit your intake of total fat to 20 to 35% of calories, limit your intake of saturated fat to no more than 10% of calories and to avoid trans fat. To achieve this, an individual consuming a 2000-calorie diet would limit their total fat intake to 65 grams per day and saturated fat intake to 20 grams per day. These are the values used when calculating the %DV for total and saturated fat. Following these guidelines will also help you lower your cholesterol intake below the 300 milligrams per day listed on the Nutrition Facts label and used to calculate its %DV.

Fibre

Fibre is not only an important contributor to the health of our intestinal system, but also confers other health benefits, including reducing the risk of heart disease, diabetes, obesity and certain types of cancer. Since these diseases are also risk factors for cognitive decline and dementia, it is likely through fibre's ability to lower risk for these diseases that higher intakes are also implicated in better cognitive health. Current recommendations for fibre suggest that an adequate intake of fibre is 25 and 38 grams per day for women and men, respectively.

Sodium

While an adequate intake of sodium in the diet is 1300 milligrams per day for adults aged 51 to 70 and 1200 milligrams per day for those over 70 years, Canadians, on average, are consuming close to three times this amount.

Current recommendations are to lower our sodium intakes such that we do not exceed 2300 milligrams per day. To help you visualize this, a teaspoon of salt contains 2300 milligrams of sodium (the other part of the salt particle is chloride). While these recommendations are predominantly aimed at heart health, one study suggests that lowering salt intake could also be beneficial for brain health, especially in those with a sedentary lifestyle.

Since over 75% of the sodium we eat is found in processed food, moving towards home-prepared meals that draw on fresh ingredients will help you achieve this sodium reduction.

Breaking the Fast:

The First Fuel Zone

You probably know that having your children eat a healthy breakfast helps support their ability to learn and grow. But as adults, we often forget that we need to feed our body and brain throughout our life. Eating a healthy breakfast not only helps us think and perform at our peak during the day, it also helps us maintain a proper body weight.

Breakfast and Body Weight

That's right: eating helps us to maintain our body weight! Individuals who regularly eat breakfast have lower body weights and lower body mass indices (BMIs) compared to those who skip breakfast. This is true not only in children and adolescents, but also in adults. For example, this benefit of breakfast intake was reported by physicians in the USA who are participating in a physician health study. Changing eating patterns to routinely include breakfast may be especially important for those who have dieted to reduce weight. Individuals who included breakfast in their lifestyle, after losing weight, were more successful in keeping the extra pounds off compared to those who were not eating breakfast.

Eating breakfast helps us control our hunger over the course of the day. Not experiencing hunger can help us avoid snacking between meals and overeating at meals. The type of foods we choose during the day can also help us control our hunger.

Controlling Your Hunger

The potential to curb appetite and reduce feelings of hunger has led many researchers to study the satiating properties of different types of food.

Protein is considered one of the most satiating of nutrients (compared to carbohydrates and fat). This means it helps us feel "full" for longer periods of time and helps us reduce the amount of food that we consume at our next meal.

The proteins found in dairy products are of special interest. While the evidence is still growing, research suggests that casein and whey, the major proteins in dairy products, are especially satiating. In addition, their metabolic processing may help us reduce the risk of developing metabolic syndrome—a health condition associated with increased risk of cognitive decline and possibly dementia.

You can easily add dairy foods at breakfast by including milk, low-fat yogurt and low-fat cheese in your breakfast pantry. Not only can this help you sustain a healthy body weight and better metabolic control, it can also help you get your recommended daily amount of calcium and vitamin D intake—two nutrients that are often lacking in the typical Canadian diet.

Have a little fun meeting your dairy requirements. For instance, try the **Parliament Hill Smoothie** (page 36)—a smoothie recipe provided by Laureen Harper. Or explore other dairy-based breakfast meals such as the **Overnight Swiss Chard, Sun-Dried Tomato and Mushroom Strata** (page 21) or **Blintz Envelopes with Blueberries** (page 9). All of these recipes have the added advantage of including fruit or vegetables and other healthy ingredients to improve their nutritional profile.

Whole grains and other high-fibre foods also help reduce your feelings of hunger. The argument here is that whole grains are slowly digested and absorbed. As a result, the glucose in these carbohydrates enters our body more gradually and helps us maintain our blood glucose levels for longer periods of time to reduce our feelings of hunger.

Also, because whole grains pass slowly through your body, the simple presence of food in your digestive system sends signals to your brain that say "I'm full." There is evidence that high-fibre foods can reduce your appetite, too.

However, there is still some debate as to which type of fibre is best. Fibre can be classified as either soluble or insoluble. Many whole grains are high in insoluble fibres, such as cellulose, which are best known for their ability to prevent constipation. Soluble fibre, on the other hand, is known for its ability to help lower blood cholesterol. Soluble fibre can be found in grains like oats, as well as in fruits and vegetables. Ultimately, we need to include both types of fibre in our diet. Draw upon recipes such as **Easy Maple Granola** (page 29), **Sweet Potato Waffles** (page 8) and **Winter Fruit Compote** (page 34) as easy and tasty ways to increase your intake of both types of fibre.

How to Use This Information

So how do you make sure that you are eating a healthy breakfast? Well, there are a number of healthy choices. Foods that are high in protein or in low-glycemic-index carbohydrates can help you control your appetite and maintain your body weight. (Find more information about the glycemic index on page 32.) Both types of foods also contribute other important nutrients that are beneficial to your overall health. The good news is that you can bring variety into your breakfast knowing you are giving your body a healthy start to the day.

Remember that maintaining a healthy body weight and controlling your cholesterol are key aspects of a brain-healthy diet. The breakfast recipes provided here were all developed to help you do this. They are low in fat and high in whole grains, fruits and vegetables. They will help contribute to your feelings of satiety throughout the day and also draw on foods that help you control your cholesterol levels and improve your overall health and metabolism.

Chapter 1

Breaking the Fast

Recipes

Whole-Wheat Oatmeal Blueberry Pancakes with Ricotta Topping   6
by Chef Dale MacKay

Sweet Potato Waffles   8

Blintz Envelopes with Blueberries   9

Shakshuka with Warmed Zaatar Pita   13

Morning Hash with Faux Poached Eggs   19

Overnight Swiss Chard, Sun-Dried Tomato and Mushroom Strata   21

Breakfast Crostini with Ricotta, Honey and Figs   27

Fruit Bruschetta   28

Easy Maple Granola   29

Breakfast Burritos   31
by Nettie Cronish

Winter Fruit Compote   34

Parliament Hill Smoothie   36
by Laureen Harper

Whole-Wheat Oatmeal Blueberry Pancakes with Ricotta Topping

By Chef Dale MacKay

Dale MacKay, who has worked with Chefs Ramsay and Boulud, was the winner of Top Chef Canada Season One

Ricotta is naturally low in fat and salt, but is still light and fluffy—making it a fantastic alternative to whipped cream.

Prep time: 15 minutes
Cook time: 20 minutes
Makes 10 servings (2 pancakes each)

PANCAKE BATTER
½ cup whole-wheat flour
½ cup all-purpose flour
3 tbsp packed light brown sugar
2 tbsp baking powder
¾ tsp salt
2 cups milk
1 cup quick rolled oats
4 eggs
¼ cup canola oil
¾ cup fresh small or wild blueberries

TOPPING
1 cup ricotta cheese
2 tbsp liquid honey
Seeds from ½ vanilla bean (or 1 tsp vanilla)

Pancake batter: In a bowl, stir together whole-wheat and all-purpose flours, brown sugar, baking powder and salt.

In a separate bowl, stir together milk and oats. Whisk eggs and 3 tbsp oil into milk mixture.

Pour milk mixture over flour mixture, stirring, just until smooth. Fold in blueberries. Let mixture stand for 10 minutes.

Lightly brush remaining oil onto a skillet or griddle set over medium heat. Using ¼ cup mixture per pancake, cook pancakes on 1 side until batter appears slightly set on the outside and small bubbles appear throughout. Flip; cook for 2 to 3 minutes or until golden. Repeat with remaining batter, taking the time to stir unused batter a few times while pancakes cook.

Topping: Meanwhile, in a bowl, combine ricotta, honey and vanilla seeds. Serve ricotta mixture spooned over warm pancakes.

NUTRITIONAL ANALYSIS PER SERVING: Calories 250; Protein 9g; Carbohydrate 29g (10%DV); Fat, total 11g (17%DV); Fat, saturated 2.5g (13%DV); Fat, trans 0g; Cholesterol 95mg (32%DV); Fibre 2g (8%DV); Sodium 500mg (21%DV).

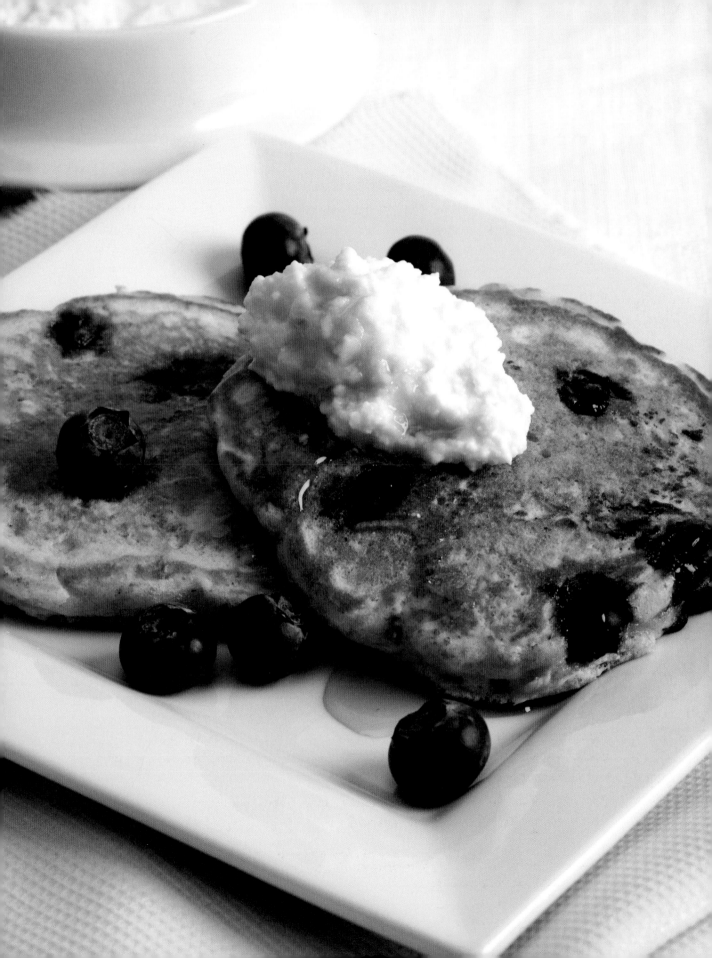

Sweet Potato Waffles

As with **Blintz Envelopes with Blueberries** (page 9), these waffles freeze beautifully. Wrap individually and reheat in the microwave or toaster oven. They're wonderful served with honey, maple-sweetened yogurt or a dried fruit compote such as **Winter Fruit Compote** (page 34).

Prep time: 10 minutes
Cook time: 15 to 20 minutes
Serves 12 (1 waffle each)

1½ cups all-purpose flour
½ cup whole-wheat flour
⅓ cup packed light brown sugar
1½ tsp baking powder
½ tsp ground cinnamon
¼ tsp salt
2 eggs
1¾ cups milk
½ cup sweet potato purée (see Tip below)
2 tbsp canola oil
1 tsp vanilla

In a large bowl, stir together all-purpose and whole-wheat flours, brown sugar, baking powder, cinnamon and salt.

In a separate bowl, whisk together eggs, milk, potato purée, oil and vanilla; pour over flour mixture. Stir until just combined.

Heat waffle maker; using ½ cup batter per waffle, cook according to manufacturer's directions.

NUTRITIONAL ANALYSIS PER WAFFLE: Calories 180; Protein 5g; Carbohydrate 29g (10%DV); Fat, total 4.5g (7%DV); Fat, saturated 1g (5%DV); Fat, trans 0g; Cholesterol 45mg (15%DV); Fibre 2g (8%DV); Sodium 135mg (6%DV).

....

TIP—Quick Sweet Potato Purée

For ½ cup sweet potato purée, boil or microwave 1 cup cubed peeled sweet potato until fork-tender. Purée until smooth in a blender or food processor.

....

Blintz Envelopes with Blueberries

Though these take a bit of time to cook and prepare for a weekday breakfast, they're perfect for keeping in the freezer to have as a last-minute breakfast. Simply wrap each one individually before freezing and then reheat in the microwave or toaster oven when needed. Feel free to substitute orange zest for the lemon zest in the filling or to add cinnamon. Make sure you buy pressed cottage cheese and not dry-pressed (which will make the filling too dry and inedible).

Prep time: 15 minutes
Cook time: 15 minutes
Serves 6 (2 blintzes each)

BLINTZES
2 eggs
4 tsp granulated sugar
¼ tsp salt
1 cup water
1 cup all-purpose flour
4 tsp canola oil

SAUCE
2 cups blueberries, fresh or frozen
2 tbsp granulated sugar
2 tbsp lemon juice
4 tsp cornstarch
¾ cup water

CHEESE FILLING
1 cup pressed cottage cheese
1 egg yolk
3 tbsp granulated sugar
3 oz light cream cheese
2 tsp grated lemon zest
½ cup blueberries, fresh or frozen
1 tbsp canola oil, for frying

Blintzes: In a blender or using an electric mixer, mix eggs, sugar, salt and water until just combined. Blend in flour until smooth. Transfer to a bowl and cover with plastic wrap; refrigerate for at least 1 hour or for up to 4 hours.

Brush 1 tsp oil in a 6-inch crepe pan set over medium-high heat. Stir batter; pour 3 to 4 tbsp into pan, tilting to spread. Cook for 45 to 60 seconds without flipping, until set and no longer moist in centre. Invert onto tea towel. Repeat with remaining oil and batter, placing waxed paper between each blintz.

Blueberry sauce: In a saucepan, combine blueberries, sugar, lemon juice, cornstarch and water. Bring to a boil over medium-high heat; boil, stirring, until blueberries have broken down and sauce has thickened, about 3 minutes. Transfer to a bowl, cover with plastic wrap and refrigerate until cooled or for up to 5 days.

Filling: In a bowl, beat cottage cheese until fluffy; beat in egg yolk, sugar, cream cheese and lemon zest. Gently fold in blueberries.

Assembly: Spoon a heaping tablespoonful of filling along centre of one blintz. Fold one edge of blintz over filling; fold opposite edge over. Fold over ends to form a package. Repeat with remaining filling and blintzes. (Blintzes can be prepared up to this point, wrapped individually in plastic wrap and frozen in an airtight container for up to 2 weeks.)

Heat oil in a non-stick skillet over medium heat; fry blintzes until warmed through, about 2 minutes per side. Serve with sauce. (Alternatively, fry frozen blintzes for 4 minutes per side or toast in 425°F toaster oven for 15 minutes.)

NUTRITIONAL ANALYSIS PER SERVING: Calories 310; Protein 12g; Carbohydrate 42g (14%DV); Fat, total 11g (17%DV); Fat, saturated 3g (15%DV); Fat, trans 0g; Cholesterol 115mg (38%DV); Fibre 2g (8%DV); Sodium 320mg (13%DV).

❧Health Savvy: Dairy Products 101

Milk We all grew up hearing the adage "Drink your milk; it's good for you." Our mothers probably said it to us, and as parents, we've probably said it to our own children. And with good reason. Milk is indeed a nutritionally sound choice: it's packed with calcium; protein; vitamins A, D, B_{12} and B_6; riboflavin; niacin; magnesium and phosphorus. No matter what your age, consuming milk is a good way to ensure overall well-being and can help to prevent certain diseases or conditions such as high blood pressure, obesity, colon cancer and osteoporosis. All the recipes in this book were tested with either 1% or 2% milk. In most baking recipes, opt for 2% milk for optimal results.

Buttermilk This is one of the most useful baking ingredients a health-conscious baker can have on hand. Made by culturing skim milk with bacteria, buttermilk produces cakes with a tender crumb, and biscuits or scones with a moist flaky interior. One important caveat: Do not use buttermilk when the recipe calls for regular milk. All recipes using buttermilk will require baking soda as their leavener, which is activated by the acid present in the buttermilk. If you're out of buttermilk, simply pour 1 tablespoon of lemon juice into a measuring cup. Top to the 1-cup mark with regular milk. Let stand for 5 minutes until milk is mottled.

Cottage cheese Cottage cheese is a fresh curd cheese made from cow's milk. It is available in whole, partly skimmed and skimmed varieties. Cottage cheese contains, per cup, roughly 25 g of protein. It also contains calcium and phosphorus, both of which contribute to healthy bones. In addition, cottage cheese is a good source of the B complex of vitamins, affiliated with nerve cell function and the body's ability to use iron. It also provides smaller amounts of B_6, pantothenic acid, thiamine, niacin and folate. Choose low-fat cottage cheese to minimize your intake of saturated fat while still benefitting from its other healthful features. However, lower-fat varieties tend to be very high in water content so they are not desirable baking allies.

Yogurt Made by adding particular strains of bacteria to whole, partly skim or skim milk, yogurt is packed with protein and calcium and can be fairly low in calories if you choose a variety made with lower-fat milk. Yogurt is also a good source of riboflavin, phosphorus and vitamin B_{12}. However, all yogurt is not created equal. If it is packed with fruit, or sweeteners, you may be getting more calories than you bargained for.

Yogurt is an excellent ingredient in baking, yielding a remarkable moistness and a lovely tang to baked goods. Be sure to use yogurt with at least a 2% fat content in baking. Shy away from non-fat yogurts when baking, since they tend to be high in sugars, stabilizers and thickeners, which can wreak havoc with recipes.

Sour cream Now available in regular, low-fat and no-fat varieties, sour cream lends a light tang to baked goods as well as a moist, tender crumb. It can often be used to replace milk or yogurt in baking recipes (and vice versa). Low-fat sour cream can be used in most baking recipes; however, do not use non-fat sour cream, due to its high water content.

Shakshuka with Warmed Zaatar Pita

This Middle Eastern dish is a spicy staple on the Gryfe breakfast table. Bold and brightly flavoured, this is the perfect way to wake up your tastebuds and your entire neighbourhood! It's also a great make-ahead dish for brunches, as the spicy tomato base can be made a day or two ahead of time. Just before serving, reheat the base on medium-low heat for 10 minutes, then add the eggs according to instructions below. This recipe can be doubled and served out of a large casserole dish for a crowd, or portioned among individual ramekins for an elegant brunch.

Prep time: 10 minutes
Cook time: 40 minutes
Serves 4

2 sweet red peppers
3 tbsp olive oil
1 large onion, coarsely chopped
6 cloves garlic, minced
¼ tsp dried red pepper flakes
¼ tsp each salt and black pepper
1 tsp tomato paste
1 can (28 oz/796 mL) crushed or diced tomatoes
4 eggs
2 whole-wheat pitas
1½ tsp zaatar
¼ cup crumbled feta cheese
½ cup coarsely torn fresh Italian parsley leaves

Turn broiler to high setting; position rack in top third of oven.

Place red peppers on an aluminum foil–lined baking sheet. Broil, turning once or twice, until skins are charred, 15 to 20 minutes. Transfer peppers to a bowl and cover with plastic wrap. Let sit until cool enough to handle, about 10 minutes. Peel and discard skin, stems and seeds. Cut peppers into bite-size pieces. Reserve.

Heat 2 tbsp oil in a large deep-set pan set over medium heat. Add onion, garlic, red pepper flakes, salt, pepper and tomato paste. Cook, stirring, until onion softens and tomato paste melts, about 4 minutes.

Add canned tomatoes (with liquid if using diced) and prepared red peppers. Increase heat to medium-high; simmer, stirring occasionally, until liquid reduces by one-third, 7 to 10 minutes.

Crack eggs on top of tomato mixture. Reduce heat to low; cook, covered, until desired doneness, 5 minutes for medium-set yolks and 7 minutes for hard-set yolks.

Meanwhile, lightly brush pitas with remaining 1 tbsp oil and sprinkle with zaatar. Toast on light setting in a toaster oven.

Uncover pan. Sprinkle with crumbled feta and parsley. Serve straight from the pan with warm zaatar pita.

NUTRITIONAL ANALYSIS PER SERVING: Calories 220; Protein 8g; Carbohydrate 26g (9%DV); Fat, total 11g (17%DV); Fat, saturated 3g (15%DV); Fat, trans 0g; Cholesterol 65mg (22%DV); Fibre 6g (24%DV); Sodium 540mg (23%DV).

TIP—How to Make Your Own Zaatar

Zaatar is the Arabic word for thyme, but actually refers to hyssop, an herb native to Syria, often combined with sesame seeds and sumac. This exotic spice can be found in Middle Eastern markets and ordered online. If you can't track it down, mix two parts each of dried thyme, oregano and marjoram with one part each sumac, sesame seeds and finely minced lemon zest.

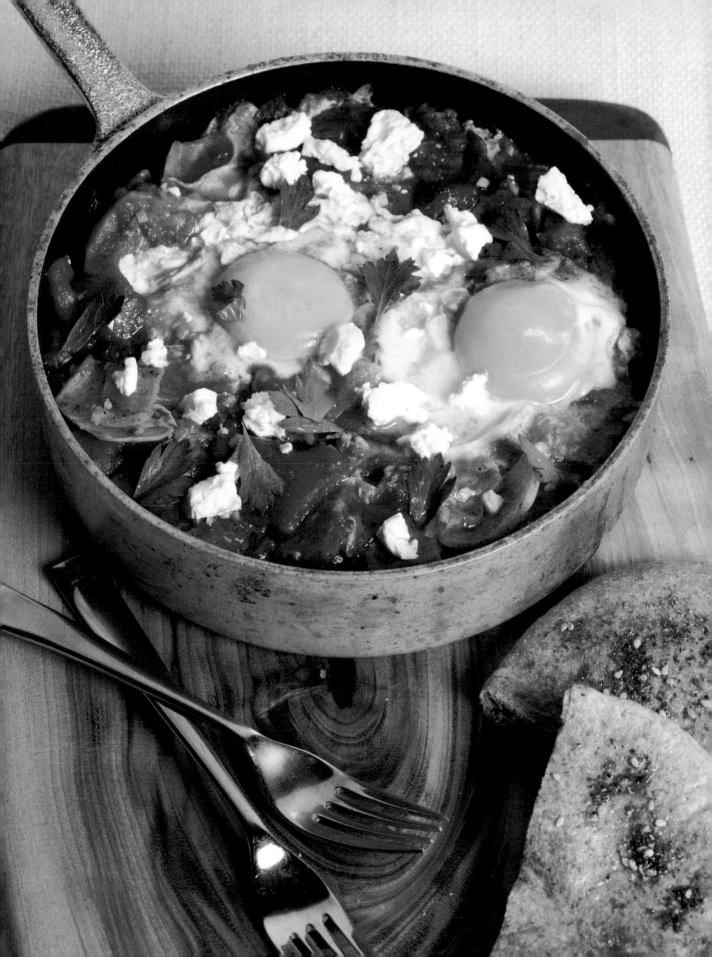

✤Health Savvy: Eggs 101

What makes this humble ingredient so eggstraordinary? Aside from being an entrée's protein or a custard's base, this baking leavener, sauce thickener and breading coater can be used for breakfast, lunch, dinner and anything in between! Here are some basic facts about the eggceptional ingredient no kitchen should be without.

Brown versus White

All eggs are made up of three basic parts: the shell, the yolk and the white. While the eggs of various birds—goose, duck and quail—are now available from gourmet grocers, chicken eggs are most commonly used in cooking to date. The shell's colour is determined by the breed of hen laying it and does not affect the egg's flavour or nutritional value. The colour of the yolk provides further insight into the laying hen; darkly coloured yolks mean the hen was wheat-fed, while those raised on grass and/or corn produce tend to make paler yolks.

Storage

Whole eggs Eggs should be refrigerated (for up to a month), as those stored at room temperature spoil seven times faster. Store eggs, large end up, in the carton they were sold in and away from pungent foods; transferring the eggs to a compartment in the fridge makes them susceptible to odours, which the shells easily absorb. Avoid keeping the carton in the refrigerator door, as constant opening of the door destabilizes the temperature and decreases shelf life.

Hard-boiled eggs last in the refrigerator for up to a week.

Yolks Cover leftover yolks with cold water and refrigerate, tightly sealed, for up to 3 days. To freeze yolks, add ⅛ teaspoon salt or 1½ teaspoons sugar or 1½ teaspoons corn syrup to every ¼ cup of yolks in an airtight container.

Whites If tightly sealed, leftover egg whites will refrigerate nicely for up to 4 days, and freeze (without the addition of salt, sugar or corn syrup) for up to 6 months. Use an ice tray for easy-to-store egg white cubes, perfectly portioned for future use.

Common Cooking Methods

Baked/shirred—cooked in oven, usually in ramekins
Fried—cooked in pan with fat (butter, oil, lard, etc.)
Poached—gently cooked, out of shell, in simmering liquid
Scrambled—yolks and whites are beaten together before cooking, and gently stirred while cooking
Shell-cooked—cooked in boiling water with the shell on

Egg Substitutes

For egg dishes (scrambled eggs, omelettes, custards, etc.): In some cases, pasteurized egg whites are blended with vegetable oils and gums, milk solids, salt, emulsifiers and vitamins. The vegetable oil and gums present replace the egg yolk, allowing the product to simulate a whole egg. Usually sold in frozen or refrigerated liquid form (e.g., Egg Beaters), these products can be substituted for equal measurements of whole eggs. Some egg substitutes are composed of 100% egg whites without any additions and are identified as such. Silken tofu is also a popular replacement among vegans.

For baking Most manufacturers will advertise that their products are equally as good as shelled eggs for baking. However, some come with stabilizers and vegetable gums that you may not want to use in your baking. They also do not generally beat up to the same volume as shelled eggs, so you may want to choose your recipes accordingly. Most egg substitute web sites can act as a guide and provide many baking recipes.

Health Concerns

Salmonella Salmonella is a type of bacterium that can be on either the inside or outside of eggs. Salmonella infection is characterized by fever, abdominal cramps and diarrhea beginning 12 to 72 hours after consuming a contaminated food or beverage. Cooking eggs destroys the bacteria; however, a lightly cooked egg with runny yolk poses a greater risk for salmonella infection compared to a hard-cooked egg. Eggs should be kept refrigerated and, once cooked, not kept at room temperature for more than 2 hours. Young children, elderly persons and persons with weakened immune systems should not eat raw or undercooked eggs. Alternatively, pasteurized eggs, which have been treated with heat to kill bacteria, are available either in or out of their shells.

Cholesterol According to the Harvard Heart Letter, eggs are not the demons they've been cracked up to be. While they are high in cholesterol (approximately 212 milligrams cholesterol in a large egg), not all of this cholesterol goes to your bloodstream—eating saturated and trans fats actually has a much greater effect on blood cholesterol levels than eating eggs. According to the Harvard Heart Letter, eating one egg per day (or seven per week) should be okay, especially if you cut back on your saturated and trans fats; these numbers are supported by the Heart and Stroke Foundation of Canada for healthy people with no history of heart disease, diabetes or high blood cholesterol. Fortunately, the recipes in this cookbook are designed to help you lower your intake of saturated and trans fats. If you prefer to minimize your cholesterol intake, you can simply omit the egg yolk (which contains all of the cholesterol) or use yolk-free egg substitutes. If you are being treated for heart disease, diabetes or high blood cholesterol levels, follow your doctor's advice as it relates to egg consumption.

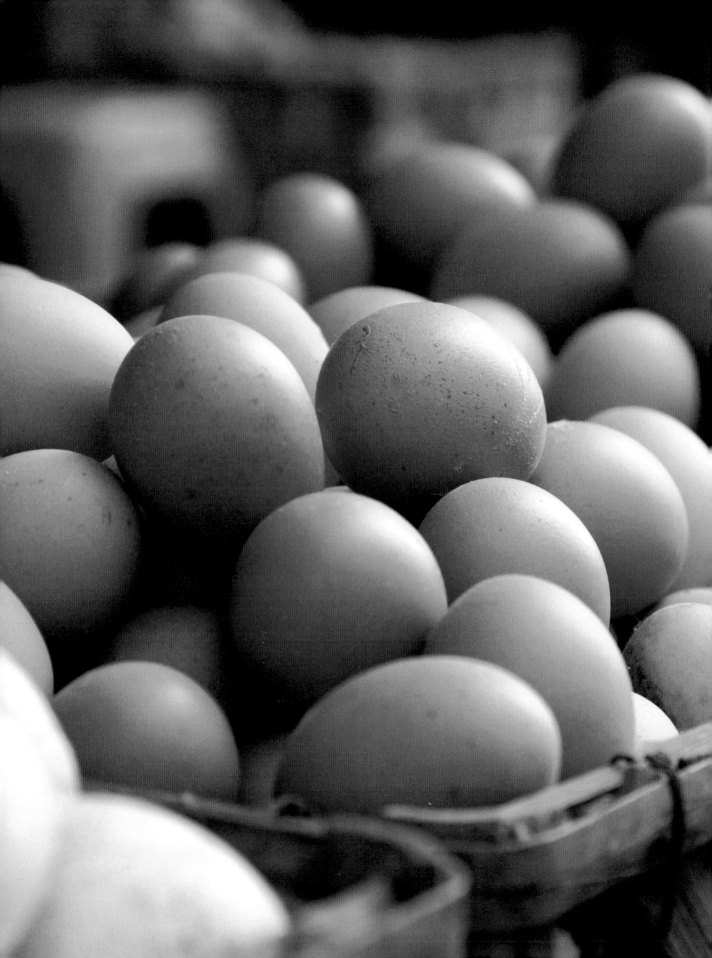

Morning Hash with Faux Poached Eggs

Sweet potatoes are a member of the morning glory family—tubers native to tropical and sub-tropical climates. Rich in vitamins A and C, this distant relative of the potato will certainly bring glory to your morning eggs and hash!

Prep time: 15 minutes
Cook time: 25 minutes
Serves 4

2 tbsp olive oil
1 large sweet potato, finely diced
1 Yukon gold potato, finely diced
½ tsp paprika
¼ tsp each salt and black pepper
1 onion, finely chopped
2½ cups finely sliced Swiss chard (both leaves and stems)
½ cup vegetable stock, preferably low-sodium
4 eggs

Heat oil in a large, deep skillet set over medium heat. Add sweet and regular potatoes; cook, stirring occasionally, until potatoes are crispy and browned on all sides, 8 to 10 minutes. Stir in paprika, salt and pepper.

Stir in onion; cook until transparent, about 2 minutes. Stir in chard; cook just until wilted, about 2 minutes.

Pour in stock, using a wooden spoon to scrape browned bits from bottom of pan. Reduce heat to low. Create 4 craters in the hash; crack 1 egg into each cavity. Cover pan immediately; cook to desired doneness, 5 minutes for medium-set eggs and 7 minutes for hard.

NUTRITIONAL ANALYSIS PER SERVING: Calories 250; Protein 9g; Carbohydrate 27g (9%DV); Fat, total 12g (18%DV); Fat, saturated 2.5g (13%DV); Fat, trans 0g; Cholesterol 215mg (72%DV); Fibre 4g (16%DV); Sodium 400mg (17%DV).

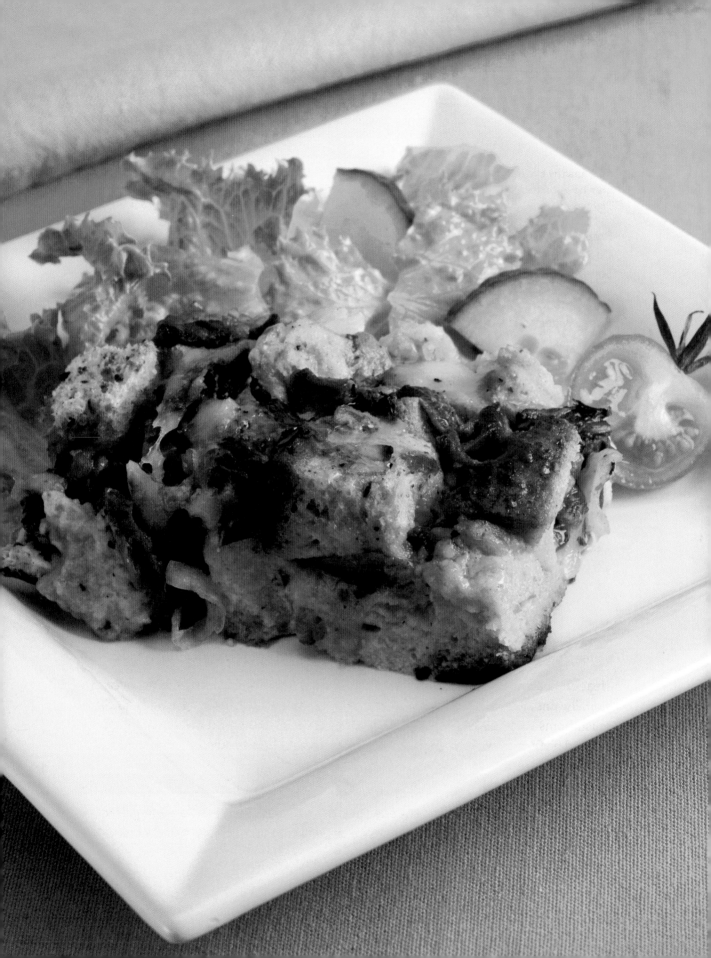

Overnight Swiss Chard, Sun-Dried Tomato and Mushroom Strata

This healthy strata solves the leftover bread dilemma and works well with any type of bread you may have on hand. Here, the brisk flavour of the sun-dried tomato complements the stronger flavour of whole-grain bread. Strata no longer needs to be a recipe reserved for white bread.

Prep time: 20 minutes plus 10 to 12 hours to soak
Cook time: 40 minutes
Serves 10

1 large bunch Swiss chard (or 2 small bunches)
2 tbsp water
2 tbsp canola oil
1½ cups finely chopped onion
2 cups sliced button mushrooms
½ tsp each salt and black pepper
¼ tsp ground nutmeg
½ cup finely sliced oil-packed sun-dried tomatoes, drained
8 cups cubed multi-grain bread (about 1 inch in diameter)
6 oz Allegro, or other fat-reduced cheese such as Swiss or Emmenthal, grated
¼ cup grated Parmesan cheese
9 eggs
2¾ cups milk
2 tbsp Dijon mustard
Pinch cayenne pepper

The night before: Tear leaves from Swiss chard, reserving stems for another use. Place leaves in a large pot with water. Cover; cook over medium-high heat, stirring once or twice, just until wilted, 3 to 4 minutes. Transfer chard to a colander; rinse under cold water. Squeeze handfuls of chard to remove as much liquid as possible; finely chop.

Heat oil in a non-stick skillet set over medium heat. Add onion; cook, stirring occasionally, until soft, 4 to 5 minutes. Add mushrooms; cook, stirring occasionally, until mushrooms have released their juices and pan is dry, 5 to 6 minutes. Add half of the salt and pepper plus the nutmeg, sun-dried tomatoes and Swiss chard. Stir to combine; remove from heat.

Coat a 3-quart (3 L) shallow baking dish with cooking spray. Add one-third of the bread cubes. Sprinkle evenly with one-third of the Swiss chard mixture and grated cheeses. Repeat layering of bread, Swiss chard mixture and cheeses twice more.

In a medium bowl, whisk together eggs, milk, mustard, cayenne pepper and remaining salt and pepper. Pour evenly over strata. Cover with plastic wrap; refrigerate overnight.

Morning: Preheat oven to 350°F. Remove strata from refrigerator; bring to room temperature for ½ hour. Bake, uncovered, in centre of preheated oven until golden brown and a knife inserted in the centre comes out clean, 40 to 50 minutes. Cool for 5 minutes before serving.

NUTRITIONAL ANALYSIS PER EACH OF 10 SERVINGS: Calories 270; Protein 18g; Carbohydrate 25g (8%DV); Fat, total 11g (17%DV); Fat, saturated 3.5g (18%DV); Fat, trans 0g; Cholesterol 205mg (68%DV); Fibre 4g (16%DV); Sodium 690mg (29%DV).

⚛Brain Savvy: Do Super Foods Exist?

These days we are bombarded by all sorts of conflicting health information. It feels like so-called "experts" are constantly declaring new "rules" or "super foods": today it's broccoli, tomorrow it's blueberries; next week it might be pomegranates. That's why it's important to understand how these scientific studies are conducted, and how to deal with this information in a way that's meaningful for your own health and well-being.

Many laboratory studies feed individual foods, one at a time, to humans or animals. Scientists do this to keep the variables down to a manageable level. But as a result, the study may only report how that one single nutrient or food affected test subjects. Even though other nutrients or foods may have similar effects, other alternatives are not discussed in the context of the study.

By only reporting on one individual food, and not the potential health benefits of food groups, studies can create the false perception that a "super food" exists and that its health benefits outweigh other similar foods. In reality, this has never been proven. When it comes to brain health, there is currently no evidence that any one single food within the same class is superior to other similar foods.

For example, in population-based studies (where we have the best evidence on high-quality diets), higher consumption of cruciferous vegetables has been associated with better preservation of cognitive function with aging. Yet, there is currently no evidence to suggest that any single cruciferous vegetable, e.g., kale, is better than another, e.g., broccoli. When overall human consumption patterns are studied in large groups of individuals, it is often impossible to isolate individual foods, rather than food classes.

Thus, you are far better off recognizing that cruciferous vegetables, in general, are part of a brain-healthy diet and wise to choose many different types of cruciferous vegetables. This approach has the added advantage that each cruciferous vegetable is somewhat unique in its composition and you are exposing yourself to the broadest possible combination of beneficial food components. (For more information on the cruciferous vegetable family, see page 84.) While the beneficial effects of these food components were originally felt to reflect their high antioxidant capabilities, emerging evidence is now suggesting that they likely play many other beneficial roles beyond that of antioxidant protection.

There Is No Convincing Evidence That Supplements Can Replace Foods

Scientists also study the active ingredients in certain foods. This helps them discover the biologic mechanism linking the healthful properties of a food to its ability to protect brain cells. In some cases, these active ingredients are then packaged and sold in isolated form as a nutritional supplement or added to other less-healthy foods.

While animal studies do suggest that consuming these isolated active components can be beneficial, there is currently no convincing evidence from human studies that supplements can benefit cognitive health. However, there are a number of studies underway in this area. One is studying the effects of omega-3 fats and is one of the more promising areas of research. Nevertheless, the National Institute of Health in the USA contends that "currently, no evidence of even moderate scientific quality exists to support the association of any modifiable factor (such as nutritional supplements, herbal preparations, dietary factors, prescription or non-prescription drugs, social or economic factors, medical conditions, toxins, or environmental exposures) with reduced risk of Alzheimer's disease."

Consuming a Wide Variety of Colourful Foods Remains the Most Prudent Advice

Nature has given us a wonderful way to find the healthiest foods. The natural pigments that give fruits and vegetables their colours also reveal foods that offer many health benefits. This includes their ability to function as antioxidants as well as supporting cell metabolism and communication. So keeping your plate as colourful as possible not only makes your meals visually appealing, it ensures that you are eating in a way that maximizes your intake of beneficial nutrients.

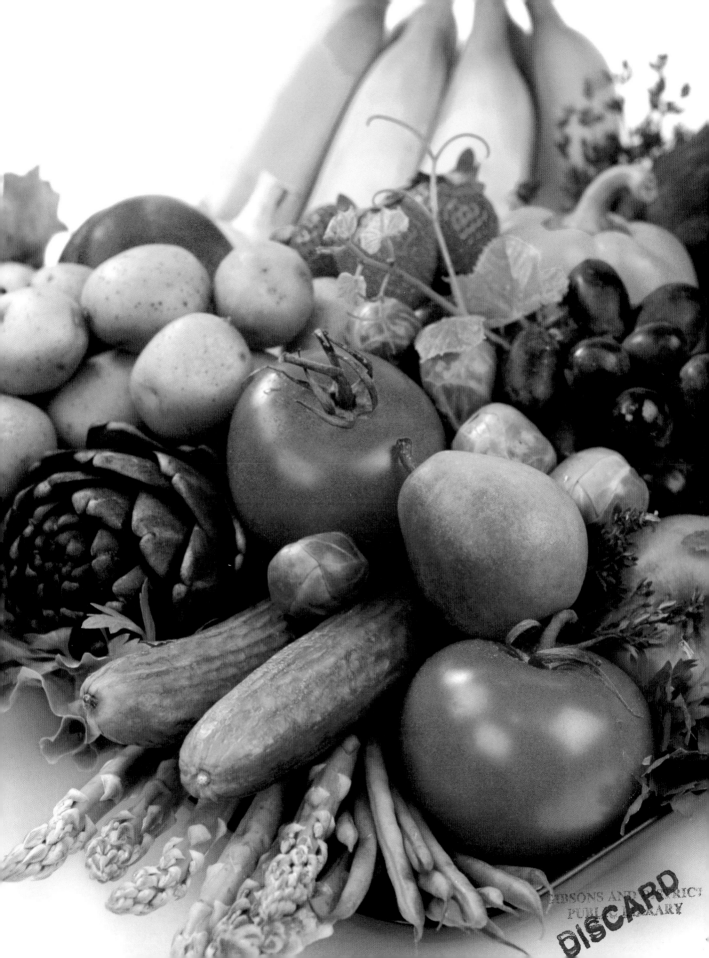

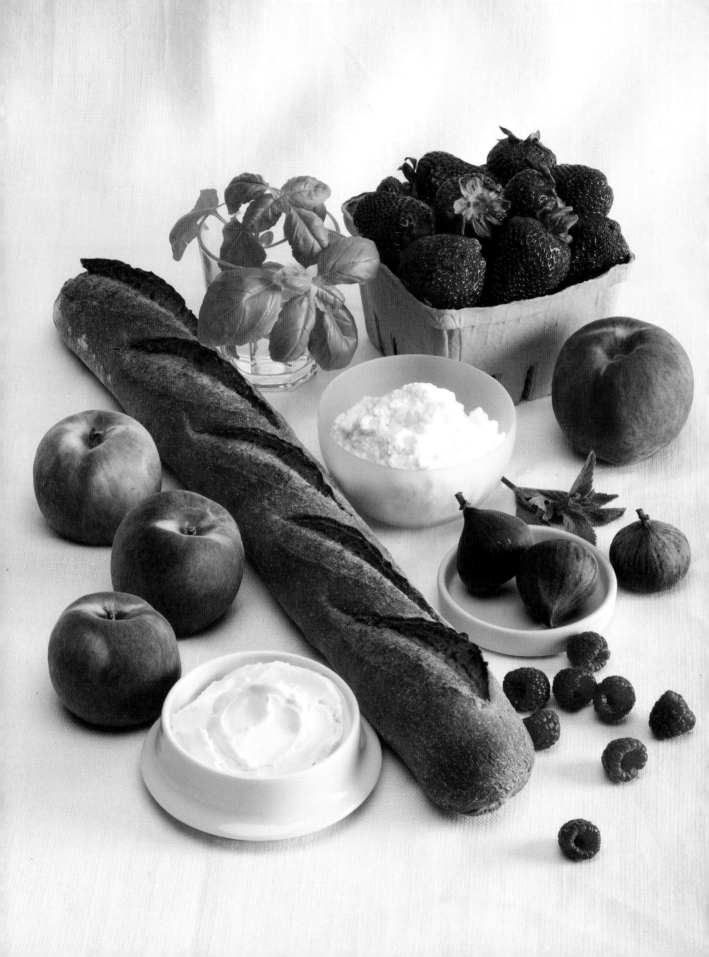

Breakfast Crostini with Ricotta, Honey and Figs

Bored of butter, jam and peanut spread? It's time to rethink your morning toast...

Prep time: 5 minutes
Serves 6

6 slices whole-wheat crusty bread
⅓ cup low-fat ricotta cheese
2 tbsp liquid honey
6 figs (fresh or dried), sliced

In a toaster oven or toaster, lightly toast bread.

In a bowl, stir together cheese and honey; spread over toast. Arrange fig slices over top.

NUTRITIONAL ANALYSIS PER SERVING: Calories 120; Protein 4g; Carbohydrate 25g (8%DV); Fat, total 2g (3%DV); Fat, saturated 0.5g (3%DV); Fat, trans 0g; Cholesterol 0mg; Fibre 3g (12%DV); Sodium 160mg (7%DV).

Fruit Bruschetta

Bruschetta needn't only precede the evening meal. Think fruit instead of tomatoes and cream cheese instead of olive oil, and you have a tasty Italian-inspired breakfast.

Prep time: 10 minutes
Serves 6

6 thin slices crusty bread (such as baguette,
    sourdough or ciabatta)
1 cup finely chopped strawberries
¾ cup finely chopped peaches
1 tbsp finely chopped fresh basil leaves
½ tsp finely chopped fresh mint leaves
1 tbsp liquid honey or agave nectar
3 tbsp light cream cheese
Whole basil and mint leaves

In a toaster oven or toaster, lightly toast bread.

In a bowl, combine strawberries, peaches, basil, mint and honey; reserve.

Arrange toast on a platter; spread cream cheese evenly on each. Spoon ¼ cup fruit onto each slice. Top with fresh basil and mint leaves.

NUTRITIONAL ANALYSIS PER SERVING: Calories 130; Protein 4g; Carbohydrate 24g (8%DV); Fat, total 2.5g (4%DV); Fat, saturated 1g (5%DV); Fat, trans 0g; Cholesterol 5mg (2%DV); Fibre 2g (8%DV); Sodium 210mg (9%DV).

Easy Maple Granola

Kasha is roasted, hulled buckwheat kernels, which are high in good-quality proteins, B vitamins, iron, calcium and fibre. It lends a nutty note to this granola that some may find overpowering; if the kasha doesn't tempt your tastebuds, simply leave it out. The nuts, spices and healthy sweeteners still make this a beneficial and flavourful yogurt topper. You can use this granola to make a scrumptious Granola Parfait: Stir together some fat-free plain or vanilla yogurt, grated dark chocolate and chopped seasonal fruit. Layer yogurt mixture and granola in a funky glass or even a coffee mug and enjoy while reading the paper. Or pack in a resealable container for an on-the-go treat.

Prep time: 5 minutes
Cook time: 25 minutes
Serves 12 (5 cups total; heaping ⅓ cup per serving)

3 tbsp canola oil

3 tbsp maple syrup

1 tbsp liquid honey

½ tsp vanilla

3½ cups large-flake rolled oats

½ cup kasha

½ tsp ground cinnamon

¼ tsp ground nutmeg

¼ tsp ground ginger

Pinch salt

½ cup unsalted raw almonds, sliced or slivered

½ cup raw walnut pieces

Preheat oven to 350°F.

In a bowl, combine oil, syrup, honey and vanilla.

In a separate bowl, toss oats with kasha, cinnamon, nutmeg, ginger, salt, almonds and walnuts. Add oil mixture to oat mixture and stir until well combined. Transfer to a parchment paper–lined baking sheet, and spread out evenly.

Bake in centre of preheated oven, stirring halfway through, until golden brown, about 25 minutes. (Granola can be stored in an airtight container for up to 1 month.)

NUTRITIONAL ANALYSIS PER SERVING: Calories 220; Protein 6g; Carbohydrate 27g (9%DV); Fat, total 10g (15%DV); Fat, saturated 1g (5%DV); Fat, trans 0g; Cholesterol 0mg; Fibre 4g (16%DV); Sodium 5mg (0%DV).

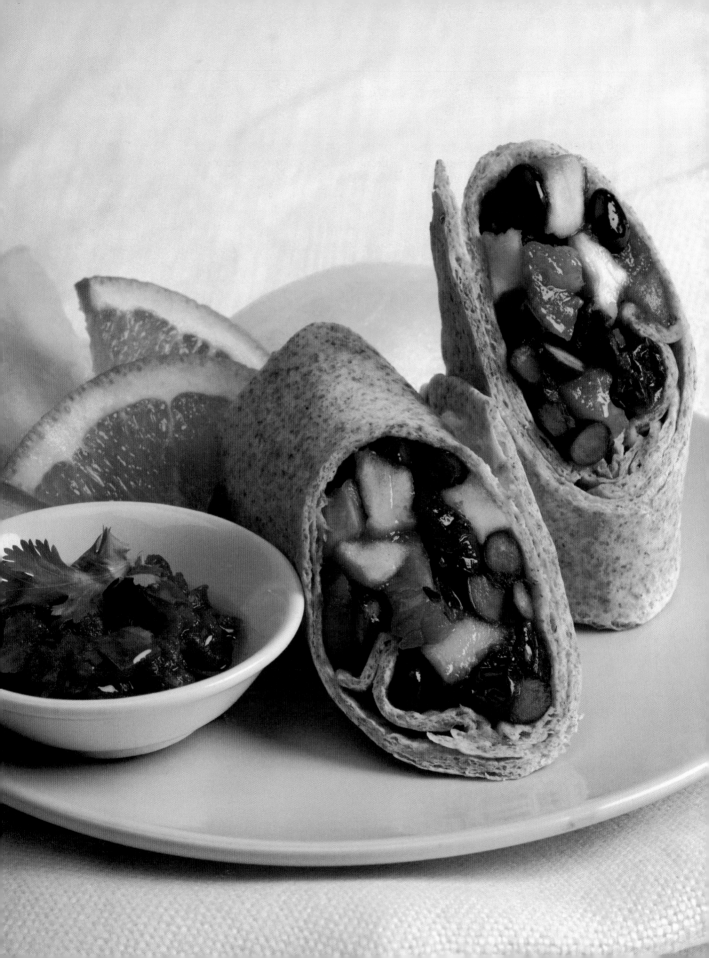

Breakfast Burritos

By Nettie Cronish

Nettie Cronish, author of more than five vegetarian cookbooks, works, cooks and teaches in Toronto.

Beans and dried fruit are delicious together. With so many tortillas to choose from, this morning meal can feed everyone—gluten-free, vegan or vegetarian. Add your own condiments: fruit or veggies, salsas, grated cheeses or vegan alternatives, or hot sauces. The choice is yours.

Prep time: 20 minutes
Cook time: 25 minutes
Serves 8 (½ burrito each)

¼ cup chopped dried apricots
¼ cup chopped dried apple or mango
¼ cup dried cranberries
1 cup apple juice
1 whole cardamom pod, cracked, or 1 small cinnamon stick
    (approx 3 inches long)
1 can (14 oz/398 mL) pinto or black beans, drained and rinsed
¼ tsp salt
4 10-inch tortillas (e.g., whole-wheat, corn, sprouted, unbleached, flax, pesto)
¼ cup salsa and/or grated cheddar cheese (optional; see Tip below)

In a saucepan, combine apricots, apples, cranberries, apple juice and cardamom; heat over low heat for 5 minutes.

Add beans; bring to a boil over medium-high heat. Reduce heat to medium-low; simmer, uncovered and stirring often, until liquid has almost evaporated (about 10 minutes). Discard cardamom. Add salt.

In a dry skillet, warm each tortilla over medium heat for about 1 minute per side.

Place ½ cup of the filling down the centre of each tortilla, leaving a 1-inch border (approx) at bottom and top. Fold bottom edge over filling; fold sides over. Roll up from bottom. Slice each tortilla in half. Serve at room temperature.

NUTRITIONAL ANALYSIS PER SERVING: Calories 180; Protein 6g; Carbohydrate 36g (12%DV); Fat, total 2g (3%DV); Fat, saturated 0.5g (3%DV); Fat, trans 0g; Cholesterol 0mg; Fibre 6g (24%DV); Sodium 330mg (14%DV).

....

TIP—Adding Extra Kick to Your Burrito

Add 1 tbsp salsa and/or grated cheese overtop each burrito. Transfer burritos to a parchment paper–lined baking sheet. Bake in a preheated 300°F oven for 5 minutes or until cheese has melted.

....

⚛Brain Savvy: Why the Glycemic Index Matters

Carbohydrates are made up of glucose bound together in long chains. These chains break down in our intestines into glucose, and the glucose is then absorbed into our bloodstream (such as with starches). Or the carbohydrate can pass through the intestinal tract, where it is used by bacteria residing in our colon (such as with fibre). In addition to starches, we also consume carbohydrates as sucrose (table sugar: glucose plus fructose) or lactose (carbohydrates in milk: glucose plus galactose). Our bodies are unable to distinguish between glucose that we eat as starch and glucose that we eat as sucrose or lactose.

In general, you don't want your blood glucose levels to rise too high after eating carbohydrates. Chronically high blood glucose levels can increase your risk of developing diabetes and high blood lipid levels (cholesterol and triglycerides). These two conditions can increase your risk of cognitive decline and dementia. The best way to keep your blood glucose levels from rising too high is to consume carbohydrates that have a low glycemic index.

The Glycemic Index

You may have heard of the glycemic index. The glycemic index, or GI, measures the effects of carbohydrates on blood glucose levels. It provides us with a good indication of which carbohydrate foods to select or avoid.

Carbohydrates that break down quickly in our intestines have a greater impact on our blood glucose levels and have a high GI score. In contrast, carbohydrates that break down slowly enter our bloodstream gradually and have less of an impact on our blood glucose levels. These have a low GI score.

In general, you want to consume foods that are within the low-to-medium GI ranges and consume high GI carbohydrate foods only in moderation. The table that follows provides some examples of foods that fall into these ranges. For example, whole grains have a lower GI value than processed grains. In general, the more processed a food, the higher the GI value.

Some carbohydrates, however, are surprisingly low in GI value. Pasta, for example, is a low GI food, and the difference in GI values between white pasta and whole-wheat pasta is small. Nevertheless, whole-wheat pasta has the advantage of helping you increase the fibre content of your diet. The best way to keep the GI value of your pasta low is to cook it only to the al dente stage. For a more detailed chart on the GI values of various foods, visit www.glycemicindex.com.

CLASSIFICATION	GI RANGE	EXAMPLES
Low GI	55 or less	Most fruits and vegetables, legumes/pulses, whole grains, nuts
Medium GI	56 to 69	Whole-wheat products, basmati rice, sweet potato, sucrose, baked potatoes (including cut and baked French fries)
High GI	70 and above	White bread, most white rice, corn flakes, extruded breakfast cereals such as puffed wheat, glucose, maltose (commonly found in processed foods)

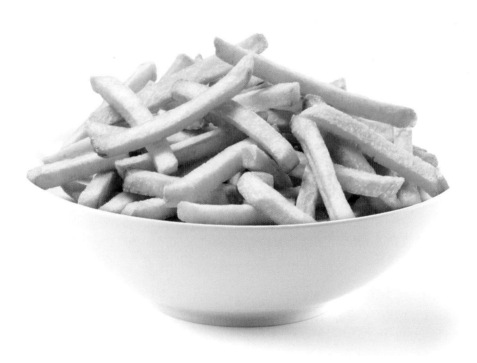

Winter Fruit Compote

Winter fruit compotes, which rely heavily on dried fruits, are a great way to include fruit in your diet during the winter months. Adding crystallized ginger brightens up the flavour; it can be found in most grocery stores, in the baking section close to the candied peels.

Prep time: 15 minutes
Cook time: 30 minutes
Serves 8 (½ cup each)

2 oranges
1 lemon
½ cup stemmed, halved dried figs
½ cup dried apricots
¼ cup dried cranberries
1 3-inch cinnamon stick (or ½ tsp ground cinnamon)
3 whole cloves
2 tbsp finely chopped crystallized ginger (or 2 tsp grated fresh gingerroot)
2½ cups water
2 tbsp (approx) liquid honey
½ cup pitted prunes
1 Granny Smith apple, peeled, cored and cut into 1/4-inch slices
1 Bosc or Bartlett pear, peeled, cored and cut into 1/4-inch slices

Using a sharp knife or vegetable peeler, cut two 3-inch strips of peel from orange and set peel aside. Juice oranges to make ¾ cup juice. Cut two 3-inch strips of peel from lemon.

Place orange and lemon peels, orange juice, figs, apricots, cranberries, cinnamon, cloves, ginger, water and honey in a medium-sized pot. Bring to a boil over high heat. Reduce heat to medium; cook, uncovered, for 20 minutes. Add prunes, apple and pear. Add more water, if necessary, to ensure that fruit is just barely covered. Cook until all fruit is softened, about 10 minutes. Remove orange and lemon rinds, cinnamon stick and cloves. Cool before serving. Taste and add more honey if necessary. (Compote can be transferred to an airtight container and refrigerated for up to 5 days.)

NUTRITIONAL ANALYSIS PER SERVING: Calories 390; Protein 3g; Carbohydrate 96g (32%DV); Fat, total 0g; Fat, saturated 0g; Fat, trans 0g; Cholesterol 0mg; Fibre 8g (32%DV); Sodium 20mg (1%DV).

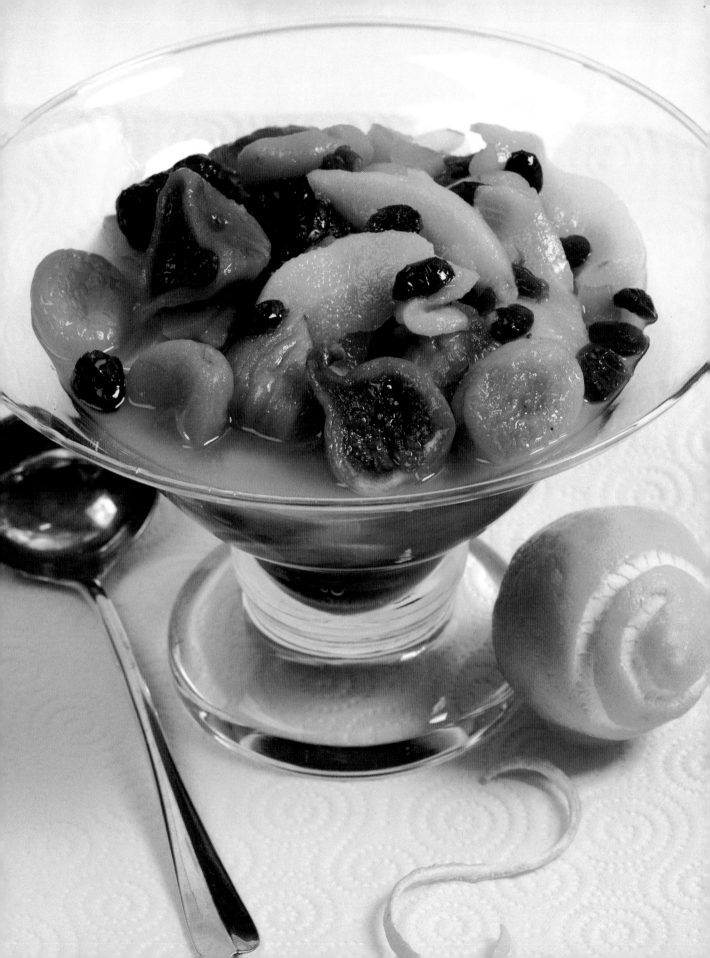

Parliament Hill Smoothie

By Laureen Harper

Ben, Rachel, Stephen and I always enjoy making a healthy breakfast to start the day off right. I feel good about helping my children make smart food choices. Like most families on the go, we love smoothies. This tasty treat is ideal after a morning workout or an afternoon hike.

Prep time: 5 minutes
Serves 2 (1 cup each)

1 small (175 g) low- or non-fat peach yogurt (or ¾ cup)
1 tsp ground flaxseed
½ banana
¾ cup (approx) milk
1 cup frozen berries

In a blender or the bowl of a food processor, combine all ingredients; purée until smooth. If mixture is too thick, add up to ¼ cup more milk.

NUTRITIONAL ANALYSIS PER SERVING: Calories 180; Protein 7g; Carbohydrate 36g (12%DV); Fat, total 2.5g (4%DV); Fat, saturated 1g (5%DV); Fat, trans 0g; Cholesterol 10mg (3%DV); Fibre 3g (12%DV); Sodium 80mg (3%DV).

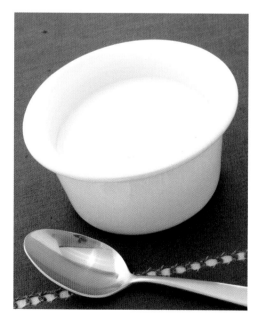

✐Kitchen Savvy: Homemade Nut Butter in Minutes

Many store-bought brands of nut butters contain excessive amounts of sodium and sugar; making your own allows you to control their levels. Also, having the flexibility to select your own blend of nuts is especially helpful for those needing peanut-free alternatives. If you opt to use peanuts in this recipe, we suggest a 1:3 peanut to other nut ratio, as these legumes contain more fat than most nut varieties and can overpower in flavour.

Prep time: 5 minutes
Makes scant 1 cup

1 cup mixed, unsalted, roasted nuts
   (peanuts, walnuts, hazelnuts, cashews, almonds, etc.)
4 tsp liquid honey or agave nectar
2 tbsp water
1½ tbsp canola oil

In the bowl of a food processor, combine all ingredients and process on high speed until puréed. Transfer to an airtight container and refrigerate for up to 1 month.

NUTRITIONAL ANALYSIS PER TABLESPOON: Calories 50; Protein 1g; Carbohydrate 3g (1%DV); Fat, total 4.5g (7%DV); Fat, saturated 0.5g (3%DV); Fat, trans 0g; Cholesterol 0mg; Fibre 0g; Sodium 0mg.

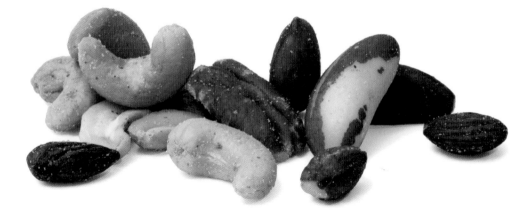

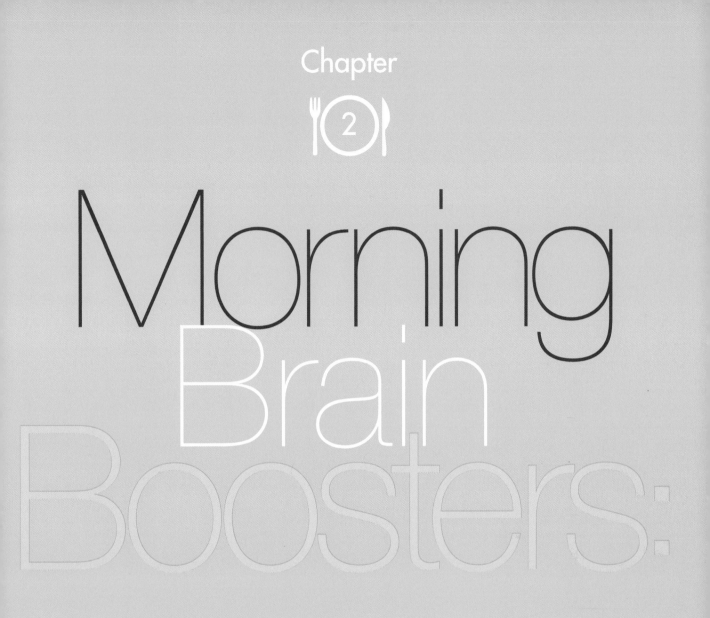

Chapter 2

Morning Brain Boosters: Fuel on the Go

As you now know,
eating breakfast
helps you maintain your
optimal weight
and helps your brain function
better during the day.

So
to get a good head
start each day,
take a few moments to eat something
truly nourishing for breakfast
rather than rushing off without
breakfast or grabbing something
on the run.
Stock your pantry with quick,
easy-to-prepare foods that you can take with you
to stay on schedule
and that also give your brain much-needed fuel.

Carbohydrates and Cognitive Function

Glucose is your brain's "preferred fuel." It is also essential for the formation of specific brain compounds, e.g., acetylcholine, needed for nerve cell communication as well as other brain functions. In healthy older adults, both refined carbohydrate foods high in the GI (e.g., white bread, bagels) or lower GI carbohydrate foods (e.g., those in the **Delicious Low-Fat, High-Fibre Blueberry Muffins** (page 44), **Granola Bites with Figs and Dates** (page 57) and **Bet-You-Can't-Eat-Just-One Cereal Cookies** (page 61) are able to boost brain function.

Giving your brain the fuel it needs improves your ability to stay focused on a task, remember things, recall specific information, maintain executive functions, and multi-task. This is especially true in older adults.

Carbohydrate Quality Counts!

Focusing on healthier carbohydrates can feed your brain even better. For example, among older adults with type 2 diabetes, eating simple, high GI carbohydrate foods can actually decrease cognitive performance, while eating lower GI carbohydrate foods does not.

While healthy individuals can fuel their brains with simple carbohydrates, the long-term consequences of this are not good. Diets high in simple carbohydrates are associated with increased risk of developing type 2 diabetes and heart disease—two diseases you need to avoid for brain health. So grabbing high-sugar snacks or fast-digesting carbs like donuts or bagels may give you a quick burst of energy, but eating them over the long term could have negative effects. Substituting complex carbs (fruits, grains, and other low GI carbs) provides both a boost in mental performance and promotes overall body health.

What About Other Nutrients?

While certain fats, especially the omega-3 fats, are essential for brain function, fats are generally not considered good fuels for the brain. Consequently, they are not likely to provide a temporary boost in brain function.

However, some amino acids in proteins do effect a direct response by the brain or are easily converted to glucose in the body and can also help fuel the brain. This is in addition to their primary role as building blocks for body proteins, including those in the brain. In the few studies that have explored the role of protein, it appears that high-protein foods may also be able to help boost brain function.

Does Caffeine Do the Trick?

Caffeine is the world's most widely consumed psychoactive substance, and many of us reach for our morning coffee or tea to increase alertness and reduce fatigue. Most research suggests that caffeine has an indirect effect on mental performance—that is, by increasing alertness it helps you to perform better. Not surprisingly, these effects are strongest in those individuals who are experiencing fatigue because of a poor night's sleep.

There is a catch-22: over-consuming caffeine can interfere with your sleep, leading you to reach for caffeine to help reduce the impact of sleep deficits. So it is important to manage your caffeine intake wisely. There is nothing wrong in reaching for a morning coffee or tea to increase your alertness, but you must not overdo it to the extent that it interferes with your sleep.

Health Canada suggests that adults should limit their intake of caffeine to 400 milligrams per day. This is equivalent to two to three 8 ounce cups of coffee or eight to ten 8 ounce cups of tea. However, most restaurants and other food service operations offer larger-sized cups, making it easy to consume this amount of caffeine in a single large serving.

You should also be aware that some energy drinks contain more caffeine than a single 8 ounce serving of coffee. Some of this caffeine may come from herbs, such as guarana and yerba maté. The label on these energy drinks would list the herbs as ingredients, but the caffeine in the herbs may not be listed as a separate ingredient. By law, caffeine does not have to be listed on labels unless it has been added to the product separately as a pure substance.

Finally, be aware of the calories and fat in prepared and blended drinks such as cappuccinos and Frappuccinos. For example, a large Iced Capp at Tim Hortons contains 470 kilocalories and includes 20 grams of fat and 12 grams of saturated fat; a Starbucks Double Chocolaty Chip Frappuccino Blended Crème contains 410 kilocalories, 20 grams of total fat and 13 grams of saturated fat; and Second Cup's large Chillatte with whipped cream has 540 kilocalories, 23 grams of total fat and 18 grams of saturated fat.

How to Use This Information

There are two aspects to optimizing our cognitive function. The first is to increase the likelihood that we will sustain our brain function as we age. A diet rich in fruits, vegetables, whole grains and sources of healthy fats is one way to help us on our journey towards healthy brain aging.

The second is to give yourself a temporary boost in cognitive function. Most research suggests that carbohydrates accomplish this best. The recipes in this section were developed to meet both of these functions. They draw heavily on fruits and complex carbohydrates and are low in fat. The carbohydrates in the fruits, grains and flour will help increase your brain function during the morning hours, while the other nutrients contribute to overall brain health. These recipes were also developed with portability in mind, so you can grab and go on those mornings when sitting down for breakfast is not possible. They also work well as desk-drawer snacks to help you avoid reaching for a less-healthy snack during the day.

Chapter 2
Morning Brain Boosters

Recipes

Delicious Low-Fat, High-Fibre Blueberry Muffins   44
by Susan Mendelson

Autumn Fruit Turnovers   46

On-the-Go Fruit Salad   49

Squash Squares with a Whole-Wheat Crust   53
by Laura Calder

Date–Pecan Oatmeal Squares   54
by Rose Reisman

Granola Bites with Figs and Dates   57

Banana Bread with Flaxseed and Wheat Germ   58

Bet-You-Can't-Eat-Just-One Cereal Cookies   61

Breakfast Pizza with Potatoes and Tomato   62
by Chef Judy Wood

Pizza Dough   63

Cheese and Herb Biscuits   64

Delicious Low-Fat, High-Fibre Blueberry Muffins

By Susan Mendelson

Susan Mendelson, author of four bestselling cookbooks, has owned The Lazy Gourmet, a gourmet cookbook store in Vancouver, since 1979, wowing locals and visitors alike with her home-spun specialties.

If you prefer small muffins, use a 24-cup mini-muffin pan and bake for 7 to 9 minutes.

Prep time: 15 minutes
Cook time: 20 minutes
Makes 12 muffins

1 cup quick rolled oats
1 cup buttermilk
2 egg whites
¼ cup melted unsalted butter
⅔ cup packed light brown sugar
½ cup + 1 tbsp all-purpose flour
½ cup spelt or whole-wheat flour
1 tsp baking powder
½ tsp baking soda
½ tsp salt
¼ tsp ground nutmeg
¼ tsp ground cinnamon
2 cups fresh or frozen blueberries

Preheat oven to 400°F. Lightly grease a 12-cup muffin pan or line with muffin cups.

In a bowl, stir together oats and buttermilk; let stand for 5 minutes. Stir in egg whites and butter.

In a separate bowl, combine brown sugar, ½ cup all-purpose flour, spelt flour, baking powder, baking soda, salt, nutmeg and cinnamon. In another bowl, gently toss blueberries with 1 tbsp all-purpose flour.

Make a well in the middle of the flour mixture; gently stir in oat mixture. Do not over-mix. Gently fold in blueberries. Spoon mixture evenly into prepared pan.

Bake in centre of preheated oven until firm to the touch, 15 to 20 minutes.

NUTRITIONAL ANALYSIS PER MUFFIN: Calories 170; Protein 4g; Carbohydrate 29g (10%DV); Fat, total 5g (8%DV); Fat, saturated 2.5g (13%DV); Fat, trans 0g; Cholesterol 10mg (3%DV); Fibre 2g (8%DV); Sodium 210mg (9%DV).

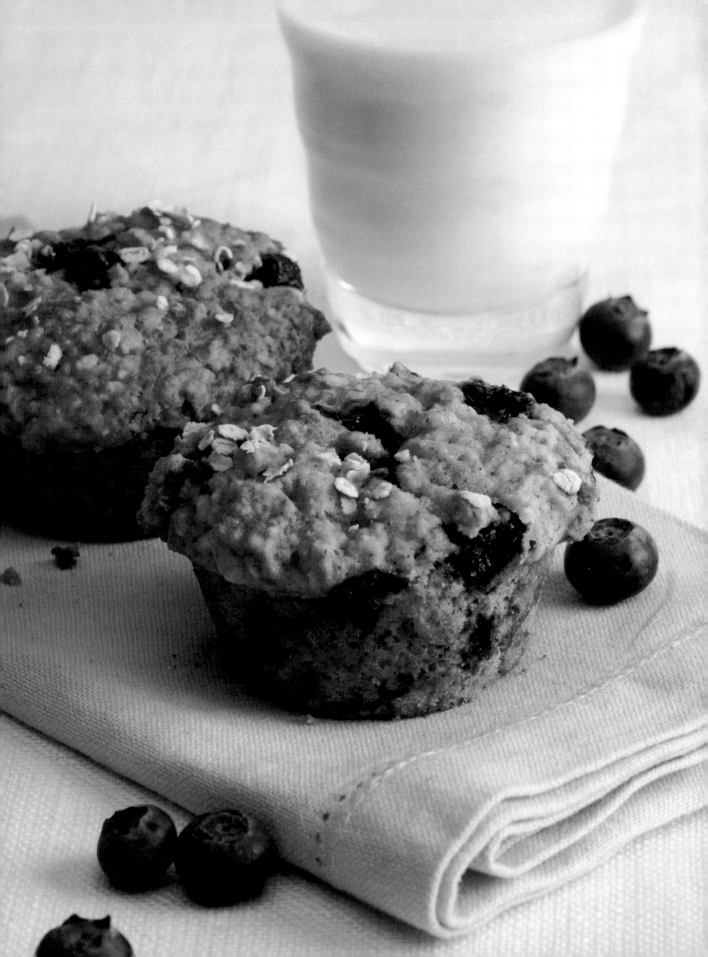

Autumn Fruit Turnovers

Apple pie gets a healthy, hand-held makeover! No deep-frying and no butter-drenched puff pastry—just wholesome goodness. For the best taste possible, use ripe fruit.

Prep time: 15 minutes
Cook time: 25 minutes
Makes 10 turnovers

1 Empire or Royal Gala apple, peeled and cored
1 Bosc pear, peeled and cored
1 tbsp canola oil or unsalted butter
1 tbsp ground cinnamon
½ tsp ground ginger
½ orange, zested and juiced
2 tbsp liquid honey or agave nectar
¼ cup raisins
¼ cup frozen or dried cranberries
1 tbsp all-purpose or whole-wheat flour
10 sheets phyllo dough, thawed
3 tbsp walnut oil or canola oil
3 tbsp granulated sugar

Preheat oven to 350°F.

Cut apple and pear into bite-size pieces.

In a saucepan set over medium-low heat, heat oil (or melt butter). Stir in cinnamon, ginger, orange zest, orange juice and honey until combined. Stir in apple, pear, raisins and cranberries until well coated. Cook for 2 minutes.

Sprinkle 1 tbsp flour over fruit, stirring to combine. Cook until mixture resembles chunky applesauce, about 5 minutes. Remove pan from heat; set aside.

Unwrap and unfold phyllo dough; cover with a damp cloth.

Lay 1 sheet of phyllo on a flat workspace. Position phyllo so the length of the sheet runs parallel to the edge of your workspace.

Lightly brush phyllo with walnut oil. Fold dough in thirds, forming a long strip. Place about ¼ cup fruit on top of the strip, in the right hand corner, leaving a 1-inch border. Fold the top left corner (farthest away from you) over and across the fruit. This will create a triangle pocket. You may have to spread the filling to accommodate the fold. Continue folding into a triangle, following the straight edge, until you get to the end of the strip. Seal the final fold with a light brush of walnut oil. Repeat using the remainder of phyllo and fruit. (Turnovers can be frozen at this point. Lightly brush with oil. Freeze on a rimmed baking sheet until completely frozen. Transfer to a freezer bag. Freeze for up to 3 months. Do not thaw before baking. Increase baking time by about 3 minutes.)

Place turnovers, seal-side down, on a parchment paper–lined baking sheet. Lightly brush each with remaining walnut oil. Sprinkle with sugar.

Bake in centre of preheated oven until golden brown, about 25 minutes.

NUTRITIONAL ANALYSIS PER TURNOVER: Calories 170; Protein 2g; Carbohydrate 26g (9%DV); Fat, total 7g (11%DV); Fat, saturated 1g (5%DV); Fat, trans 0g; Cholesterol 0mg; Fibre 2g (8%DV); Sodium 95mg (4%DV).

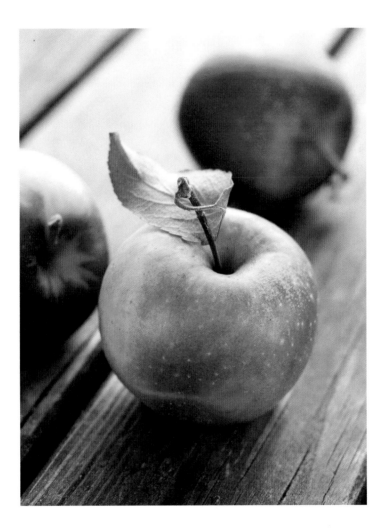

❧Health Savvy: How Do You Like Them Apples?

Be certain to include apples and other white fruit, such as pears, in your diet. In terms of brain health, there has been much emphasis on darkly coloured fruit, especially berries, because of their high antioxidant content. However, a recent study showed that consumption of white fruit (apples and pears) is associated with a decreased risk of stroke. While the protective component of apples and pears has not been identified, this study strongly supports the recommendation that we should draw on a wide and diverse variety of fruit to maximize their health benefits.

Galas and Grannies and Goldens, oh my! When you have a long list of varieties and even more recipes to choose from, it's difficult to know which apple is best for different purposes. Here's a quick guide:

PURPOSE	CHARACTERISTIC REQUIRED	RECOMMENDED VARIETIES
Raw	Bright flavour Balanced sweetness Crisp texture	Fuji, Gala, Macoun, Red Delicious
Cooked	Balance of sweet, tart and spicy Holds shape when cooked	Golden Delicious, Granny Smith, Ida Red, Jonathan, Northern Spy
Multi-purpose	Good balance of firm and mealy texture	Braeburn, Cortland, Empire, Honeycrisp, Jonagold, McIntosh, Mutsu (Crispin), Pink Lady

On-the-Go Fruit Salad

Carol says one of the benefits of working on this cookbook is that it gave her the opportunity to ask one of her graduate students, Tupur Rahman, to share her recipe for this nutrient- and antioxidant-packed fruit salad. Tupur makes a large quantity, packs it in small- to medium-sized plastic containers and freezes it. Grabbing a container from the freezer in the morning is an easy way for her to ensure that she has a healthy meal while at work. The mango's natural acid keeps the apples crisp and prevents them from turning brown.

Prep time: 10 minutes
Serves 4 (1 cup each)

2 Granny Smith apples
1 large mango, peeled
1 large pomegranate, seeded

Cut apples and mango into bite-size pieces; combine with pomegranate seeds.

Transfer to portioned-sized airtight containers and refrigerate for up to 4 days or freeze for up to 2 weeks.

NUTRITIONAL ANALYSIS PER SERVING: Calories 70; Protein 1g; Carbohydrate 18g (6%DV); Fat, total 0g; Fat, saturated 0g; Fat, trans 0g; Cholesterol 0mg; Fibre 3g (12%DV); Sodium 0mg.

....

TIP—Seeding Pomegranates

Consider the pomegranate a laborious ingredient no more! Here are two easy techniques for coaxing out those seeds in record time:

1. Water bath: Quarter pomegranate. Working with one piece at a time, submerge segments in a large bowl of cold or room-temperature water. Use your fingers to gently scrape the seeds out of the membrane. The pith will naturally rise to the top while the seeds fall to the bottom of the bowl, for easy separation and absolutely no mess.

2. Spoon spank: Halve pomegranate lengthwise. Hold the cut-side of the pomegranate over a large bowl and whack the skin-side with a wooden spoon. This is a slightly messier option, as you might get sprayed, but it's a great stress reliever!

....

❦Health Savvy: Fats Deconstructed

It is important to make wise choices when it comes to fat selection, since many studies show that diets high in fat (and particularly in saturated fat) are associated with an increased risk of cognitive decline with aging. One benefit of eating healthful fats, such as poly- and monounsaturated fats as found in avocados and canola oil, is that these lower our risk of heart disease and atherosclerosis. This helps to keep our brain arteries and veins healthy, and allows our vascular system to deliver much-needed nutrients and oxygen to the brain and eliminate the brain's waste material. Ensuring that you are consuming enough omega-3 fats is important for brain health; however, we encourage you to do this by consuming a diet rich in nuts, seeds (such as flax) and fish.

Solid Fats

Butter (unsalted) There really is no substitute for the delicious taste of butter, which makes so many baked goods sublime. But—and this is a big but—butter is high in saturated fats, so it's unhealthy to eat in large quantities. For healthy baking, it's optimal to reduce the butter a bit: keep some in for flavour, but replace the rest with canola oil. Other techniques include heating whatever butter that is called for to a nutty brown; this intensifies the flavour and allows you to use somewhat less. (For a tip on browning butter, see page 260.)

Margarine For dietary, kosher or other reasons, sometimes margarine can be substituted for butter. Use only the hard stick variety, if you must absolutely use margarine. The problem with margarine is that to make margarine potentially beneficial polyunsaturated fats need to be hydrogenated—to transform them from a liquid to a solid—turning them into harmful saturated fats. In addition, often artificial colour, flavour, stabilizers, emulsifiers and gums are added to make margarine appear and taste more like butter. When you purchase margarine, be certain to look for "non-hydrogenated" on the label, as these margarines do not contain the harmful trans fats.

Shortening Like margarine, shortening has undergone a process of hydrogenation, negating any of the benefits the vegetable oils may have had in their original state. Use sparingly, mainly for flaky pie crusts.

Liquid Fats

Vegetable, nut and seed oils Vegetable, nut and seed oils are used in baking primarily for one of two reasons: for their fat content and for their flavour. They cannot be used for recipes that need creaming to lighten a batter since they cannot retain air or be creamed. Always try to buy cold-pressed oils, which enables the oils to retain their vitamin E content; hot processing and purification processing destroy the vitamin E found naturally in these oils, as well as a great deal of their inherent flavour. Heat, light and oxygen promote deterioration of all oils, so be sure to store them in an airtight container in a cool, dry, dark place.

Olive oil Known as the healthiest oil due to its high monounsaturated content, olive oil contains polyphenols, flavonoids and antioxidants. It has been linked with reducing heart disease and certain cancers such as colon and breast. It is a great cooking oil, wonderful for frying, cooking, salad dressings and the like. Its naturally exuberant flavour, however, renders it less than ideal for baking. Unless you want a pronounced fruity or peppery flavour to your baking, it's best not to use olive oil. The one exception to this is extra light olive oil. This is not a "light" oil per se. It still has the same grams of fat (9 calories per gram or 120 calories per tablespoon) as extra virgin, but it has been specially filtered and refined to make it mild flavoured so it can be used more generally in baking.

Canola oil The next healthiest oil after olive oil, canola oil is extremely low in saturated fat and quite high in monounsaturated fats. This makes it an excellent choice for low-fat baking. Of course, you can't aerate it for cakes as is possible with butter, but it is flavourless, which makes it an ideal option.

Flavoured oils These are a great option for introducing moisture and high amounts of flavour into your baking or cooking. Hazelnut oil is an amber-hued oil, rich in flavour and aroma. It's best used in cooking at the end of a recipe since, as with all oils, heating robs it of its delicate flavour. Try adding a few drops into pancake batter, nut-filled coffee cake or hazelnut cookies. Sesame oil, either the pale-coloured variety or the darker golden variety made from toasted sesame seeds, is wonderful for cooking, marinades and salads. It can also be used to great effect in baking, introducing a deep nutty overtone to cakes and cookies. Pumpkin seed oil is very dark coloured, almost a grass green in some cases. It has a very strong flavour and so should mostly be confined to savoury dishes. Walnut oil, like the specialty oils mentioned above, is expensive, but a little goes a long way. It has a relatively low smoking point, making it ideal for sautés and stir-frying. It is a wonderful addition to cookies, yeast breads and some cakes.

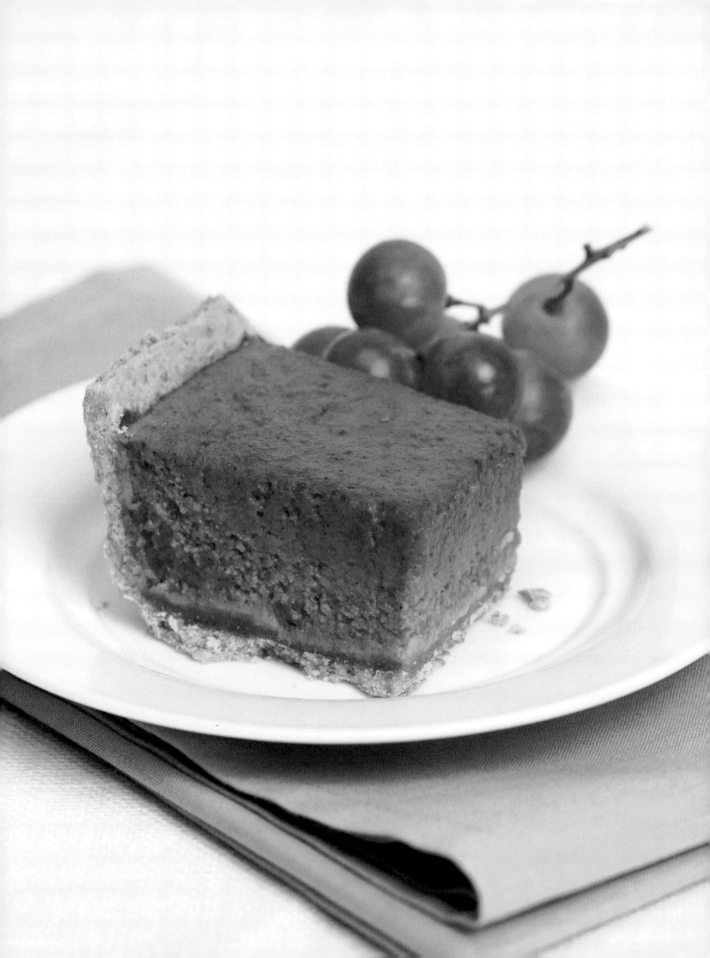

Squash Squares with a Whole-Wheat Crust

By Laura Calder

Host of French Food at Home *on the Food Network, Laura Calder is also the acclaimed author of three books on French cuisine,* French Food at Home, French Taste *and* Dinner Chez Moi.

At home, we never made pumpkin pie, always squash, which we rather self-righteously preferred. It's not just the squash that makes this so tasty, though—the whole-wheat crust, too, lends a pleasant nuttiness, and the honey in place of sugar adds natural warm depth to the taste. This recipe is also great made in a 9-inch pie shell.

Prep time: 20 minutes
Cook time: 45 minutes
Makes 16 squares

CRUST

1¼ cups whole-wheat flour

Pinch salt

6 tbsp cold unsalted butter,
    cut into pieces

2 tbsp ice-cold water

FILLING

2 cups puréed squash

1 cup milk

3 eggs

½ cup liquid honey (preferably organic)

1¼ tsp ground cinnamon

¼ tsp ground cloves

¼ tsp ground ginger

¼ tsp ground nutmeg

Pinch salt

Preheat oven to 450°F.

Crust: In the bowl of a food processor, combine flour, salt and butter; pulse to fine crumbs. Add water; pulse just until dough comes together. Gather dough into a ball. Transfer to a lightly floured surface. Roll out dough to an 11 x 11-inch square. Fit into an 8-inch square baking pan.

Filling: In a bowl, whisk together squash, milk, eggs, honey, cinnamon, cloves, ginger, nutmeg and salt until smooth; pour into pastry-lined pan.

Bake in centre of preheated oven for 10 minutes. Reduce oven temperature to 375°F; bake until top is set, about 35 minutes. Let cool completely in pan on rack before cutting into squares.

NUTRITIONAL ANALYSIS PER SQUARE: Calories 130; Protein 3g; Carbohydrate 19g (6%DV); Fat, total 6g (9%DV); Fat, saturated 3g (15%DV); Fat, trans 0g; Cholesterol 50mg (17%DV); Fibre 2g (8%DV); Sodium 25mg (1%DV).

Date–Pecan Oatmeal Squares

By Rose Reisman

Rose Reisman, author of over 17 cookbooks on nutrition and wellness, has long been known for her passion for low-fat cooking. She not only teaches and makes several media appearances per month, but she has also recently launched, along with her personal food delivery service, a line of frozen food products as well.

Date squares, often known as matrimonial squares, have been a classic for decades, but the oatmeal crust often contains a cup or more of butter or vegetable shortening. My version only uses ⅓ cup of oil, yet it's incredibly delicious and rich tasting. Dates are an excellent source of energy and carbohydrates, as well as protein and iron. I buy my pitted dates at a bulk food store and keep them in the freezer. To chop dried fruits, I use scissors, which is easier than a knife.

Prep time: 15 minutes
Cook time: 35 minutes
Makes 12 squares

2 cups chopped pitted dates
2 tbsp granulated sugar
1 cup orange juice
1 tsp grated orange zest
1¼ cups quick rolled oats

1 cup all-purpose flour
¾ cup packed light brown sugar
¼ cup chopped toasted pecans
1 tsp ground cinnamon
⅓ cup vegetable oil
¼ cup water

Preheat oven to 350°F. Lightly grease an 8-inch square baking pan.

In a saucepan, combine dates, sugar and orange juice; bring to a boil over medium-high heat. Reduce heat to medium; simmer until dates are soft and liquid is absorbed, 10 to 15 minutes. Mash mixture; let cool.

In a bowl, stir together orange zest, oats, flour, brown sugar, pecans, cinnamon, oil and water until combined. Pat half the mixture onto bottom of prepared pan. Spread a thin layer of date mixture overtop. Sprinkle remaining oat mixture on top of dates.

Bake in centre of preheated oven until golden, 25 to 35 minutes. Cool to room temperature on rack before slicing and serving. (Squares can be stored at room temperature for up to 2 days or frozen for 2 weeks.)

NUTRITIONAL ANALYSIS PER SQUARE: Calories 280; Protein 3g; Carbohydrate 50g (17%DV); Fat, total 8g (12%DV); Fat, saturated 0.5g (3%DV); Fat, trans 0g; Cholesterol 0mg; Fibre 4g (16%DV); Sodium 5mg (0%DV).

TIP—Are You a Date Lover?

If you really love dates, feel free to use up to 1 lb in the filling!

❧ Health Savvy: Stocking Your Baking Pantry

All-purpose flour Available both bleached and unbleached, this is, as its name implies, the workhorse of flours. With its moderate protein content, it can be used successfully in most cakes, cookies, biscuits and scones. Unless the recipe specifically requests that you do so, *do not* sift the flour before you measure, as this will throw off the ratio of ingredients. All-purpose flour should be measured by the dip-and-sweep method. (Dip the measuring cup into the flour so that the flour is mounded on top; then using the blunt edge of a table knife or your fingers, sweep off the excess flour.) All-purpose flour has had the bran and germ removed during milling. Bleached flour is made when chemicals such as chlorine dioxide, benzoyl peroxide or acetone peroxide are used to treat the flour, providing it with an ivory white colour as well as a slightly more delicate flavour and texture. Unbleached flour has been aged naturally, with no added colours or chemicals. Some people prefer this variety, stating they prefer a flour with no minute bitterness from the bleaching. Bleached and unbleached flour can be used interchangeably.

Whole-wheat flour For whole-wheat flour, the entire grain is milled, including the bran and the germ. As a result, the flour has a speckled appearance and a coarser texture than all-purpose flour. It is rich in fibre and highly nutritious. However, it can go rancid quickly, so purchase small bags and store them in your freezer. The flour can be measured and used right from the freezer. Baked goods made with whole-wheat flour will be chewier and heavier than those made with all-purpose flour. Don't be tempted to substitute all of the all-purpose flour in a recipe with whole-wheat flour. The general rule of thumb, for yeast breads, is to use 60% whole-wheat flour and 40% white all-purpose flour. For cakes, cookies and quick breads, replace no more than half of the white flour with whole-wheat flour.

Wheat germ Wheat germ, the isolated germ of the wheat grain, is highly nutritious. It can be added to almost any cake, quick bread, cookie or bread to boost the nutritional value. It will, of course, add a distinctly nutty, whole-grain taste (so choose wisely what you add it to!). Wheat germ is highly perishable, so store it in the refrigerator or in the freezer.

Wheat bran Wheat bran is the outer layer of the wheat kernel and is very high in carbohydrates, calcium and fibre. Coarser and darker than wheat germ, it too can be added to muffins, cookies and quick breads to increase their fibre content and nutritional value. Highly prone to rancidity, wheat bran should be stored in the refrigerator or freezer.

Oats These are whole-grain oats (or groats) that have been steamed and then rolled flat. Steel-cut oats are whole-grain oats that have been cut with steel cutters, resulting in coarse, unevenly shaped oats. Oat bran is the outer husk of the whole-grain oat. It contains most of the fibre and some of the fat. Oats are especially known for their high content of soluble fibres, which help to reduce blood cholesterol levels.

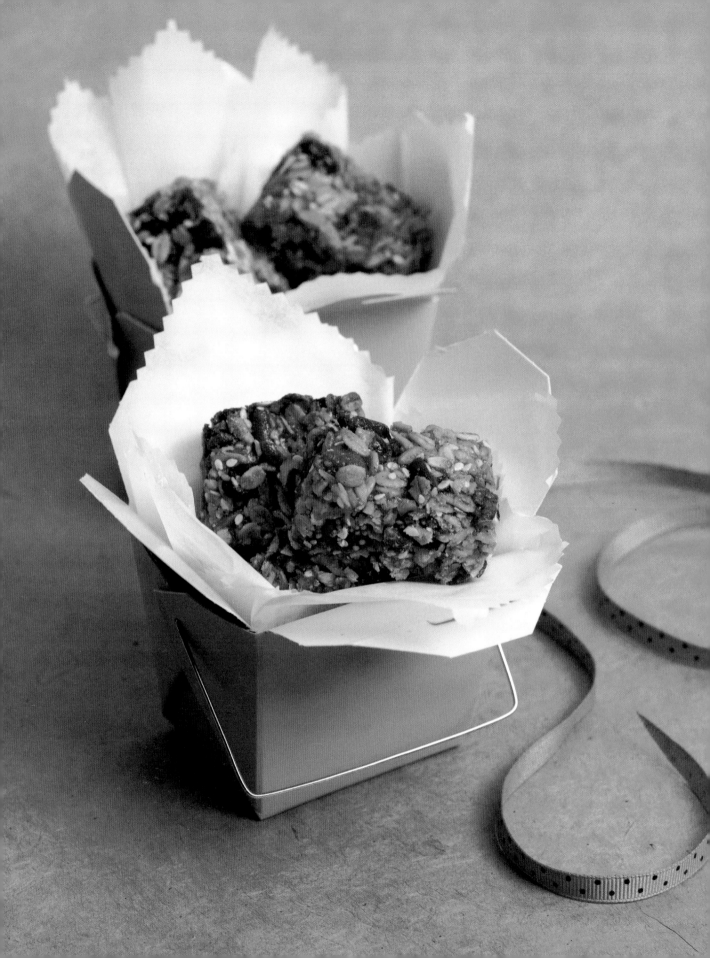

Granola Bites with Figs and Dates

Sticky, crunchy and sweet—**Easy Maple Granola** (page 29) does double duty in this recipe, but it can easily be swapped with your favourite store-bought brand.

Prep time: 15 minutes
Cook time: 25 minutes
Makes 24 bites

⅓ cup unsalted butter, melted
¼ cup each liquid honey and pure maple syrup
2 tbsp packed light brown sugar
1½ tsp vanilla
1 egg
2 cups Easy Maple Granola (page 29)
¾ cup chopped dates
⅔ cup chopped pecans
⅓ cup raisins
¼ cup chopped figs
¼ cup all-purpose flour
2 tbsp sesame seeds
¼ tsp each ground cinnamon and salt

Preheat oven to 350°F. Lightly grease an 8-inch square baking pan. Line with parchment paper, leaving a 2-inch overhang on two sides to facilitate later removal of slab.

In a bowl, stir together butter, honey, maple syrup, brown sugar, vanilla and egg.

In a separate large bowl, combine granola, dates, pecans, raisins, figs, flour, sesame seeds, cinnamon and salt. Stir into egg mixture until well blended. Transfer mixture to prepared pan, smoothing and pressing down top.

Bake in centre of preheated oven until set and top seems dry, 20 to 25 minutes. Let cool in pan on rack. Refrigerate for at least 1 hour or for up to 1 day before cutting into bite-size pieces. (Can be stored in an airtight container at room temperature for up to 5 days.)

NUTRITIONAL ANALYSIS PER BITE: Calories 190; Protein 3g; Carbohydrate 26g (9%DV); Fat, total 9g (14%DV); Fat, saturated 2g (10%DV); Fat, trans 0g; Cholesterol 15mg (5%DV); Fibre 3g (12%DV); Sodium 30mg (1%DV).

Banana Bread with Flaxseed and Wheat Germ

This quick bread uses the slightly different method of beating the eggs with the sugar and then adding the oil, resulting in a lighter texture and colour when fully baked. One slice gives you nutty flavours, great banana overtones, and the goodness of flaxseeds and wheat germ.

Prep time: 15 minutes
Cook time: 70 minutes
Makes 16 slices

1½ cups all-purpose flour
¼ cup flaxseeds
¼ cup toasted wheat germ
1 tsp baking soda
¼ tsp each ground cinnamon and salt
2 eggs
1 cup granulated sugar
⅓ cup canola oil
1½ cups mashed ripe bananas (about 4 bananas)
2 tbsp light sour cream or yogurt
1 tsp vanilla
½ cup toasted chopped walnuts

Preheat oven to 325°F. Lightly grease a 9 x 5-inch loaf pan.

In a bowl, combine flour, flaxseeds, wheat germ, baking soda, cinnamon and salt.

In a separate bowl, using electric beaters (or stand-up mixer), beat together eggs and sugar until light and fluffy, about 5 minutes. Gradually, in a slow, steady stream, pour in oil until thoroughly incorporated. On low speed, add bananas, sour cream and vanilla.

Using a wooden spoon, stir flour mixture into banana mixture until combined. Fold in walnuts. Transfer mixture to prepared pan; smooth top.

Bake in centre of preheated oven until golden brown and top of loaf springs back when lightly pressed, 65 to 70 minutes. Let cool in pan on wire rack. Invert pan to remove. (Loaf can be wrapped in plastic wrap and stored at room temperature for 3 days or frozen for up to 2 weeks.)

NUTRITIONAL ANALYSIS PER SLICE: Calories 200; Protein 4g; Carbohydrate 29g (10%DV); Fat, total 9g (14%DV); Fat, saturated 1g (5%DV); Fat, trans 0g; Cholesterol 30mg (10%DV); Fibre 2g (8%DV); Sodium 125mg (5%DV).

❧Health Savvy: Dried Fruit 101

Raisins Raisins are one of the most nutritious dried fruits in the world. They are free of cholesterol and fat, and are low in sodium. They provide many necessary vitamins and minerals, including iron, potassium, calcium and certain B vitamins. Raisins are a good source of fibre and are rich in antioxidants. As well, they are 70% pure fructose (a natural form of sugar), which is easily digested for quick energy!

The most popular raisin is, of course, the Thompson seedless variety, but there are many different varieties. No matter what the variety, the process is the same: grapes are harvested when they reach a minimum sugar content of 19% or higher, usually sometime around the end of August. After picking, the grapes are laid out on paper trays to sun-dry. This takes on average about 3 weeks. Raisins can only be labelled as such once their moisture content has been reduced to about 15%. Four pounds of fresh grapes yield one pound of raisins.

Raisin colours vary according to the drying process used. For example, a dark purplish/black raisin is sun-dried. A light to medium brown raisin is mechanically dehydrated in special drying tunnels. A golden to bright yellow raisin is mechanically dried and treated with sulphur.

Dates Dates are among the sweetest, richest and most flavourful dried fruits available. They are equally as great in sweet baked goods as they are in Middle Eastern savoury fare. There are many varieties but, by far, the Medjool date stands out as the reigning queen of flavour. Plump, powerfully sweet and rich, Medjool dates are fruity and marvellously moist. Dates provide a good source of fibre and potassium, a mineral that helps keep blood pressure in check. Although they initially contain a fair amount of vitamin C, this vitamin is lost during the drying process. Like most dried fruit, dried dates also contain iron.

As with raisins, dried currants and apricots, dates lend themselves to a variety of sweet and savoury dishes. Don't relegate them just to the filling found in date squares. Moroccan tagines often contain dates, as do many Middle Eastern beef and lamb dishes.

Dried cranberries Dried cranberries are sweeter than fresh cranberries and can double for raisins in most recipes, including salads, baked goods and cereals. They are portable, store well and, like raisins, contain fibre and antioxidants. Depending on whether they are purchased in bulk or under a brand name, there may be slight nutritional differences. For example, dried cranberries can differ in the amount of calories and carbohydrates they have since different companies will add varying levels of sugar to their product. (Adding some sugar is important not only to the taste of the dried cranberry but to its texture as well.) In addition, the amount of fibre can be different.

Manufacturers also add varying amounts of oil during the processing of dried cranberries—to maintain a certain texture—which may alter their nutritional profiles.

Currants Currants are the dried version of the Zante or Corinthe grape, a beautiful wild grape with a sweet, tart intense flavour and a dark blue, almost black skin. They are one of the oldest-known raisins. Currants contain a healthy amount of dietary fibre (both soluble and insoluble), iron, potassium and B vitamins.

Dried figs Dried figs are one of the best plant sources of calcium and fibre. According to USDA (United States Department of Agriculture) data for the Mission variety, dried figs are among the richest of dried fruits in fibre, copper, manganese, magnesium, potassium, calcium, and vitamin K, relative to human needs. They have smaller amounts of many other nutrients. Figs have a laxative effect and contain many antioxidants.

Dried apricots Dried apricots are the pitted, unpeeled, dried half of a fresh apricot. Dried apricots are rich in vitamin A and are a source of iron and calcium. The bright orange ones most commonly available in grocery stores have been treated with sulphur dioxide to preserve their colour. Increasingly, unsulphured dried apricots are available; they're just as firm and plump as their chemically treated brethren, but are more likely to be brown or caramel coloured. They are intensely flavoured. If using the unsulphured variety in baking, add a touch of lemon juice to your recipe to equal the amount of acid required, which is found in the bright orange variety.

Prunes Now known as dried plums (thanks to a conscientious marketing board), prunes are a powerhouse of nutrients, including B vitamins, potassium, magnesium and boron. They contain both soluble and insoluble fibre. A single serving of prunes (about 5 prunes) has 3 grams of fibre. They also contain phenolic compounds that promote good health. When buying prunes, regardless of the variety, look for very plump, moist fruit and avoid any shrivelled or dry-looking fruit. Try to buy from a store with a high turnover rate.

Other options In addition to the dried fruits mentioned here, you can also indulge in dried mangoes, papaya, apples, pears, pineapple and peaches when you're looking for a snack, baking accessory or savoury accompaniment. However, be careful when purchasing dried bananas—they are sometimes fried in coconut oil, which increases their content of both total fat and saturated fat.

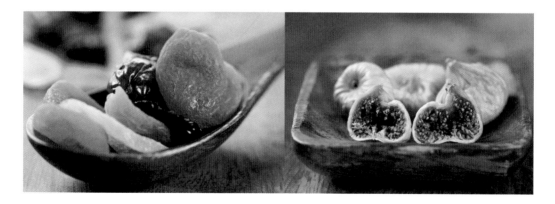

Bet-You-Can't-Eat-Just-One Cereal Cookies

Talk about a mouthful! These are highly addictive; don't be surprised if they're gone before you can say "Bet-You-Can't-Eat-Just-One Cereal Cookies!" If you're a chocoholic, feel free to add ¼ cup mini chocolate chips.

Prep time: 15 minutes
Cook time: 12 minutes per batch
Makes 36 cookies

2 eggs
½ cup packed light brown sugar
¼ cup unsalted butter, melted
1 tsp vanilla
½ cup shredded carrots
⅓ cup coarsely chopped walnuts
1 cup golden raisins
½ cup chopped apricots
½ cup dried cranberries

¼ cup pumpkin seeds
1 cup all-purpose flour
1 cup quick rolled oats
½ tsp each ground cinnamon and baking soda
¼ tsp salt
1½ cups oat cereal rounds (such as Cheerios)

Preheat oven to 350°F.

In a large bowl, whisk together eggs, brown sugar, butter and vanilla. Stir in carrots, walnuts, raisins, apricots, cranberries and pumpkin seeds.

In a separate bowl, combine flour, oats, cinnamon, baking soda and salt. Add flour mixture to fruit mixture and stir just until combined. Stir in cereal. Batter will be loose.

Drop by heaping tablespoonfuls onto parchment paper–lined cookie sheets, 12 per tray.

Bake in centre of preheated oven until golden and firm when lightly pressed, about 12 minutes. Cool pans on rack for 5 minutes. Transfer cookies to racks to cool completely. Repeat with remaining batter.

(Cookies can be stored in an airtight container at room temperature for up to 5 days or frozen for up to 2 months.)

NUTRITIONAL ANALYSIS PER COOKIE: Calories 90; Protein 2g; Carbohydrate 13g (4%DV); Fat, total 3g (5%DV); Fat, saturated 1g (5%DV); Fat, trans 0g; Cholesterol 15mg (5%DV); Fibre 1g (4%DV); Sodium 55mg (2%DV).

Breakfast Pizza with Potatoes and Tomato

By Chef Judy Wood

Currently the chef at Meez Fast Home Cuisine in Calgary, Judy Wood has worked at The Four Seasons Hotel in Calgary, as the head chef at Buchanan's Chop House in Calgary and more recently became founder and executive chef of the successful Savoury Cafe and Catering.

An altogether novel approach to morning dining, this grab-and-go is full of complex carbs to keep you feeling satiated for hours.

Prep time: 60 minutes
Cook time: 25 minutes
Makes 24 slices

1 whole-wheat Pizza Dough (page 63)
1 red-skinned potato, sliced ¼ inch thick
1 small unpeeled sweet potato,
    sliced ¼ inch thick
4 oz prosciutto, trimmed of any excess fat
¼ cup (approx) cornmeal
4 tsp olive oil
¼ tsp salt

½ tsp black pepper
1 tomato, sliced
1¼ cups shredded aged cheddar
    (about 4 oz)
1 tbsp finely chopped fresh rosemary
    (optional)
2 green onions (white and light
    green parts only), slivered

Preheat oven to 400°F.

Prepare pizza dough according to directions on page 63. (Alternatively, use store-bought whole-wheat pizza dough.)

In a large pot of boiling salted water, cook red-skinned and sweet potatoes until tender, about 5 minutes. Drain. Set aside.

Place prosciutto on a parchment paper–lined baking sheet; bake until crispy, 5 to 10 minutes. Let cool.

Divide dough in half. On a floured surface, roll out each piece of dough until quite thin, about 9 x 12 inches. Sprinkle two rimmed baking sheets with cornmeal; transfer dough to prepared baking sheets. Brush with half the oil; sprinkle with ¼ tsp each salt and pepper. Bake in centre of preheated oven until very lightly golden, about 5 minutes. Remove from oven; increase oven temperature to 450°F.

On each precooked pizza dough base, layer half the cooked potatoes, sweet potatoes, prosciutto and tomatoes. Sprinkle with cheese, rosemary (if using) and remaining ¼ tsp pepper. Bake until pizza is browned, about 10 minutes. Garnish with green onion. Let rest for 5 to 10 minutes before slicing into pieces.

NUTRITIONAL ANALYSIS PER SLICE: Calories 110; Protein 5g; Carbohydrate 13g (4%DV); Fat, total 5g (8%DV); Fat, saturated 1.5g (8%DV); Fat, trans 0g; Cholesterol 10mg (3%DV); Fibre 2g (8%DV); Sodium 350mg (15%DV).

Pizza Dough

Prep time: 10 minutes
Makes enough for 2 pizzas

1 tbsp active dry yeast
1 tsp liquid honey
1¼ cups warm water
2½ to 3 cups whole-wheat bread flour
1 tsp salt
2 tbsp olive oil

In a small bowl, dissolve yeast and honey in ¼ cup warm water. Let stand until mixture begins to froth, about 5 minutes.

In a stand-up mixer fitted with the dough hook, combine 1½ cups flour with salt. Add olive oil and yeast mixture. Stir in remaining 1 cup water and gradually add remaining flour, ¼ cup at a time, until a soft dough forms. Knead until dough is smooth and firm and pulls away from the side of the bowl. Transfer to an oiled bowl, cover with plastic wrap and let rise until doubled, about 30 minutes.

....

TIP—No Mixer? No Problem.

In a food processor fitted with the dough hook or metal blade, combine 2 cups flour with salt. Add olive oil, yeast mixture and remaining 1 cup water and process on low speed until a soft dough forms. Gradually add remaining flour, ¼ cup at a time, until dough is smooth and firm and pulls away from the side of the bowl. Process on low speed for an additional 2 to 3 minutes to knead the dough. Proceed with recipe above.

....

Cheese and Herb Biscuits

A savoury snack that's crave-worthy morning, noon and night! These freeze beautifully in a resealable bag for up to 3 months. When you're ready to enjoy them, simply pop them in the microwave for 30 seconds or bake at 350°F for 10 to 12 minutes.

Prep time: 10 minutes
Cook time: 25 minutes
Makes 12 biscuits

2 cups all-purpose flour
½ cup whole-wheat flour
1½ tsp baking powder
¾ tsp salt
½ tsp baking soda
⅓ cup cold unsalted butter, cubed
½ cup finely grated reduced-fat cheddar cheese
2 tbsp finely chopped fresh chives
4 tsp finely chopped fresh rosemary
1 cup buttermilk
1 egg

Preheat oven to 350°F.

In a large bowl, combine all-purpose and whole-wheat flours, baking powder, salt and baking soda. Using two knives or a pastry cutter, cut in butter until mixture resembles coarse meal. Stir in cheese, chives and rosemary.

In a separate bowl, stir together buttermilk and egg. Pour all at once over flour mixture, and stir with a fork until mixture holds together in a soft sticky ball. Transfer to a lightly floured work surface.

Knead dough a couple of times. Using floured hands, pat into layer about 1 inch thick. Using 2- or 2½-inch round cookie cutters, cut out biscuits, rerolling scraps (once only) to get an even dozen. Place on a parchment paper–lined baking sheet.

Bake in centre of preheated oven until puffed and golden, 20 to 25 minutes.

NUTRITIONAL ANALYSIS PER BISCUIT: Calories 160; Protein 5g; Carbohydrate 21g (12%DV); Fat, total 6g (9%DV); Fat, saturated 4g (20%DV); Fat, trans 0g; Cholesterol 35mg (12%DV); Fibre 1g (4%DV); Sodium 300mg (13%DV).

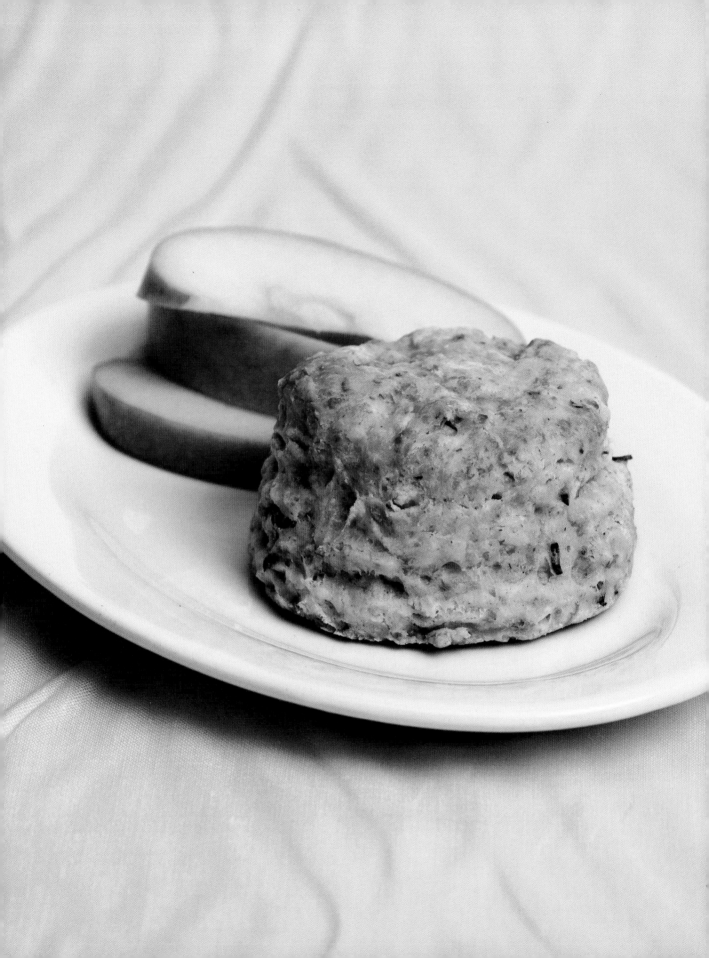

Chapter

3

Lunch for All:

Mid-Day Mindfullness

Who would have thought that lunch is a sunrise story? Well, in some ways it is. Many of us remember the days when we saw the sunrise as we were heading home from a night of festivities. However, nowadays we are more likely to be sitting quietly with our morning coffee watching the sunrise after a good night's sleep. That's because we naturally wake up earlier as we age. However, this also means that lunch may be the best time of day to plan those multi-generational meals: adolescents are finally out of bed, and the older generation is awake and fully engaged in the day's activities.

Circadian Rhythms

"Circadian rhythms" refers to our internal biologic clock that controls our 24-hour daily cycle. This biologic timekeeper is primarily orchestrated by neurons in a region of the brain called the suprachiasmatic nucleus, or SCN. SCN brain cells communicate with other areas of the brain and help control our sleep–wake cycle, body temperature, hormone release, eating behaviour, and energy metabolism.

The integration of biologic processes by the SCN is one of the ways that we ensure that our body is ready to metabolize the foods we eat and ready to draw upon body stores to provide energy when we are asleep. We know that allowing the body to maintain its own natural circadian rhythm is important. Disruptions to these rhythms, such as those experienced in shift workers, can not only lead to sleep disorders but can also lead to obesity, diabetes and metabolic syndrome. All of these disorders contribute to increased rates of cognitive decline with aging.

Changes in Circadian Rhythms with Aging

With aging, our circadian rhythm slowly shifts towards the morning, in that we naturally go to bed earlier at night and rise earlier the next morning, relative to when we were younger. We also change our eating patterns to match our times of wakefulness.

During youth, it is common that our largest meal of the day is supper. The opposite is true as we age. For many older adults, the largest meal of the day is breakfast. The old adage of "tea and toast" for dinner in older adults is partly true and can reflect a smaller appetite as the day progresses. The key is to ensure that food and nutrient needs are met during the day when our appetites are naturally the strongest, and to make sure even small meals draw on healthy foods.

How to Use This Information

Keep in mind that changes to your daily eating patterns are a natural and normal part of aging. However, it can put additional pressure on those preparing meals for adolescents and older adults living in the same household. That's why lunch is a good time of day, from an appetite perspective, for individuals of all ages. So this chapter concentrates on those foods lacking in the diet of many North Americans. The overall goal is to enrich lunch with healthy foods that everyone can enjoy, regardless of age.

Chapter 3

Lunch for All

Recipes

Argentinean Steak Sandwich   73

Saag Paneer Sandwich   74

Four-Season Frittata   77

Caramelized Onion and Tomato Phyllo Tart   78

Pesto Orzo with Roasted Trout and Peas   80

Chicken with Rhubarb Chutney over Dark Greens   83

Shaved Green Salad with Spicy Grilled Shrimp   86

Asian Greens and Rice Noodle Salad   87

Scallop Niçoise Salad   88
by Chef Mark McEwan

Chickpea and Herb Salad with Warm Lemon Dressing   93

Grilled Salmon with Green Salad and Apple Vinaigrette   95
by Chef Chuck Hughes

Corn, Black Bean and Tomato Salad   97

Ceviche Lettuce Wraps   98

Cream of Broccoli Soup   100

Roasted Tomato and Garlic Soup with Rice   101

Mediterranean Stuffed Peppers   102

Curried Lentil and Wheatberry Salad with Mango   105

Wild Rice Salad   108

Golden Quinoa with Raisins and Almonds   109

Sweet Pepper and Barley Risotto Tart with Spinach and Pine Nuts   111

Thin-Crust Pizza with Balsamic-Glazed Tomatoes
and Pesto   113

Pear, Spinach and Blue Cheese Flatbread with Onion Jam   115

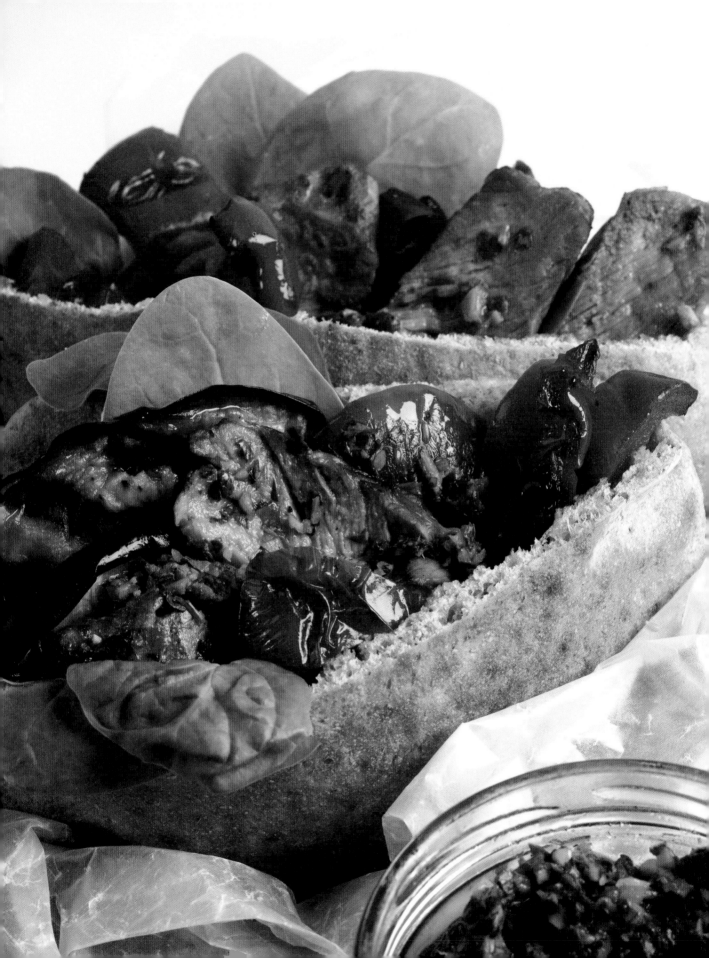

Argentinean Steak Sandwich

Chimichurri is a flavour-packed condiment from Argentina and a fantastic way to use up the fresh herbs hanging around your fridge! Leave the ketchup and mustard behind—this is the ultimate topper for grilled meat.

Prep time: 15 minutes
Cook time: 30 minutes
Serves 4 (½ pita sandwich each)

CHIMICHURRI SAUCE
5 cloves garlic
1 small shallot
2 cups loosely packed fresh Italian parsley
   (stems and leaves)
1 cup loosely packed fresh coriander
   (stems and leaves)
¼ tsp dried red pepper flakes
¼ cup olive oil
3 tbsp red wine vinegar
¼ tsp each salt and black pepper

SANDWICH
1 strip loin steak (about 8 oz)
Pinch each salt and black pepper
½ Italian eggplant, trimmed
1 sweet red pepper, cored and seeded
½ red onion, trimmed
2 6-inch whole-wheat pitas, halved
2 cups loosely packed fresh baby spinach,
   trimmed

Chimichurri sauce: In a blender or the bowl of a food processor, purée all chimichurri ingredients until smooth. Cover with plastic wrap and refrigerate until ready to use (or refrigerate in an airtight container for up to 2 weeks).

Sandwich: To make sandwich, heat a grill pan or cast-iron skillet over high heat. Sprinkle steak lightly with salt and pepper; sear until a golden brown crust is formed, 4 to 5 minutes per side. Remove steak from pan and cover with tin foil.

Meanwhile, slice eggplant lengthwise into 6 to 8 slices, each about ¼ inch thick. Cut red pepper into 8 slices. Slice onion into ½-inch-thick rings.

Arrange eggplant slices around pan. Cook 2 minutes per side or until softened with char marks; remove and set aside. Add peppers. Cook 5 minutes per side or until charred and softened; remove and set aside. Add onion; cook 3 minutes per side or until softened.

Slice steak against the grain into thin strips. Stuff each pita half with ½ cup spinach. Layer 2 pieces each of red pepper and eggplant with 3 to 4 slices of steak. Top with red onions. Drizzle with 2 tbsp chimichurri sauce.

NUTRITIONAL ANALYSIS PER SERVING: Calories 350; Protein 22g; Carbohydrate 29g (10%DV); Fat, total 17g (26%DV); Fat, saturated 4.5g (23%DV); Fat, trans 0g; Cholesterol 40mg (13%DV); Fibre 5g (20%DV); Sodium 370mg (15%DV).

Saag Paneer Sandwich

This recipe makes more saag spread than you will need for this sandwich—about 2 cups total. Stir a couple of tablespoons of the leftover spread into a risotto, use as a dip with pita and vegetables, toss with roasted potatoes, or simmer with chickpeas, cauliflower and fresh tomatoes. The saag spread can also be frozen for up to 3 months.

Prep time: 10 minutes
Cook time: 10 minutes
Serves 4 (½ pita sandwich each)

1 tbsp olive oil
½ tsp each ground cumin, ground coriander, ground cinnamon, turmeric, curry powder
   (or 2 tbsp garam masala)
1 small onion, coarsely chopped
1 fresh red hot chili pepper, stemmed, seeded and finely chopped (or ¼ tsp dried red
   pepper flakes, crushed)
3 cloves garlic, coarsely chopped
1 tsp grated fresh ginger (or ½ tsp ground ginger)
1 package (300 g) frozen chopped spinach, thawed
2 tbsp low-fat plain yogurt
¼ tsp each salt and black pepper
2 large whole-wheat pitas, halved
4 Bibb or Boston lettuce leaves
8 thin slices of paneer, halumi or mozzarella cheese
1 large Roma tomato (or 2 small), sliced
¼ cup thinly sliced red onion

Heat oil in a non-stick pan set over medium heat; stir in cumin, coriander, cinnamon, turmeric and curry powder. Cook, stirring, until fragrant and toasted, about 1 minute.

Add onion, chili, garlic and ginger; cook until softened, about 3 minutes.

Using a wooden spoon, stir in spinach to combine with onion mixture, scraping any browned bits from bottom of pan. Cook for 2 minutes.

Pour spinach mixture into a blender or the bowl of a food processor; purée until smooth. Add yogurt, salt and pepper; pulse to combine.

Spread 2 tbsp spinach mixture inside each pita half. Stuff with lettuce; layer with cheese, tomato slices and a few thin slices of red onion.

NUTRITIONAL ANALYSIS PER SERVING: Calories 250; Protein 12g; Carbohydrate 26g (9%DV); Fat, total 11g (17%DV); Fat, saturated 5g (25%DV); Fat, trans 0g; Cholesterol 25mg (8%DV); Fibre 4g (16%DV); Sodium 430mg (18%DV).

❦ Health Savvy: A World of Sandwiches

Although this lunchtime staple can be traced back to religious scripture—the Jewish Passover feast requires that herbs, a paste of fruit and nuts, and/or horseradish be consumed between two pieces of matzah—it was during a late-night cribbage game that it essentially took hold. It was cribbage night in the 18th century and John Montagu, the fourth Earl of Sandwich, couldn't be bothered to interrupt his game for dinner. Instead, he requested some meat be brought to him between two slices of bread—allowing him to dine without dirtying his fingers or cards. Culinary history was made, and the sandwich has been circling the globe ever since.

The handy concept was canonized as the ultimate convenience food during the Industrial Revolution. The daily exodus of workers from the home demanded an inexpensive and portable meal, and sandwiches quickly became the lunch of choice.

The "sammie" has been adopted and acculturated by practically every nation. If you are looking for new flavours between your bread, here is a small collection of international sandwich ideas to inspire the Montagu in you:

Falafel A Middle Eastern pita sandwich stuffed with deep-fried chickpea fritters and a variety of cold salads (beets, eggplant, parsley, cabbage), and traditionally topped with hummus, tahini and spicy harissa. Replace the fritters with spit-roasted spiced chicken or lamb for a shawarma.

Panini Italian ciabatta rolls are sliced horizontally, layered with meats—salami, prosciutto, sopressata, etc.—and cheese before being roasted on a warm grill.

Tartine For this open-faced sandwich of France, a thin slice of bread is topped with a luxurious spread. From butter to melted brie, the options are endless.

Quesadilla Melted cheese and stewed beans are folded up in the centre of a corn tortilla for this Mexican "sandwich." Heartier siblings of this hand-held meal include the fajita, burrito and taco—all of which add different combinations of rice, salsas and meat to the quesadilla's filling.

Bánh mì This Vietnamese sandwich marries southeast Asian flavour with French colonial history. It's traditionally made on a French baguette (introduced to the region by colonizers); savoury roasted meats or pâté, usually pork, are layered with refreshing pickled salads of cucumber, carrots, daikon and cilantro, and topped with hot chili sauces.

Baozi Chinese steamed buns are leavened and cooked in bamboo steamers over simmering water. Stuffed with roasted or ground meat, vegetable and/or bean paste fillings, this Asian take on the sandwich is served alongside soy sauce, vinegar and chili paste for dipping.

Kitchen Savvy: Alternatives to Mayonnaise

Here is an array of delicious, lighter alternatives to mayonnaise that will pep up any sandwich.

- Baba ghanouj
- **Chimichurri sauce** (see recipe on page 73)
- Chutney—mango, tomato, apple, etc.
- Cranberry sauce
- Greek yogurt/tzatziki
- Guacamole
- **Harissa** (see recipe on page 204)
- Homemade barbecue sauce
- Hummus—plain, roasted red pepper, garlic, etc.
- Infused oil—chili, herb, garlic, etc.
- Mustard
- **Nut butters**—peanut, almond, cashew, etc. (For a nut butter recipe, see page 37)
- **Onion jam** (see recipe on page 115)
- **Pesto**—basil, sun-dried tomato, cilantro, etc. (For a recipe for basil pesto, see page 80)
- Ratatouille
- Salsa—tomato, corn, mango, etc.
- Salsa verde
- Sriracha
- Tapenade—olive, sun-dried tomato, artichoke, etc.

Four-Season Frittata

Frittatas are dependable dinner and lunch allies since they involve staples you're most likely to have on hand: eggs, onions, garlic, a little milk and any cheese or veggie. When imagination fails and appetites rumble, a frittata is the easy answer to any season's mealtime woes.

Prep time: 15 minutes
Cook time: 20 minutes
Serves 6

MASTER RECIPE
1 tbsp vegetable oil
1 onion, chopped
2 cloves garlic, minced
8 eggs
¼ cup milk
¼ tsp black pepper
Pinch salt

WINTER FILLING
1 cup cooked whole-wheat fusilli or macaroni
1½ cups cooked broccoli florets
4 oz smoked chicken breast, julienned
½ cup shredded cheddar cheese

SPRING FILLING
1½ cups cooked asparagus pieces
4 oz smoked turkey breast, julienned
½ cup shredded Emmenthal or Swiss cheese

SUMMER FILLING
1 large tomato, seeded and diced
1 cup cooked peas or chopped fresh green beans
2 tbsp chopped fresh basil or mint leaves
½ cup shredded fontina cheese

AUTUMN FILLING
1 cup diced zucchini
1 cup diced sweet red pepper
½ cup cooked fresh corn kernels
½ cup shredded smoked Gouda cheese

Heat oil in 9- or 10-inch ovenproof skillet set over medium heat. Add onion and garlic; cook, stirring, for 3 minutes, until softened. Preheat broiler.

Whisk together eggs, milk, pepper, salt and choice of filling, excluding cheese. Pour into skillet, stirring well. Top with cheese. Reduce heat to medium-low; cook, without stirring, until sides and bottom are set, about 8 to 10 minutes. Broil until golden brown and set, about 3 minutes. Let sit for 3 minutes. Remove to platter to serve in wedges.

NUTRITIONAL ANALYSIS PER EACH OF 6 SERVINGS (BASED ON MASTER RECIPE): Calories 140; Protein 9g; Carbohydrate 3g (1%DV); Fat, total 9g (14%DV); Fat, saturated 2.5g (13%DV); Fat, trans 0g; Cholesterol 290mg (97%DV); Fibre 0g; Sodium 95mg (4%DV).

Caramelized Onion and Tomato Phyllo Tart

Alternating layers of butter or oil with mustard is an excellent way to reduce fat when using phyllo. (This is especially good when phyllo is wrapped around stuffed chicken breasts!) Asiago cheese can be replaced with fontina or Edam.

Prep time: 40 minutes
Cook time: 45 minutes
Serves 8

3 tbsp olive oil
3 onions, thinly sliced
4 sheets phyllo pastry
¼ cup unsalted butter, melted
¼ cup Dijon mustard
1½ cups shredded Asiago cheese
2 tomatoes, sliced
1 large clove garlic, minced
1 tbsp chopped fresh basil leaves
¼ tsp black pepper

Preheat oven to 375°F.

Heat 2 tbsp oil in a large non-stick skillet set over medium-low heat. Add onion; cook, stirring often, until golden and caramelized, 30 to 45 minutes.

Meanwhile, cut each sheet of phyllo in half crosswise. Place one half on tea towel, keeping the rest covered with a damp towel. Lightly brush sheet with melted butter; place another sheet on top, a little askew so they are not perfectly aligned. Brush top phyllo with 1 tbsp mustard. Keeping phyllo slightly askew, repeat layers, alternating brushing with butter and mustard until all the phyllo has been used. Transfer to a 14 x 4½-inch French tart pan with removable bottom. Fold phyllo edges under to fit.

Place onions on prepared tart; sprinkle with cheese. Top with overlapping slices of tomatoes. Sprinkle with garlic, basil and pepper. Drizzle remaining 1 tbsp oil overtop.

Bake in centre of preheated oven until phyllo is golden, 30 to 45 minutes.

NUTRITIONAL ANALYSIS PER EACH OF 8 SERVINGS: Calories 240; Protein 6g; Carbohydrate 14g (5%DV); Fat, total 18g (28%DV); Fat, saturated 8g (40%DV); Fat, trans 0g; Cholesterol 35mg (12%DV); Fibre 2g (8%DV); Sodium 430mg (18%DV).

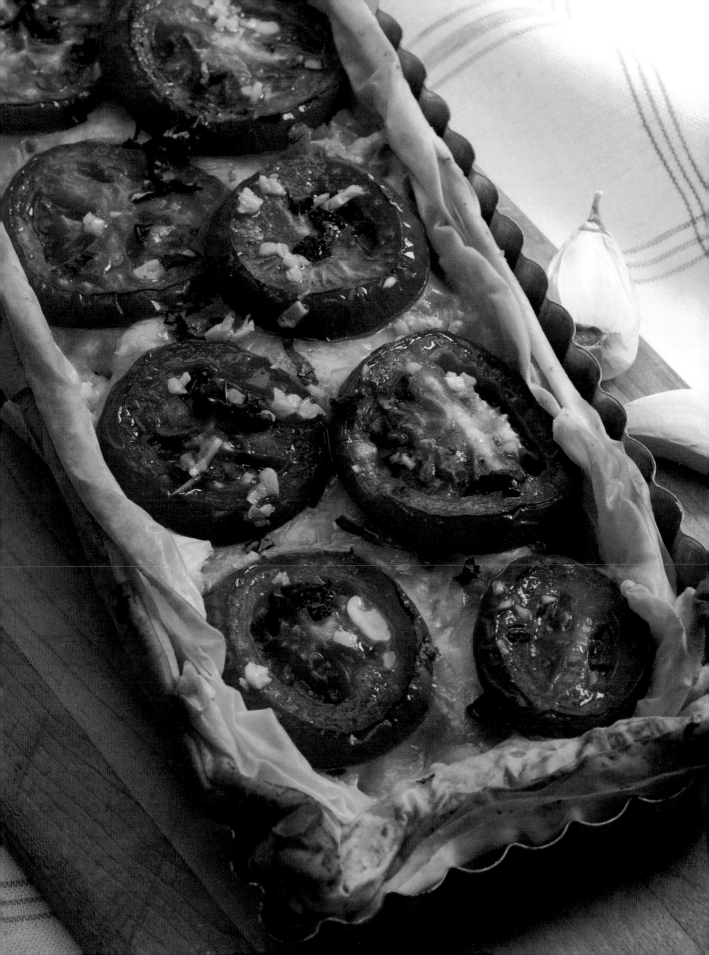

Pesto Orzo with Roasted Trout and Peas

If you prefer a smoky flavour or need to save time, replace the roasted trout with your favourite store-bought smoked trout.

Prep time: 10 minutes
Cook time: 15 minutes
Serves 6 (1⅓ cups each)

FISH
2 rainbow trout fillets (about 6 oz each)
¼ tsp each salt and black pepper

PESTO SAUCE
2 cups packed fresh basil leaves (2 to 3 bunches)
¼ cup toasted walnut pieces
3 tbsp grated Parmesan cheese
1 tbsp finely grated lemon zest
3 tbsp olive oil
2 tbsp water
2 cloves garlic, coarsely chopped
¼ tsp each salt and black pepper

PASTA
2 cups uncooked orzo
1½ cups frozen peas (or 1 lb asparagus, trimmed and cut into 1-inch lengths)

Preheat oven to 350°F.

Fish: Place trout, skin-side down, on a parchment paper–lined baking sheet. Sprinkle with salt and pepper. Bake in centre of preheated oven for 10 minutes.

Pesto sauce: Meanwhile, place all ingredients for pesto sauce in the bowl of a food processor. Purée, scraping down sides of bowl a few times, until fairly smooth or desired consistency is reached.

Pasta: In a large pot of boiling salted water, cook orzo until al dente, about 8 minutes. Add peas; cook for 1 to 2 minutes more or until peas are tender. Reserving 1 cup pasta water, drain well. Transfer pasta and peas to a bowl. Flake fish, discarding skin. Add to pasta. Stir pesto into pasta, stirring gently until both pasta and fish are well coated, thinning out with reserved pasta cooking water as necessary.

NUTRITIONAL ANALYSIS PER SERVING: Calories 400; Protein 24g; Carbohydrate 45g (15%DV); Fat, total 15g (23%DV); Fat, saturated 2.5g (13%DV); Fat, trans 0g; Cholesterol 40mg (13%DV); Fibre 5g (20%DV); Sodium 300mg (13%DV).

TIP—Add Variety to Your Pesto Sauce

If you're feeling adventurous, feel free to replace the basil in the pesto with arugula or coriander, or use half mint and half basil.

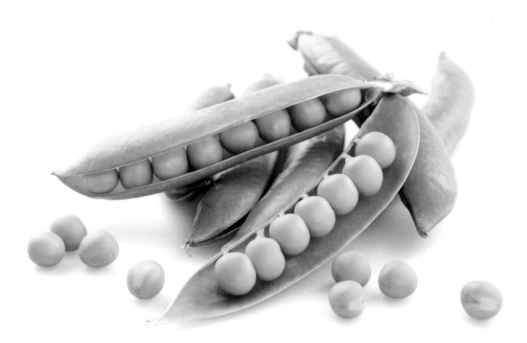

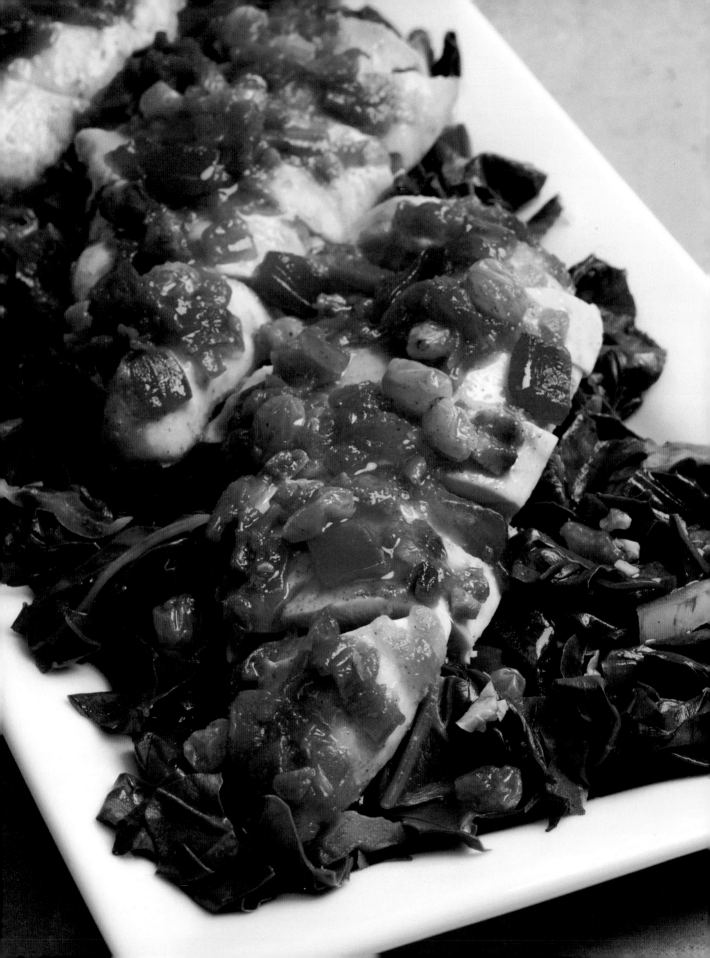

Chicken with Rhubarb Chutney over Dark Greens

Rhubarb, which is a source of calcium, vitamin C and potassium, was known only for its medicinal properties until about 200 years ago. Thankfully, someone finally realized that it's also delicious! Rhubarb pairs wonderfully well with both sweet and savoury foods, especially with fresh ginger.

Prep time: 30 minutes
Cook time: 30 minutes
Serves 4 (about 1 cup each)

CHUTNEY
3 cups chopped rhubarb, fresh or frozen
1 apple, peeled, cored and shredded
½ cup granulated sugar
¼ cup cider vinegar
1 tbsp minced fresh ginger
2 cloves garlic, minced
1 tsp ground cumin
½ tsp ground cinnamon
¼ tsp salt
½ cup diced red onion
½ cup golden raisins
2 tbsp orange juice

SALAD
3 small boneless skinless chicken breasts
1 tbsp olive oil
2 cloves garlic, minced
1 bunch Swiss chard, washed well and drained, coarsely chopped, stems included

Preheat oven to 400°F.

Chutney: In a large heavy saucepan, combine rhubarb, apple, sugar, vinegar, ginger, garlic, cumin, cinnamon, salt and red onion. Cook, covered, over medium heat, stirring often, until rhubarb has fallen apart and mixture has thickened, about 10 minutes. Stir in raisins and orange juice. Cool slightly. (Chutney can be refrigerated in an airtight container for up to 3 days. Bring to room temperature before using.)

Salad: Place chicken breasts on an aluminum foil–lined baking sheet and spread 1 cup chutney over chicken. Bake in centre of preheated oven until chicken is no longer pink inside, about 20 minutes.

Meanwhile, heat oil in a skillet set over medium-high heat. Add garlic; cook, stirring, for 2 minutes. Add Swiss chard and 2 tbsp water; cook, stirring, until wilted and tender, 7 to 10 minutes.

Divide greens among four plates. Drizzle with chicken juices. Slice chicken into thin strips and divide equally among plates. Top with remaining chutney.

NUTRITIONAL ANALYSIS PER SERVING: Calories 200; Protein 1g; Carbohydrate 50g (17%DV); Fat, total 0g; Fat, saturated 0g; Fat, trans 0g; Cholesterol 0mg; Fibre 4g (16%DV); Sodium 150mg (6%DV).

🌾Health Savvy: Cruciferous Vegetables

Consuming a diet rich in cruciferous vegetables is associated with greater preservation of cognitive function with aging. This should not be surprising, since vegetables provide us with a rich array of brain-healthy nutrients. Not only can they be high in fibre, vitamins and minerals, they can also contain compounds, generally referred to as plant polyphenols, which both protect against tissue damage and help sustain an overall healthy metabolic profile.

Want to get into the healthy habit of eating more vegetables? When grocery shopping, the most important principle is to select vegetables that you and your family enjoy, and then expand your repertoire so that you are eating the broadest variety possible. Since different classes of vegetables differ in the types and amounts of nutrients and polyphenols they contain, variety is an easy way to ensure that you are exposing yourself to all of these compounds. Don't look for the "super food"—it does not exist. While individual vegetables may be high in one specific compound (e.g., an antioxidant), other vegetables may rank higher in different compounds (e.g., fibre). Indeed, there is currently no evidence from human studies that any one vegetable outweighs the brain-health benefits of another. The best adage is: Variety is the spice of life—and the best route to supporting brain health.

TYPE	CHARACTERISTICS	SUBSTITUTIONS	PERFECT PAIRINGS
Arugula	Has a strong, peppery, spicy flavour. Resembles dandelion greens. Also known as rocket, rucola, rugula.	Watercress, dandelion greens, baby spinach, radicchio	Salads, grilled meats, wilted in pastas, with citrus flavours and hearty mains
Bok choy	Has a mild, sweet cabbagey flavour. The leaves have a distinct nutty taste that intensifies when cooked.	Choy sum, napa cabbage	Soy sauce, ginger, sherry, garlic, hoisin sauce, oyster sauce, chilies, sesame oil, mushrooms
Broccoli	Long stalks with tightly closed dark green florets. Sweet and crunchy.	Broccolini, broccoflower, Chinese broccoli	Cheese, citrus, Asian flavours, fresh herbs, all nuts, flavoured butters
Brussels sprouts	Strong cabbage flavour. Tightly packed light green leaves usually arranged around a long tapering stalk.	Fresh broccoli florets	Flavoured butters, all nuts, mushrooms, cheese sauces
Cabbage	Available in green, red and Savoy varieties. Has a sweet, crunchy nuttiness.	Usually another cabbage of a different colour or napa cabbage	Vinegars, ciders, fruit

TYPE	CHARACTERISTICS	SUBSTITUTIONS	PERFECT PAIRINGS
Cauliflower	Most common variety is white but also available in purple, green and orange (the latter developed in Canada!). Mild, sweet.	Broccoli, broccoflower	Herbed butters, cheese, honey, Asian flavourings
Chinese cabbage	Fairly mild, crunchy, retains its texture well when cooked.	Bok choy, choy sum, regular cabbage	Hoisin sauce, vinegars, sesame oil
Collard greens	Mild flavoured. Smaller leaves tend to be more flavourful. Look for crisp dark green leaves.	Mustard greens, kale, bok choy	Great for adding to soups, for sautéing, terrific with garlic and citrus
Daikon	A large Oriental radish with a sweet, tangy flavour. Interior is crisp, juicy and white. Skin can be either creamy white or black. Choose firm, smooth roots that have a luminous gleam.	White radish	Asian seasonings, vinegars, fresh herbs
Kale	Available in regular, black and curly. Has a mild cabbagey flavour. Best bought in the winter months in small bunches.	Spinach, Swiss chard	Garlic, fresh ginger, hearty spices, herbs
Mustard greens	Has a peppery flavour, reminiscent of mustard. Look for crisp young leaves with a rich green colour.	Turnip greens, kale	Onion, garlic, fresh ginger, earthy spices
Rutabaga	A pleasantly mild and sweet flavour.	Turnip, butternut squash	All manner of herbs and spices, garlic
Turnip	Slightly sweet, nutty.	Rutabaga	Garlic, herbs, onions, Mediterranean spices

Broccoli and kale rank highest when it comes to fighting cancer, although all members of the cruciferous family contain potent anti-cancer compounds. These little warriors can break down free radicals and stop malicious entrepreneurs of disease.

Shaved Green Salad with Spicy Grilled Shrimp

A light and refreshing salad is the perfect companion to spicy shrimp.

Prep time: 15 minutes
Cook time: 6 minutes
Serves 4 (2 cups each)

TARRAGON VINAIGRETTE
2 tbsp canola oil
1 tbsp walnut oil
2 tbsp sherry vinegar
1½ tsp minced or grated shallot
1 tbsp finely chopped fresh tarragon
1 tsp liquid honey or agave nectar
¼ tsp each salt and black pepper

SALAD
1 bulb fennel
4 large celery stalks
1 large English cucumber

¼ cup loosely packed Italian parsley
   leaves, roughly torn

SHRIMP
½ tsp paprika
¼ tsp cayenne pepper
1 clove garlic, minced
1 tbsp olive oil
½ tsp lemon zest
1 tsp lemon juice
Pinch each salt and black pepper
12 jumbo shrimp (or 20 large shrimp),
   peeled and deveined

Vinaigrette: In a bowl, whisk together all vinaigrette ingredients until well combined. Set aside.

Salad: Cut off and discard bottom "stump" of fennel bulb. Cut bulb in half lengthwise; remove tough inner core. Reserve fennel fronds for garnish. Using a mandolin or sharp chef's knife, thinly slice half-moon shavings of fennel. Continue until entire bulb and stems are shaved.

Cut about an inch off each end of the celery stalks; slice, as you did the fennel, until entire stalk is thinly shaved. Cut cucumber in half lengthwise, producing two long sides of cucumber. Shave to produce half-moon slices. Repeat for second half of cucumber. Toss shaved vegetables together with parsley.

Shrimp: Heat a grill pan over medium heat; grease lightly. In a bowl, combine paprika, cayenne pepper, garlic, oil, lemon zest and juice, salt and pepper. Toss shrimp in spice mixture until well coated. Grill shrimp in prepared pan until pink, 2 to 3 minutes per side.

Assembly: Lightly dress salad with vinaigrette. Stack shrimp on top of salad; serve warm or cold.

NUTRITIONAL ANALYSIS PER SERVING: Calories 220; Protein 12g; Carbohydrate 12g (4%DV); Fat, total 15g (23%DV); Fat, saturated 1.5g (8%DV); Fat, trans 0g; Cholesterol 95mg (32%DV); Fibre 3g (12%DV); Sodium 330mg (14%DV).

Asian Greens and Rice Noodle Salad

Forget sodium-saturated chow mein! Making this food-court favourite at home allows you to control the salt levels and increase vegetable portions.

Prep time: 20 minutes
Cook time: 10 minutes
Serves 6 (1⅓ cups each)

1 nest dried rice vermicelli (or 5 oz rice noodles)
1 tbsp toasted sesame oil
1 tbsp canola oil
6 bundles baby bok choy (each about 4 inches long), leaves separated
1 cup frozen shelled edamame
2 cloves garlic, thinly sliced
1 piece fresh ginger (about 1 inch), grated
1 cup loosely packed snow peas, ends trimmed, halved
1 large carrot, peeled and thinly sliced
1 tsp hot sauce, such as sriracha (optional)
3 tbsp low-sodium soy sauce or tamari
¼ cup vegetable stock, preferably low-sodium
1 lime, juiced
2 green onions (white and light green parts only), finely sliced
¼ cup fresh whole coriander leaves
1 tbsp toasted white or black sesame seeds

Place dried rice vermicelli in a large bowl; cover with boiling water and let stand for 5 minutes or until softened.

Heat sesame and canola oils in a large deep-set pan or wok set over medium-high heat. Add bok choy; gently stir-fry until slightly softened, about 3 minutes.

Add frozen edamame, garlic and ginger; stir-fry until fragrant, about 1 minute. Stir in snow peas, carrot, hot sauce (if using), soy sauce and stock. Cook, covered, for 2 minutes.

Meanwhile, drain rice noodles. Toss with lime juice, green onions and coriander. Add vegetable medley to noodles; toss to combine. Sprinkle with sesame seeds and serve hot, room temperature or cold.

NUTRITIONAL ANALYSIS PER SERVING: Calories 210; Protein 7g; Carbohydrate 28g (9%DV); Fat, total 7g (11%DV); Fat, saturated 0.5g (3%DV); Fat, trans 0g; Cholesterol 0mg; Fibre 3g (12%DV); Sodium 310mg (13%DV).

Scallop Niçoise Salad

By Chef Mark McEwan

Mark is well known across the country not only because he's a judge for Top Chef *on the Food Network, but also because his three restaurants continue to entice patrons on all occasions. He is also author of* Great Food at Home.

This elegant salad is ideal for an al fresco lunch in the spring or summer. Champagne vinegar, with its subtle acidity, not only complements the scallops but helps round out the peppery notes of the arugula as well. This salad will also work well with lobster, poached halibut or grilled chicken breast.

Prep time: 10 minutes
Cook time: 35 minutes
Serves 6 (1⅓ cups plus 2 scallops each)

8 fingerling potatoes, scrubbed (about ½ lb)
1 lb French green beans
3 tbsp white wine vinegar
2 tbsp champagne vinegar (or additional white wine vinegar)
2 tsp freshly grated horseradish (or bottled prepared horseradish)
¾ tsp Dijon mustard
⅓ cup + 1 tbsp olive oil
¼ tsp each salt and black pepper
12 dry-packed sea scallops
1 tbsp butter
½ lb Brussels sprouts, shredded
1 can (19 oz/540 mL) navy beans, drained and rinsed
¼ bunch Italian parsley sprigs, roughly chopped
3 cups arugula leaves, loosely packed

Preheat oven to 450°F.

In a large pot of boiling salted water, boil potatoes until fork-tender, 15 to 20 minutes. Using a slotted spoon, remove potatoes from water; set aside. In same pot, blanch French beans for 2 minutes. Immediately remove beans from pot; rinse under cold running water to stop the cooking process.

In a separate bowl, combine white wine and champagne vinegars, horseradish, mustard, ⅓ cup oil and a pinch each salt and pepper; whisk thoroughly.

Slice potatoes into quarter-inch coins and cut French beans in half on bias; toss together with one-third of dressing. Let stand for 10 minutes to allow potatoes to absorb some of the dressing.

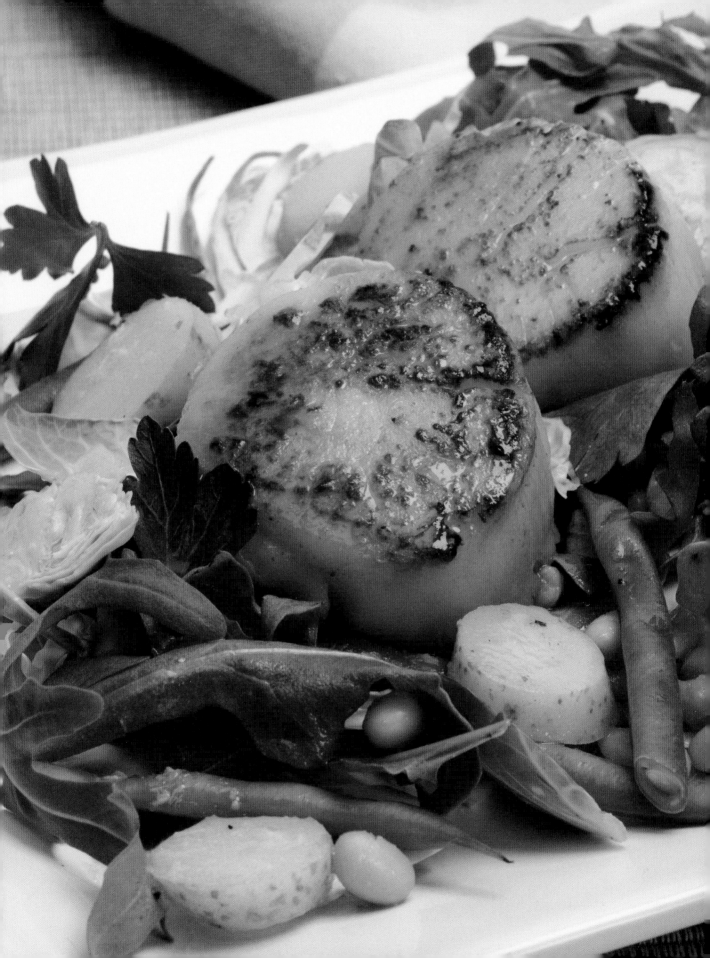

Meanwhile, pat scallops dry; sprinkle with a pinch of salt.

Thoroughly heat an ovenproof non-stick skillet set over medium-high heat. Place scallops in pan; sear until bronzed at base, 2 to 3 minutes. Add butter and remaining 1 tbsp oil. Turn scallops over; immediately transfer pan to preheated oven. Cook until bronzed on the other side, 7 to 8 minutes.

Add Brussels sprouts, navy beans, parsley and a pinch each salt and pepper to potatoes. Divide potato mixture evenly among 6 plates; top with arugula and 2 scallops. Drizzle with remaining dressing.

NUTRITIONAL ANALYSIS PER SERVING: Calories 350; Protein 24g; Carbohydrate 25g (8%DV); Fat, total 17g (26%DV); Fat, saturated 3g (15%DV); Fat, trans 0g; Cholesterol 45mg (15%DV); Fibre 7g (28%DV); Sodium 370mg (15%DV).

❦ Health Savvy: Rah Rah for Roots!

Look underground for more ways to boost your physical and mental well-being. Turnips, beets, parsnips, carrots, sweet and regular potatoes, as well as garlic, leeks and onions are all high in complex carbohydrates and full of fibre and folate. Most contain essential minerals such as potassium, phosphorus, magnesium and small amounts of iron.

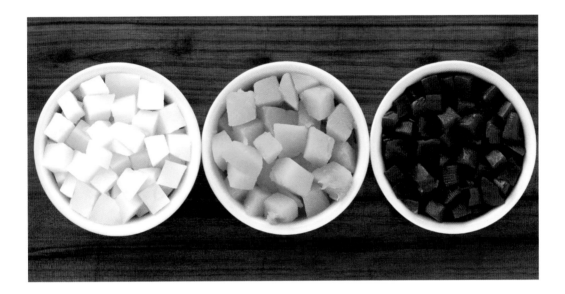

✎ Kitchen Savvy: A Trio of Vinaigrettes

SUN-DRIED TOMATO VINAIGRETTE
2 tbsp finely chopped sun-dried tomatoes
2 tbsp balsamic vinegar
1 tsp Dijon mustard
1 clove garlic, minced
Pinch each salt and black pepper
⅓ cup extra virgin olive oil

In a small bowl, whisk together first five ingredients. Gradually whisk in oil. Can be stored in an airtight container in the refrigerator for up to 1 week.

GREEK-STYLE VINAIGRETTE
2 tbsp red wine vinegar
1 clove garlic, finely minced
¼ tsp dried oregano
Pinch each salt and black pepper
¼ cup extra virgin olive oil
2 tbsp crumbled feta cheese

In a small bowl, whisk together first four ingredients. Gradually whisk in oil. Can be stored in an airtight container in the refrigerator for up to 1 week. Just before serving, whisk in feta cheese.

CITRUS VINAIGRETTE
1 tbsp each lime, lemon and orange juice
1 tbsp liquid honey
1 tsp poppy seeds
Pinch each salt and black pepper
¼ cup extra virgin olive oil

In a small bowl, whisk together first four ingredients. Gradually whisk in oil. Can be stored in an airtight container in the refrigerator for up to 1 week.

Chickpea and Herb Salad with Warm Lemon Dressing

All the flavours of Italy with none of the guilt! Lightly caramelizing the lemon mellows its acidic punch and lends a smoky sweetness to this delicious dish.

Prep time: 10 minutes
Cook time: 7 minutes
Serves 4 (1½ cups each)

2 tbsp olive oil
1 lemon, halved
3 cloves garlic, coarsely chopped
2 cups packed arugula leaves
¼ cup finely chopped fresh basil leaves
¼ cup finely chopped fresh Italian parsley leaves
1 can (15 oz/443 mL) chickpeas, drained and rinsed
Pinch each salt and black pepper
4 thin shavings of Parmesan cheese

Heat oil in a small non-stick pan set over medium heat. Add lemon halves, cut-side down; sear until lightly caramelized, 5 to 7 minutes. Remove lemon halves from pan. Add the garlic and cook until fragrant and softened, about 1 minute. Remove from heat.

In a bowl, toss arugula with basil, parsley and chickpeas.

Squeeze caramelized lemon over salad. Drizzle with garlic-infused oil.

Season salad with salt and pepper. Top with shaved pieces of Parmesan.

NUTRITIONAL ANALYSIS PER SERVING: Calories 230; Protein 11g; Carbohydrate 20g (7%DV); Fat, total 12g (18%DV); Fat, saturated 3.5g (18%DV); Fat, trans 0g; Cholesterol 10mg (3%DV); Fibre 3g (12%DV); Sodium 260mg (11%DV).

....

TIP—How to Shave Parmesan
A vegetable peeler is the best tool for shaving thin ribbons of Parmesan.

....

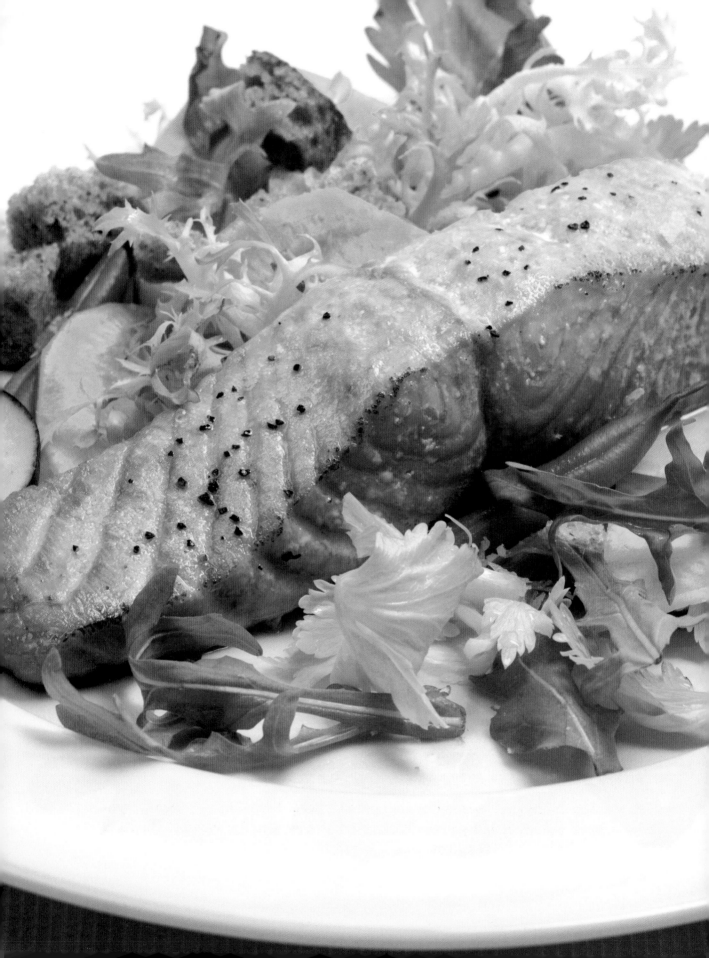

Grilled Salmon with Green Salad and Apple Vinaigrette

By Chef Chuck Hughes

Chuck Hughes is the chef and co-owner of two restaurants, Garde Manger and Le Bremner in Montreal, the acclaimed author of Garde Manger, *and host of Food Network Canada and the Cooking Channel's* Chuck's Day Off *and* Chuck's Week Off.

This light apple juice–based vinaigrette is a perfect accompaniment to this dish—it livens up the salad greens and complements the fish beautifully, making it a perfect mid-day meal.

Prep time: 15 minutes
Cook time: 35 minutes
Serves 2 (2½ cups salad and 1 salmon fillet each)

2 salmon fillets (4 oz/125 g each)
Pinch each salt and black pepper

APPLE VINAIGRETTE
1 cup apple juice
1 tbsp cider vinegar
1 tsp Dijon mustard
Pinch each salt and black pepper
3 tbsp canola oil

GREEN SALAD
6 sprigs frisée lettuce
1 handful baby arugula leaves
1 handful blanched baby green beans
1 handful celery leaves
1 small yellow beet, peeled and thinly sliced
2 large radishes, trimmed and thinly sliced
⅓ cup slightly crushed toasted croutons
2 tsp grated lemon zest

Apple vinaigrette: Place apple juice in a small pot. Bring to a boil over high heat; boil until juice is reduced by half. Transfer to a bowl; let cool slightly. Whisk in vinegar, mustard, salt and pepper. Whisk in oil.

Salmon: Lightly sprinkle salmon with salt and pepper. Place skin-side down in a grill pan set over medium-high heat. Cook, without flipping, until opaque and fish flakes easily with a fork, about 10 minutes.

Green salad: In a large bowl, toss together frisée, arugula, green beans, celery leaves, beets and radishes. Stir in one-third of vinaigrette, tossing gently until well coated. Add crushed croutons. Add lemon zest; toss again. Divide evenly between two plates. Top each plate with salmon. Drizzle with remaining vinaigrette, if desired.

NUTRITIONAL ANALYSIS PER SERVING: Calories 330; Protein 28g; Carbohydrate 15g (5%DV); Fat, total 17g (26%DV); Fat, saturated 3g (15%DV); Fat, trans 0g; Cholesterol 70mg (23%DV); Fibre 5g (20%DV); Sodium 190mg (8%DV).

TIP—To Make Your Own Smoked Salmon

Chuck loves to serve this salad with smoked salmon. To make your own smoked salmon, stir together 1 cup each packed light brown sugar and granulated sugar, ¼ cup salt and 3 cups hot water. Add 8 oz raw salmon, pressing the salmon until submerged. Cover with plastic wrap and refrigerate overnight. The next day, remove salmon from brine; discard brine. Rinse salmon to remove any excess salt. Place salmon, skin-side down, on a rack; let stand until salmon is dry to the touch, about 1 hour. Layer 2 pieces of aluminum foil in the bottom of a wok. Add 2 handfuls of hickory or alderwood chips to the wok, and place over high heat. Add ½ cup water. Position a bamboo steamer on top of chips and place salmon inside. Cover with lid or aluminum foil. Smoke until salmon is firm to the touch and the edges are a little brown and crusty, 20 to 30 minutes. Let cool. Slice and serve over green salad.

Corn, Black Bean and Tomato Salad

This summer favourite has all the bells and whistles: antioxidant-rich black beans, crunchy jicama and fresh juicy tomatoes. The zing in the dressing comes from fresh lime juice. If you can, slice the kernels off fresh corn for an even livelier salad.

Prep time: 15 minutes
Serves 6 (1⅓ cups each)

SALAD
2 cups cooked corn kernels (fresh or canned)
1 can (19 oz/540 mL) black beans, drained and rinsed
2 tomatoes, seeded and diced
1 ripe avocado, pitted and diced
½ cup chopped red onion
½ cup chopped jicama or red radish
⅔ cup chopped fresh coriander leaves

DRESSING
3 tbsp lime juice
1 tbsp each Dijon mustard and liquid honey
2 cloves garlic, minced
½ tsp each ground cumin, ground coriander and black pepper
¼ tsp salt
Dash hot pepper sauce
¼ cup olive oil

Salad: In a large bowl, gently toss together corn, black beans, tomatoes, avocado, red onion, jicama and coriander.

Dressing: In a small bowl, whisk together lime juice, mustard, honey, garlic, cumin, coriander, pepper, salt and hot pepper sauce. In thin stream, gradually whisk in oil until emulsified. Pour over salad, tossing gently until well coated. Serve at room temperature.

NUTRITIONAL ANALYSIS PER SERVING: Calories 320; Protein 10g; Carbohydrate 44g (15%DV); Fat, total 14g (22%DV); Fat, saturated 2g (10%DV); Fat, trans 0g; Cholesterol 0mg; Fibre 10g (40%DV); Sodium 260mg (11%DV).

Ceviche Lettuce Wraps

Ceviche is a popular Latin American dish of raw fish that has been marinated in citrus juice (usually lime) just long enough for the acid in the juice to "cook" the fish. Only very fresh fish should be used in this recipe.

Prep time: 35 minutes
Serves 6

4 sole fillets or any buttery white-flesh fish (about 12 oz total)
6 large limes, juiced
1 nest dried rice vermicelli
½ papaya
2 tbsp finely chopped fresh mint leaves
2 tbsp finely chopped fresh coriander leaves
2 fresh red hot chili peppers, seeded and finely chopped
1½ tsp minced or grated shallot
½ tsp each salt and black pepper
1 tbsp olive oil
6 radicchio, Bibb or Boston lettuce leaves

Slice sole lengthwise into thin strips; cut across strips into small cubes. Place in a bowl and pour lime juice overtop (there should be just enough juice to cover the fish). Cover bowl with plastic wrap; refrigerate until fish turns opaque, 25 to 30 minutes.

Place nest of rice vermicelli in a large bowl; cover with boiling water and let stand until softened, about 5 minutes.

Meanwhile, finely dice papaya. In a bowl, combine papaya with half of the chopped mint and coriander plus chili, shallots, salt, pepper and oil.

Drain vermicelli; return to bowl and add remaining tablespoon of each herb, tossing to combine.

Drain fish well; discard lime juice. Gently stir fish into papaya mixture.

Arrange lettuce leaves on a platter. Divide vermicelli equally among lettuce leaves. Top with equal portions of ceviche. Roll up lettuce leaf around filling.

NUTRITIONAL ANALYSIS PER SERVING: Calories 150; Protein 14g; Carbohydrate 15g (5%DV); Fat, total 3g (5%DV); Fat, saturated 0.5g (3%DV); Fat, trans 0g; Cholesterol 35mg (12%DV); Fibre 1g (4%DV); Sodium 250mg (10%DV).

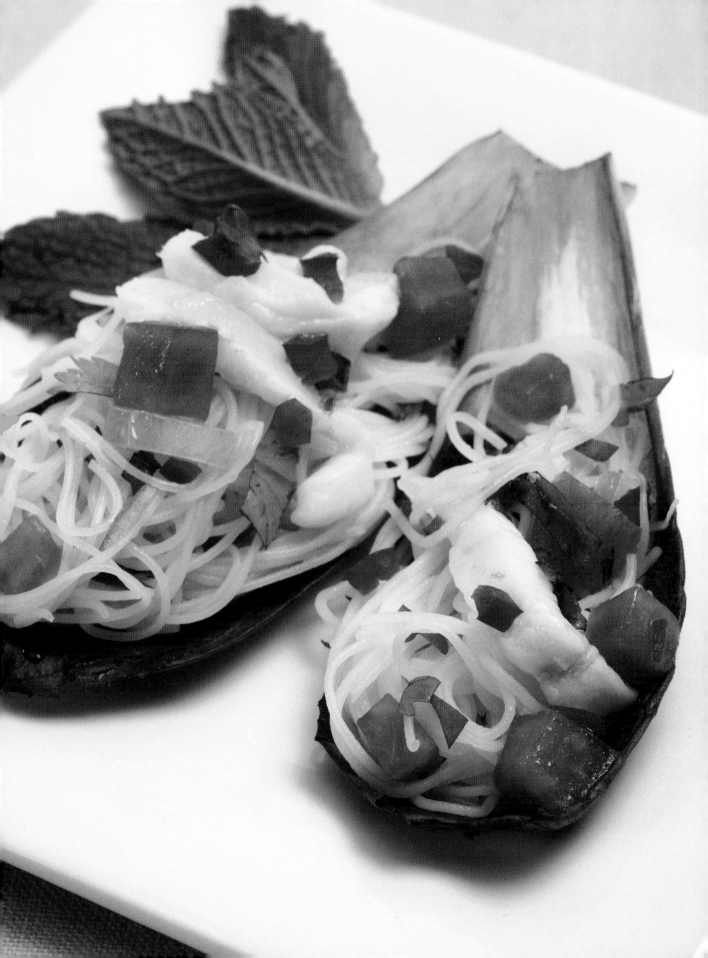

Cream of Broccoli Soup

"Creamed" soups, made without any cream or milk, are one of the easiest dishes to prepare. Adding a potato along with the vegetable of your choice adds the requisite creaminess that cream would otherwise provide. Consider this a master recipe and substitute cauliflower, squash, zucchini or another vegetable of your choice for the broccoli.

Prep time: 15 minutes
Cook time: 20 minutes
Serves 4 (1 cup each)

2 tbsp vegetable oil
1 onion, chopped
2 cloves garlic, minced
½ tsp curry powder
¼ tsp each salt and black pepper
6 cups chopped broccoli (florets and peeled stems)
1 large potato, peeled and cubed
2 to 2½ cups vegetable or chicken stock, preferably low-sodium
1 cup water

Heat oil in a heavy saucepan set over medium heat. Add onion and garlic; cook, stirring, until softened, about 5 minutes. Stir in curry powder, salt and pepper. Stir in broccoli and potato, stirring until well coated. Pour in stock and water. Bring to a boil; reduce heat and simmer, covered, until vegetables are tender, about 15 minutes.

In batches, transfer soup to a blender or the bowl of a food processor; purée until smooth. (Soup can be covered and refrigerated for up to 3 days. Reheat over low heat, adding up to ½ cup more stock to thin, if necessary.)

NUTRITIONAL ANALYSIS PER SERVING: Calories 210; Protein 10g; Carbohydrate 32g (11%DV); Fat, total 8g (12%DV); Fat, saturated 0.5g (3%DV); Fat, trans 0g; Cholesterol 0mg; Fibre 9g (36%DV); Sodium 420mg (18%DV).

Roasted Tomato and Garlic Soup with Rice

This is a personal favourite of Daphna's. She notes: I adore the way roasting coaxes the flavour out of vegetables, adorning them with a sweetness and intensity they would not otherwise have. The jalapeño adds depth, and the herbs lend a light headiness to the mix. Feel free to forego the rice if you like. You can serve this on its own as a meal with some hearty whole-wheat ciabattas and a green salad. It's also delicious served at room temperature.

Prep time: 70 minutes
Cook time: 30 minutes
Serves 6 (1 cup each)

2½ lb plum tomatoes
1 whole head garlic
2 onions, peeled, halved and quartered
1 jalapeño, halved and seeded
2 tbsp olive oil
¼ tsp salt

¼ tsp each black pepper, dried oregano and dried basil
2 cups (approx) vegetable stock, preferably low-sodium
1 cup water
¼ cup long-grain rice

Preheat oven to 400°F.

Cut stem end off tomatoes; halve lengthwise. Place cut-side up on a large aluminum foil–lined baking sheet. Trim ¼ inch off top of garlic without disturbing cloves; place on baking sheet along with onions and jalapeño, making sure all vegetables are in a single layer and not overlapping. Brush with olive oil. Combine half of the salt and all of the pepper, oregano and basil; sprinkle evenly over vegetables.

Roast in centre of preheated oven until tomatoes are browned and onions and garlic are softened, about 1 hour. Let cool slightly. Squeeze garlic cloves out of skins, discarding skins.

In a blender or the bowl of a food processor, in three batches, purée tomatoes, onions, jalapeño and garlic, adding about ½ cup stock to each batch, until very smooth. Transfer mixture to a saucepan, adding water and remaining salt. Bring to a boil over medium-high heat; stir in rice. Simmer, covered and stirring occasionally, until rice is tender, 20 to 25 minutes. (Soup can be cooled and refrigerated for up to 2 days. Reheat over low heat. If soup thickens too much, stir in another ½ cup stock.)

NUTRITIONAL ANALYSIS PER SERVING: Calories 130; Protein 3g; Carbohydrate 19g (6%DV); Fat, total 5g (8%DV); Fat, saturated 0.5g (3%DV); Fat, trans 0g; Cholesterol 0mg; Fibre 4g (16%DV); Sodium 270mg (11%DV).

Mediterranean Stuffed Peppers

All the flavours of Greece wrapped up in one neat little package! Lima and fava beans are lean sources of protein and are readily available year-round in the canned and frozen sections of the grocery store. A hearty main for vegans and vegetarians; for everyone else, the perfect side to a mild-flavoured fish fillet!

Prep time: 15 minutes
Cook time: 60 minutes
Serves 6

2 tbsp olive oil
1 onion, finely chopped
4 cloves garlic, minced
¼ tsp dried red pepper flakes, crushed
1 tbsp dried oregano
1 tbsp dried thyme
1 tbsp grated lemon zest
1 Italian eggplant, finely diced
   (about 5 cups)

½ tsp each salt and black pepper
1 can (28 oz/796 mL) no-salt-added
   diced tomatoes
1 can (14 oz/398 mL) lima or fava beans,
   drained and rinsed
6 red, yellow or orange peppers
¼ cup finely chopped fresh mint leaves

Preheat oven to 425°F.

Heat oil in a large deep-set pan set over medium heat. Add onion and garlic; cook, stirring, until softened, about 2 minutes. Stir in red pepper flakes, oregano, thyme and lemon zest until onion and garlic are well coated.

Add eggplant; cook, stirring often, until softened and lightly browned, about 6 minutes. Stir in salt and pepper.

Using a wooden spoon, stir in tomatoes along with their liquid, scraping up any browned bits from bottom of pan. Stir in beans. Bring to a boil over high heat. Reduce heat to medium; boil gently, uncovered, stirring often, until liquid in pan has reduced by half, 15 to 20 minutes.

Meanwhile, cut tops off peppers, reserving "cap"; discard seeds. Place peppers in a 12 x 8-inch rectangular glass baking dish.

Stir mint into stewed vegetables. Spoon mixture into peppers. Top each stuffed pepper with cap of pepper, slightly askew. Bake in centre of preheated oven for 30 minutes. Serve hot, cold or room temperature.

NUTRITIONAL ANALYSIS PER SERVING: Calories 190; Protein 6g; Carbohydrate 33g (11%DV); Fat, total 5g (8%DV); Fat, saturated 1g (5%DV); Fat, trans 0g; Cholesterol 0mg; Fibre 9g (36%DV); Sodium 240mg (10%DV).

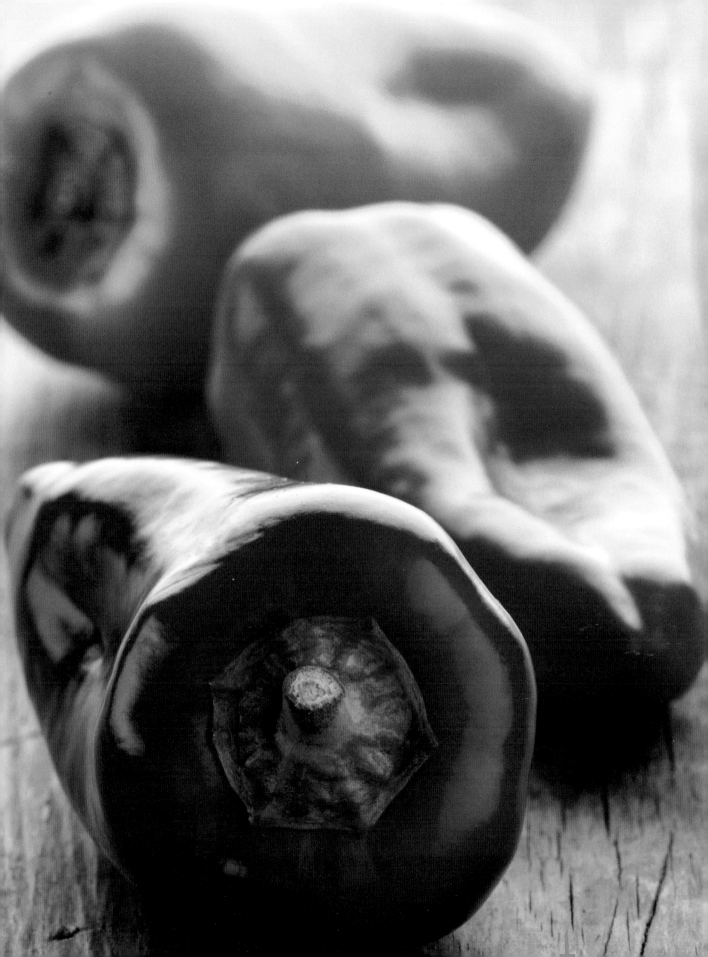

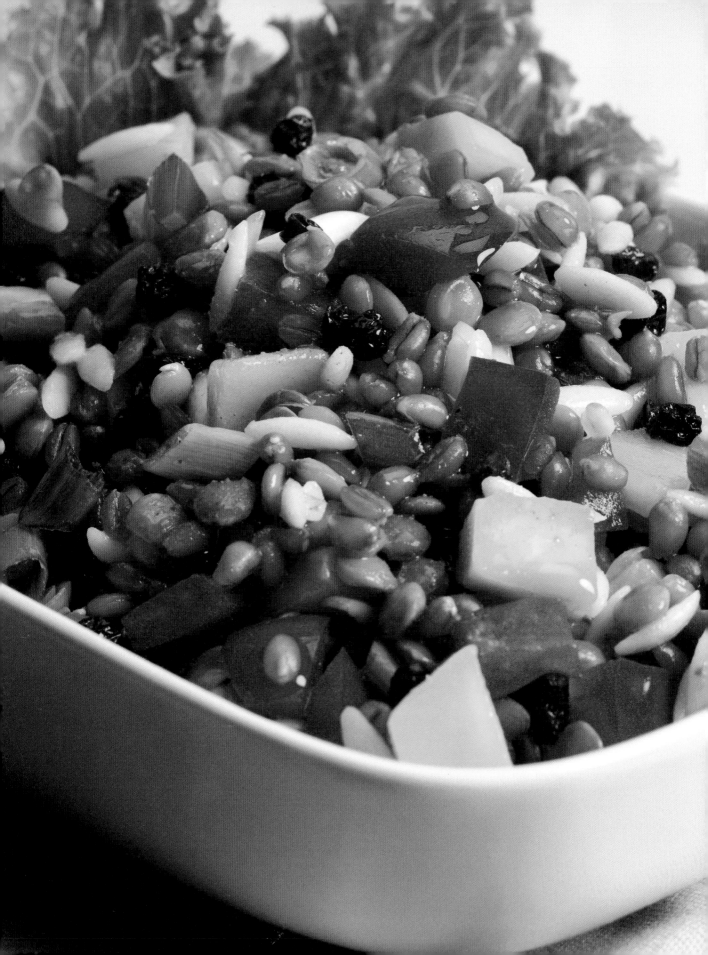

Curried Lentil and Wheatberry Salad with Mango

Wheatberries are the whole, unprocessed wheat kernel. This means they contain all three parts of the grain: the germ, bran and starchy endosperm. Only the hull, the inedible outer layer of the grain, has been removed. Consequently, wheatberries retain all of the grain's vitamins, minerals and phytochemicals. Wheatberries have an exceptional nutrient profile; they're high in fibre, low in calories, and packed with vitamins and minerals. A half-cup serving of cooked wheatberries is a great source of manganese, selenium, phosphorus and magnesium.

Prep time: 20 minutes
Cook time: 70 minutes
Serves 8 (1⅓ cups each)

SALAD

⅔ cup wheatberries
½ cup green lentils
⅓ cup orzo pasta
½ cup dried currants
6 green onions (white and light green parts only), sliced
1 ripe mango, peeled and diced
1 sweet red pepper, seeded and diced

DRESSING

¼ cup cider vinegar
2 tsp liquid honey
1½ tsp ground cumin
1 tsp Dijon mustard
½ tsp each ground coriander and salt
¼ tsp each paprika, turmeric and ground cardamom
Pinch each cayenne and black pepper
⅓ cup canola oil

Salad: Add wheatberries to a large pot of boiling salted water. Boil for 40 minutes. Add lentils; cook for 20 minutes. Add orzo; cook for 10 minutes. Stir in currants. Drain well; transfer to a large mixing bowl. Cool slightly, about 10 minutes. Stir in green onions, mango and red pepper.

Dressing: Meanwhile, in a small bowl, whisk together vinegar, honey, cumin, mustard, coriander, salt, paprika, turmeric, cardamom, cayenne and pepper. Gradually whisk in oil. Pour dressing over salad, tossing gently but thoroughly until well coated. (Salad can be covered with plastic wrap and refrigerated for up to 2 days. Bring to room temperature before serving.)

NUTRITIONAL ANALYSIS PER SERVING: Calories 380; Protein 14g; Carbohydrate 63g (21%DV); Fat, total 9g (14%DV); Fat, saturated 0.5g (3%DV); Fat, trans 0g; Cholesterol 0mg; Fibre 9g (36%DV); Sodium 170mg (7%DV).

❦Health Savvy: Grains

Our new mantra should be "Go for the whole grain!" Like so many fruits and vegetables, whole grains contain a complex web of disease-fighting compounds. They are rich complex carbohydrates, providing much necessary fibre and resistant starch. They lower cholesterol, contain potent antioxidants and improve insulin sensitivity.

Barley is an exceptionally versatile grain. It can be used as a stuffing, as part of a pilaf, in a soup or as the base for a risotto. It is an excellent source of soluble fibre, which can be beneficial in lowering blood cholesterol levels.

In general, the more intact barley kernels are, the more nutritious they are, since a great deal of the nutrients and fibre is located in the outer layers. Hulled barley, the most complete whole-grain variety since the bran and germ are left intact, is high in thiamine and fibre as well as numerous vitamins and minerals, including calcium, magnesium, phosphorus, potassium, vitamin A, vitamin E, niacin and folate. Pearl barley, which is most widely available, is a more refined version of the grain. Although it has less iron, manganese, phosphorus and thiamine than regular barley, it is still quite nutritious.

Regular barley will take about 2 hours to cook, pot barley about 1 hour and pearl barley about 45 minutes.

Bulgur is the parched, steamed and dried berries of the wheat. Highly nutritious, bulgur contains protein, calcium, iron, riboflavin and niacin. It comes in three grades: coarse grind (which has a rice-like texture and is best used for pilafs and stuffings), medium grind (best for side dishes) and fine grind (best for desserts and breads).

Cornmeal is available in a variety of colours: white, yellow and blue. It is made up of dried ground corn kernels and can be purchased in a coarse, medium or fine grind. If you are trying to increase your intake of carbohydrates, cornmeal is a good place to start. It also contains protein and is low in fat. As well, cornmeal contains thiamine, folate and vitamin B_6, as well as selenium, manganese, magnesium and iron.

Couscous Made from semolina, couscous is one of the easiest side dishes to prepare. In general, the rule of thumb is 1⅓ cups liquid (water or stock) to 1 cup dry couscous. To prepare, bring liquid to a boil over high or medium-high heat. Stir in couscous. Cover tightly, remove from heat and let stand for 5 minutes. Fluff with fork; season to taste with salt and black pepper. For extra flavour, try whole-wheat couscous or toast regular couscous in a small dry skillet.

Farro Unlike some of the more popular grains (with the exception of cracked wheat and bulgur), farro needs to be soaked before cooking. One of the oldest grains on the planet, it is blessed with an attractive nutrient profile. An excellent source of complex carbohydrates, farro has twice the fibre and protein of modern wheat. Cook farro as you would rice. Use a ratio of 2 parts water to 1 part farro. Bring to a boil over high heat; reduce heat and simmer over low heat for about 25 minutes. Once tender, farro will remain chewy (discard any remaining water).

Quinoa Actually a seed, quinoa is a dynamo on the nutritional runway. It is a rich source of protein. Since quinoa contains all nine essential amino acids, its protein profile is similar to that found in meat, fish, eggs and poultry. It is also high in lysine, an amino acid essential for tissue growth and repair. Quinoa's high-quality protein and unique amino acid profile make it an important staple for vegetarians and vegans, who rely on plant sources to meet their dietary requirements. It also contains potassium, riboflavin, magnesium, zinc and copper.

You can buy regular, red or black quinoa. All come coated with a bitter resin called saponin. This should be rinsed away by washing the quinoa before you cook it. Sometimes, this resin is removed by mechanical polishing. However, polishing also removes the germ, making it less nutritious.

To prepare quinoa, rinse it under cool running water. Combine 1 part quinoa and 2 parts water (such as 1 cup quinoa and 2 cups water) in a small saucepan and place over high heat. When water comes to a boil, cover with a lid and reduce to a simmer over low heat. Continue to cook for 12 to 15 minutes, until all of the liquid has been absorbed and the quinoa is translucent. Remove from heat and fluff with a fork. Quinoa triples in size when cooked; 1 cup dry quinoa yields 3 cups cooked.

Dry-roasting the quinoa in a skillet before cooking it will lend a distinct nuttiness to your dish.

Rice In general, enriched rice is a good source of B vitamins, such as thiamine and niacin, and also provides some iron, phosphorus, magnesium and folate. Brown rice, which has only the outer hull removed, retains many vitamins and minerals, including niacin, vitamin B6, magnesium, manganese, phosphorus, selenium and vitamin E. It also has four times the insoluble fibre found in white rice. Wild rice has more protein than either brown or white rice, and also supplies good amounts of potassium, zinc, folate and fibre.

Rice can be classified many ways: according to size (long, medium and short grain), according to how it's processed (enriched, converted and instant rice) and by variety (such as arborio, aromatic, basmati, red, sticky or sweet, Texmati, Thai Jasmine, Wehani and wild pecan or popcorn rice).

Depending on the variety and size, 1 cup of rice will generally yield between 3 and 4 cups cooked rice, take between 15 and 50 minutes to cook and require from 1¼ to 2½ cups liquid. Store rice in an airtight container in a cool, dark, dry place.

Wheatberries are decidedly the king of the whole-grain castle. They are the whole, unprocessed wheat kernels and contain all three parts of the grain, including the germ, bran and starchy endosperm. Only the hull (the inedible outer layer of the grain) has been removed. Wheatberries retain all of the grain's vitamins, minerals and phytochemicals. They are high in fibre and a good source of manganese, selenium, phosphorus and magnesium. Wheatberries also contain lignans, phytochemicals thought to guard against breast and prostate cancers.

Wheatberries are an ideal sidekick served as a salad, as a pilaf or as part of a stuffing. They lend a nutty chewiness to breads and can also be toasted for a quick snack.

Wild Rice Salad

Full of grains, nuts and fruit and low in fat, this colourful salad makes a perfect addition to your brain-healthy repertoire. Its high fibre content can be attributed to the outer case on the wild rice, which is retained after harvesting. While called rice, wild rice is actually an edible grass and known for its nutty, smoky taste. This recipe can easily be switched up by replacing the wild rice with wheatberries, the pecans with almonds and the cranberries with other dried fruit or fresh pomegranate.

Before cooking, be sure to rinse the rice thoroughly to remove any debris. Place rice in a large bowl filled with water, stir once or twice and set bowl aside for 5 to 10 minutes. Any debris will float and can then be strained off.

Prep time: 20 minutes
Cook time: 40 minutes
Serves 8 (1 cup each)

6 cups water
2 cups wild rice
1½ tsp salt
1 cup chopped toasted pecans
1 cup dried cranberries
¼ cup chopped fresh Italian parsley leaves
1 tbsp olive oil
1 orange, zested
¼ tsp black pepper

In a large saucepan, bring water, wild rice and 1 tsp salt to a boil over medium-high heat. Boil, covered, until rice is tender but not mushy, 35 to 40 minutes. Drain well. Transfer to a bowl and refrigerate, uncovered, until cool.

Add pecans, cranberries, parsley, olive oil, orange zest and remaining ½ tsp salt plus pepper to wild rice. Toss thoroughly. (Salad can be covered with plastic wrap and refrigerated for up to 24 hours.) Serve cool or at room temperature.

NUTRITIONAL ANALYSIS PER SERVING: Calories 280; Protein 6g; Carbohydrate 41g (14%DV); Fat, total 12g (18%DV); Fat, saturated 1g (5%DV); Fat, trans 0g; Cholesterol 0mg; Fibre 5g (20%DV); Sodium 150mg (6%DV).

Golden Quinoa
with Raisins and Almonds

The South American seed gets a Moroccan spin in this recipe. While reasonably rich in protein in its own right, this salad is the perfect complement to Moroccan-spiced chicken or lamb.

Prep time: 20 minutes
Cook time: 20 minutes
Serves 6 (1 cup each)

2 tbsp olive oil
1 red onion, finely chopped
1 tbsp ground turmeric
1 cup quinoa
2 cups chicken or vegetable stock, preferably low-sodium
Pinch saffron threads (about 8 small threads)
1 cup golden raisins
¼ tsp each salt and black pepper
½ cup sliced almonds

Heat oil in a pot set over medium heat. Add onion; cook until softened and translucent but not browned, about 3 minutes. Stir in turmeric until onions are well coated; cook for 2 minutes.

Meanwhile, rinse quinoa in a sieve; drain well. (If you skip this step, the quinoa might have a slightly bitter taste.)

Add quinoa to pot, stirring to coat with infused oil. Cook, stirring, until quinoa has turned a golden yellow, about 1 minute. Add stock. Bring to a boil over high heat; add saffron and raisins. Reduce heat to low and cook, leaving the lid slightly ajar so steam can escape. Cook, without disturbing, until liquid has been completely absorbed and quinoa has puffed, about 15 minutes or according to package directions.

Fluff quinoa with a fork. Stir in salt and pepper. If there is still liquid in the pot, turn off burner and allow the pot to sit on a warm burner, uncovered, for a few minutes. The quinoa will dry up with stirring. Adjust seasoning to taste.

Transfer quinoa to serving dish; top with almonds.

NUTRITIONAL ANALYSIS PER SERVING: Calories 260; Protein 5g; Carbohydrate 40g (13%DV); Fat, total 9g (14%DV); Fat, saturated 1g (5%DV); Fat, trans 0g; Cholesterol 0mg; Fibre 5g (20%DV); Sodium 160mg (7%DV).

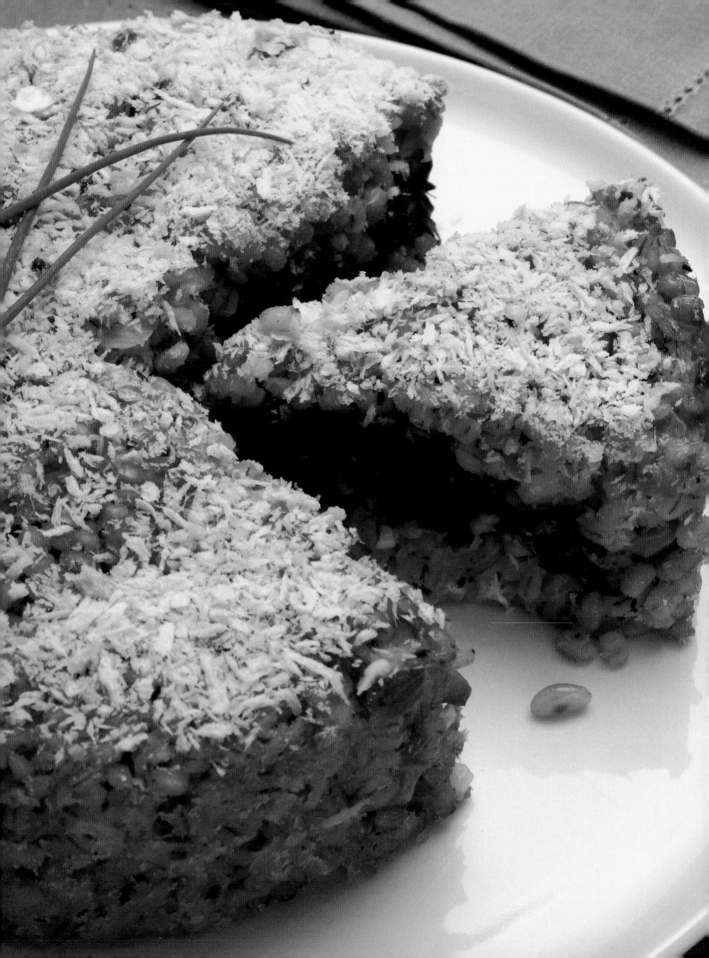

Sweet Pepper and Barley Risotto Tart with Spinach and Pine Nuts

Barley has one of the lowest glycemic indices of all foods and is exceptionally rich in fibre. Its nutty flavour combines well with the peppers and spinach used in this recipe. While it takes a bit longer than other grains to cook, this recipe allows you to prepare the dish in advance and simply reheat in the oven when ready to serve.

Prep time: 30 minutes
Cook time: 85 minutes
Serves 8

RISOTTO

2 tbsp olive oil
1 small onion, chopped
2 large cloves garlic, minced
1½ cups pot barley
½ cup white wine
5 cups chicken or vegetable stock, preferably low-sodium
½ sweet red pepper, finely chopped
½ sweet yellow or orange pepper, finely chopped
2 tbsp chopped fresh oregano leaves
2 tbsp chopped fresh chives
¼ tsp black pepper
½ cup grated Parmesan cheese

SPINACH

8 cups baby spinach (about 1 bunch or 2 300-g packages frozen spinach, thawed)
¼ cup pine nuts
2 tbsp olive oil
2 cloves garlic, finely minced
1 tsp lemon juice
¾ cup bread crumbs, preferably panko

Risotto: Heat oil in a pot set over medium heat. Add onion and garlic; cook, stirring until soft but not browned, about 5 minutes. Stir in barley for 1 minute.

Pour in white wine; cook, stirring, until wine has been absorbed by barley. Add 2 cups stock. Bring to a boil over medium heat. Cook, stirring occasionally, until most of the stock has been absorbed. Add 2 more cups stock and return to boil, stirring occasionally, until stock has been absorbed. Add last cup stock; when most of stock has been absorbed, add red and yellow peppers, oregano, chives and pepper. Cook until all stock has been absorbed. Taste barley; add more water or stock if still too crunchy and continue cooking until the liquid has been completely absorbed. Stir in cheese until melted; set aside to cool.

Spinach: Place spinach and ½ cup water in a large pot; cook, covered, over high heat until wilted, 3 to 4 minutes. Transfer spinach to colander; cool immediately under cold running water. When cool enough to handle, squeeze out excess water. Chop spinach coarsely.

Heat a small frying pan over medium heat. Add pine nuts; cook, stirring frequently, until lightly browned and toasted, 3 to 4 minutes. Remove from hot pan immediately to prevent further browning.

Heat oil in frying pan set over medium heat. Add garlic; cook for 1 minute. Add spinach, pine nuts and lemon juice. Stir until well mixed. Remove from heat and set aside.

Assembly: Preheat oven to 375°F.

Lightly grease an 8-inch springform pan with cooking spray. Add ½ cup bread crumbs; shake pan until bread crumbs are stuck to bottom and sides. Shake out excess. Add half of barley risotto to pan, smoothing surface. Top with spinach, spreading evenly, leaving an edge of ½ to 1 inch around outside of pan. Cover with remaining risotto, spreading out evenly and smoothing surface. Sprinkle with remaining ¼ cup bread crumbs. (Risotto can be covered with plastic wrap and refrigerated for up to 12 hours. Bring to room temperature for 2 to 3 hours before heating.)

Bake risotto in centre of preheated oven until top is lightly browned, about 45 minutes. Remove ring from springform pan; transfer to a serving plate. Cut into wedges and serve.

NUTRITIONAL ANALYSIS PER EACH OF 8 SERVINGS: Calories 310; Protein 7g; Carbohydrate 43g (14%DV); Fat, total 12g (18%DV); Fat, saturated 2.5g (13%DV); Fat, trans 0g; Cholesterol 5mg (2%DV); Fibre 5g (20%DV); Sodium 240mg (10%DV).

Thin-Crust Pizza with Balsamic-Glazed Tomatoes and Pesto

Everyone loves pizza, so this single-serving thin-crust version was developed to provide you with a much healthier option. Sodium has been dramatically lowered by reducing the amount of dough and by relying on full-flavoured ingredients such as balsamic-glazed tomatoes and pesto sauce to up the flavour. We've also dramatically lowered the total fat and saturated fat content by replacing much of the mozzarella with smaller portions of the more richly flavoured low-fat goat cheese, and the sausage or pepperoni with roast chicken. It's not perfect; this version still comes with close to one-third of your day's allowance for sodium and fat. However, as long as you are attending to your overall diet, there is lots of room to include this pizza. The key is to prepare your meals as healthily as you can but not abstain from treats or favoured foods—this could lead to cravings, which make it more difficult to stay on course.

If you don't have any leftover chicken in the fridge, simply roast chicken breasts (skin on and bone in) at the same time you are roasting the balsamic-glazed tomatoes. Be sure to discard the skin before adding the chicken to the pizza.

Prep time: 30 minutes
Cook time: 60 minutes
Serves 8 (one 6-inch pizza)

BALSAMIC-GLAZED TOMATOES
1 pint cherry tomatoes, halved
1 tsp olive oil
1 tbsp balsamic vinegar
8 to 10 sprigs fresh thyme
Pinch black pepper

PIZZA
¼ cup yellow cornmeal
¼ cup all-purpose or whole-wheat flour
1 bag (340 g) prepared whole-wheat pizza dough, or refer to Pizza Dough recipe (page 63)
½ cup pesto sauce (page 80)
2 cloves garlic, finely sliced
2 roasted skinless chicken breasts, shredded
¼ cup black olives, pitted and quartered
1 whole roasted red pepper, skin and seeds removed, cut in strips
3 oz fat-reduced soft goat cheese
Pinch black pepper

Balsamic-glazed tomatoes: Preheat oven to 350°F. Place tomato halves on a parchment paper–lined baking sheet and sprinkle with olive oil, balsamic vinegar and thyme sprigs. Gently toss, then spread in a single layer, cut-side up, and season with pepper. Roast in preheated oven until semi-dried, about 40 minutes. Remove from oven and set aside. (Can be made up to a day in advance and refrigerated.)

Pizza: Increase oven temperature to 450°F. Sprinkle 1 tbsp cornmeal over a parchment paper–lined baking sheet.

Sprinkle a clean, flat workspace with flour. Divide pizza dough into 8 pieces and roll out each piece into a 6- to 7-inch round. Transfer 2 pieces of dough to prepared baking sheet. (Alternatively, divide dough in half, roll each piece into a 12-inch round and place on baking sheet. Increase cooking time by 1 minute if making a larger pizza.)

Place 1 tbsp pesto sauce on each pizza round (4 tbsp if making larger pizzas) and spread over the dough to within ¼ inch of the edge. Divide remaining ingredients into 8 equal portions (2 portions for larger pizzas). For each pizza, evenly arrange garlic slices on dough. Spread shredded chicken, olives, roasted tomato and pepper strips evenly across dough. Scatter pieces of goat cheese overtop and season generously with pepper. Bake in centre of preheated oven until edges of pizza are a dark golden brown, 10 or 11 minutes. Repeat with remaining pieces of dough and toppings.

NUTRITIONAL ANALYSIS PER EACH OF 8 SERVINGS: Calories 380; Protein 22g; Carbohydrate 35g (12%DV); Fat, total 18g (28%DV); Fat, saturated 4.5g (23%DV); Fat, trans 0g; Cholesterol 40mg (13%DV); Fibre 5g (20%DV); Sodium 680mg (28%DV).

TIP—Roasting Peppers

When buying roasted red peppers, be certain to select a low-sodium variety. However, if you prefer to avoid the sodium altogether, simply roast your own. Place pepper under broiler for 12 minutes, turning 2 or 3 times to ensure all sides are blackened. Transfer to a bowl and cover immediately with plastic wrap, or place in a parchment bag. After 10 minutes, the charred skin will easily pull away from the soft, sweet and smoky flesh.

TIP—Pitting Olives

While pitted olives are widely available, pitting them yourself is easy, especially if you plan to chop them afterwards. Simply place the olives on a cutting board and press down on them using the flat side of a knife. The flesh will easily separate from the pit.

Pear, Spinach and Blue Cheese Flatbread with Onion Jam

Strongly flavoured cheese is a great ingredient for adding a ton of flavour without a lot of fat. The stronger the cheese, the less you'll need to pack a punch in this dish. Roquefort and Gorgonzola are great options, but play around with your favourites to find the blue that's right for you!

Prep time: 10 minutes
Cook time: 25 minutes
Serves 4

ONION JAM
¼ cup olive oil
1 clove garlic, minced or thinly sliced
1 tbsp fresh thyme leaves (or ½ tsp dried)
1 red onion, finely chopped
½ cup red wine
2 tbsp liquid honey or agave nectar
¼ tsp each salt and black pepper

FLATBREAD
¼ cup yellow cornmeal
¼ cup all-purpose or whole-wheat flour
1 bag (340 g) prepared whole-wheat pizza dough, or refer to Pizza Dough recipe (page 63)
2 cups loosely packed fresh baby spinach
3 tbsp crumbled blue cheese or feta cheese
2 Bosc pears, peeled, cored and thinly sliced

Preheat oven to 450°F. Sprinkle cornmeal over a parchment paper–lined baking sheet.

Onion jam: Heat 2 tbsp oil in a non-stick pan over medium heat. Add garlic and thyme; cook until fragrant, about 1 minute. Add onion; cook until softened and slightly caramelized, about 10 minutes. Add wine and honey. Bring to a boil over high heat; reduce heat to medium and cook, stirring occasionally, until onions have absorbed the wine and turned deep purple, 8 to 10 minutes. Stir in salt and pepper.

Flatbread: Meanwhile, sprinkle a clean, flat workspace with flour. Roll out pizza dough into a narrow strip (roughly 5 x 15 inches), about ¼ inch thick. Transfer dough to prepared baking sheet. Lightly brush dough with 1 tbsp oil. Bake in centre of preheated oven until golden, 10 to 12 minutes.

Assembly: Combine spinach, cheese and pears in a bowl. Drizzle with remaining oil; season with salt and pepper.

Spread onion jam on baked dough. Top with spinach mixture. Cut into even pieces.

NUTRITIONAL ANALYSIS PER EACH OF 4 SERVINGS: Calories 320; Protein 6g; Carbohydrate 41g (14%DV); Fat, total 14g (22%DV); Fat, saturated 2.5g (13%DV); Fat, trans 0g; Cholesterol 5mg (2%DV); Fibre 5g (20%DV); Sodium 450mg (19%DV).

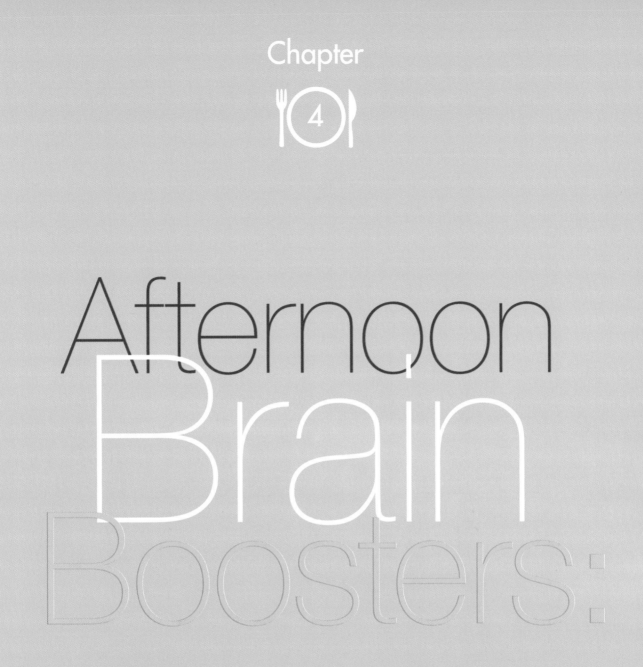

Chapter 4

Afternoon Brain Boosters:

Slump Ye Not

Many of us experience an afternoon slump in our energy and cognitive function. This can be especially true for middle-aged and older adults. Imagine a meeting room filled with young people performing at their peak while you are feeling that you have just landed from an overseas flight and are fighting jet lag. Well, read on! Armed with these brain-boosting foods, you'll be able to lift your performance and minimize the age differences.

Circadian Rhythms in Cognitive Function

Not only do our circadian patterns impact when we eat, but they also influence the time of day when we are performing at our cognitive peak. These shifts in cognitive performance parallel the changes in our circadian cycle, with older adults performing at their cognitive peak early in the morning. In contrast, younger adults are often at their cognitive peak later in the afternoon and their nadir (low) early in the morning. Therefore, late in the afternoon, there is a reasonably large age-related difference in cognitive function when youth are at their peak and older adults at their circadian low.

There has been some research exploring the ability of foods or nutrients to help boost cognitive performance at this time of day. A study conducted at Baycrest examined the impact of consuming a glucose drink. Glucose was able to boost performance in the late afternoon in older adults and reduce the differences in cognitive performance between younger and older adults by about 50%.

In the Baycrest study, participants were given 50 grams of glucose, an amount just slightly higher than in a normal soft drink—however, there are healthier ways to obtain glucose if you want to boost cognitive performance. The recipes in this chapter offer many suggestions, drawing on the potential brain-boosting effects of carbohydrates, e.g., **Cranberry Pumpkin Seed Crunchy Snack** (page 124) and **Fennel-Spiced Asiago Biscotti** (page 123).

Afternoon Snacks—Be Certain to Reach for Low-Sodium Snacks!

As you may know, there is a worldwide effort to encourage people to reduce their sodium intake as a way of helping to control blood pressure. This can help reduce the risk of cardiovascular disease and stroke.

But did you know high sodium intake may also increase the rate of cognitive decline in older adults? A study shows this is particularly true among older adults who had both high sodium intake and low levels of physical activity. In other words, the proverbial "couch potato" reaching for the high-salt snack while watching television!

The recipes in this chapter, however, are designed to give you a burst of flavour without relying on salt; e.g., **Indian-Spiced Chickpeas** (page 127) and **Southwestern-Spiced Nuts** (page 128).

You will also discover how to prepare foods with flavour substitutes for salt. That's important because up to 80% of our sodium intake comes from packaged and prepared foods and not the salt you add to your food. There's nothing better than home-cooked meals as a way of replacing the flavour you may now get from salty processed foods.

How to Use This Information

As we've seen, our peak levels of cognitive function slowly shift from later in the day to early morning as we age. This is a normal and natural shift in our circadian pattern that comes with aging. But it appears that we can temporarily boost our cognitive function during periods of low performance by consuming carbohydrates. However, many of the carbohydrate choices available to us are either high in fat or salt. So this chapter offers you many tasty, low-fat and low-salt alternatives. Many of these can easily be taken with you to work or to appointments. **Roasted Edamame Bean Dip** (page 138) and **Thai-Inspired Almond and Peanut Dipping Sauce** (page 140) can be eaten with fresh vegetables; **Bite-Size Nut Scones** (page 141) can be eaten on their own. If you prefer a sweet rather than savoury food in the afternoons, simply reach for one of the portable recipes in Chapter 2.

Chapter 4
Afternoon Brain Boosters

Recipes

Fennel-Spiced Asiago Biscotti   123

Cranberry Pumpkin Seed Crunchy Snack   124
by Susan Mendelson

Chili Chocolate Bark with Cherries and Pistachios   125

Indian-Spiced Chickpeas   127

Southwestern-Spiced Nuts   128

Seaweed and Sesame Wonton Crackers   133

Parmesan and Pepper Wonton Crackers   134

Roasted Edamame Bean Dip   138

Thai-Inspired Almond and Peanut Dipping Sauce   140

Bite-Size Nut Scones   141

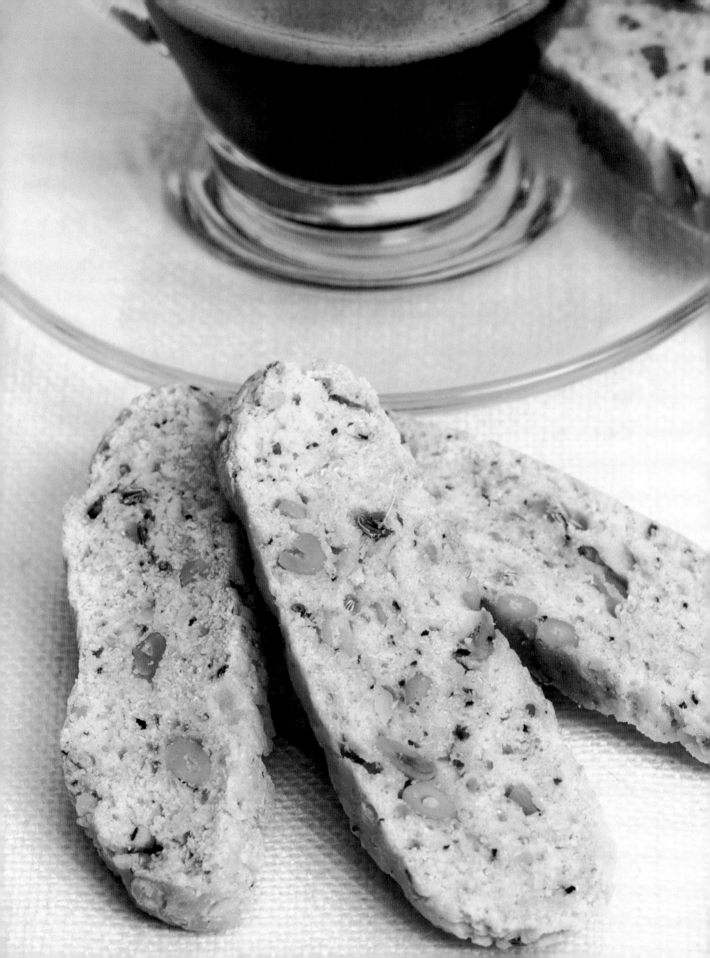

Fennel-Spiced Asiago Biscotti

Not just a sweet dessert cookie, these biscotti combine the earthy flavour of Asiago cheese with the freshness of fennel seeds and tartness of black pepper.

Prep time: 15 minutes plus 15 minutes resting time
Cook time: 45 minutes
Makes about 42 biscotti

½ cup pine nuts
2 cups all-purpose flour
¼ cup cornmeal, fine or medium ground
1 tsp baking powder
1 tsp salt
1 tsp black pepper
½ tsp dry mustard

⅛ tsp baking soda
⅛ tsp cayenne pepper (optional)
¾ cup finely grated Asiago cheese
2 tsp fennel seeds, crushed
2 eggs, lightly beaten
½ cup buttermilk

Preheat oven to 350°F.

Arrange pine nuts on a baking sheet in a single layer. Bake in centre of preheated oven, stirring once or twice, until lightly toasted, 5 to 8 minutes. Cool; chop coarsely.

In a bowl, stir together flour, cornmeal, baking powder, salt, pepper, mustard, baking soda and cayenne pepper (if using). Add Asiago, pine nuts and fennel seeds.

In a small bowl, whisk together eggs and buttermilk; add to the flour mixture, stirring until dough starts to cling together. Turn out onto a lightly floured work surface; gently knead until a smooth, somewhat sticky, dough forms. Shape into a ball; cover with plastic wrap. Let stand at room temperature for 15 minutes.

Divide dough into thirds. Shape each third into a 7-inch-long log. Place on a parchment paper–lined cookie sheet; flatten slightly.

Bake in centre of preheated oven until golden brown, about 25 minutes. Cool on cookie sheet for 5 minutes. Transfer to a wire rack; cool for 20 minutes.

Reduce oven temperature to 325°F. Using a serrated knife, slice logs diagonally into ¼-inch thick slices. Return slices to cookie sheet; bake for 6 minutes. Turn slices over; bake until crisp and dry, about 6 minutes (do not overbake). Cool on wire racks.

NUTRITIONAL ANALYSIS PER BISCOTTI: Calories 45; Protein 1g; Carbohydrate 6g (2%DV); Fat, total 1.5g (2%DV); Fat, saturated 0g; Fat, trans 0g; Cholesterol 0mg; Fibre 0g; Sodium 30mg (1%DV).

TIP—How to Replace Buttermilk in Recipes

If you do not have buttermilk, simply combine ½ cup low-fat milk and ½ tsp white vinegar, and let stand for 5 minutes before using.

Cranberry Pumpkin Seed Crunchy Snack

By Susan Mendelson

Always wondering what to do with the jack-o'-lantern's insides after Halloween? Are you guilty of discarding those seeds after Thanksgiving's pumpkin pie? It's time to start putting these gems to good—healthy and spicy and sweet—use!

Prep time: 15 minutes
Cook time: 25 minutes
Makes 6½ cups (2 tbsp per serving)

1 cup whole rolled oats
2 cups raw, hulled, unsalted pumpkin seeds
1 tbsp canola oil
½ cup pecan pieces
¼ cup maple syrup
1 tsp ground cinnamon
½ tsp ground nutmeg
½ tsp ground allspice
½ tsp salt
3 cups dried cranberries
½ cup dried blueberries

Preheat oven to 350°F.

In a bowl, stir together oats, pumpkin seeds and oil. Spread onto a lightly greased baking sheet. Bake in centre of preheated oven, stirring once, until mixture starts to crisp, about 15 minutes. Transfer mixture to a bowl; stir in pecans and maple syrup, tossing gently to coat well. Stir in cinnamon, nutmeg, allspice and salt, stirring to coat well.

Return mixture to baking sheet. Bake until dry and crisp, 8 to 10 minutes. Cool in pan on rack for 20 minutes.

Stir in cranberries and blueberries, mixing well. (Store in an airtight container for up to 2 weeks.)

NUTRITIONAL ANALYSIS PER SERVING: Calories 70; Protein 2g; Carbohydrate 10g (3%DV); Fat, total 3g (5%DV); Fat, saturated 0g; Fat, trans 0g; Cholesterol 10mg; Fibre 1g (4%DV); Sodium 25mg (1%DV).

Chili Chocolate Bark with Cherries and Pistachios

This snack is as rich in antioxidants as it is in flavour! Sweet, salty, spicy and smooth—there's no palate this bark won't satisfy.

Prep time: 10 minutes
Cook time: 3 minutes
Makes 1½ lb (12 2-oz servings)

1½ cups bittersweet chocolate chips
1½ cups pure semi-sweet chocolate chips (or additional bittersweet chocolate chips)
¼ tsp cayenne pepper
¾ cup dried cherries
¾ cup raw, shelled, unsalted pistachio nuts

Place bittersweet and semi-sweet chocolate chips in a microwave-safe bowl; microwave on high for 30 seconds. Using a rubber spatula, stir chocolate chips for 20 seconds. Repeat microwaving and stirring two more times. Microwave for 15 seconds. Remove from microwave; stir chocolate until completely melted, smooth and silky. Stir in cayenne pepper until well combined. Stir in cherries and pistachios.

Pour mixture onto a parchment paper–lined 10 x 15-inch baking sheet, spreading evenly.

Refrigerate until hardened, about 25 minutes. Break into uneven, jagged pieces. (Can be stored, well wrapped, in refrigerator for up to 2 months.)

NUTRITIONAL ANALYSIS PER SERVING: Calories 260; Protein 4g; Carbohydrate 34g (11%DV); Fat, total 15g (23%DV); Fat, saturated 8g (40%DV); Fat, trans 0g; Cholesterol 0mg; Fibre 4g (16%DV); Sodium 5mg (0%DV).

Kitchen Savvy: Flavour without the Salt

Too much salt does more than just bloat you.

High intake of this mineral is linked with hastened cognitive decline in healthy older adults and is largely responsible for skyrocketing blood pressure—a major risk factor for stroke and vascular dementia. Dried spices are fantastic for helping you amp up flavour while cutting down salt, so stop limiting your seasoning to white salt and explore the seemingly endless spice options available in your local grocery store. When it comes to slashing sodium, variety really is the spice of life!

Use: Spices can be used to add sweet or savoury notes to dishes, but should never be added just before serving. Spices can taste like dry, mealy cardboard if they are not toasted. Warm spices in a dry pan over medium heat until fragrant or in a 375°F oven for 3 to 5 minutes to arouse the essential oils, refreshing them and maximizing the flavour they can impart to your dish.

Storage: Spices should be sealed in airtight containers, tucked into a cool, dry environment for up to 6 months. Do not store near the heat of the oven.

Varieties: Allspice, anise, caraway seed, cardamom, cayenne pepper, celery seed, chili powder, cinnamon, cloves, coriander, cumin, fennel, ginger, mace, mastic, mustard, nutmeg, paprika, pepper, red pepper, saffron, sumac, Szechuan pepper, turmeric.

Blends: Chinese five spice, curry powder, dukka, Garam masala, herbes de Provence, lemon pepper, zaatar.

Indian-Spiced Chickpeas

Also known as garbanzo beans, chickpeas are creamy and soft, but turn super-crunchy when baked. If Indian flavours are not for you, the Southwest spice mix in **Southwestern-Spiced Nuts** (page 128) would work here, too.

Prep time: 5 minutes
Cook time: 50 minutes
Makes about 1½ cups (2 tbsp per serving)

½ tsp each ground cinnamon, ground cardamom and ground cloves
½ tsp each ground coriander, ground ginger, ground nutmeg and paprika
¼ tsp salt
1 tbsp olive oil
1 can (19 oz/540 mL) chickpeas

Preheat oven to 350°F.

In a large bowl, combine spices and salt. Place oil in a separate bowl.

Drain and rinse chickpeas; dry well. Place in a bowl with oil and toss to coat. Add to spice mixture and toss until evenly coated. Arrange in a single layer on a parchment paper–lined baking sheet. Bake in centre of preheated oven until chickpeas are golden and make a rattling sound when tray is shaken, about 50 minutes. (Chickpeas can be stored in an airtight container at room temperature for up to 3 months.)

NUTRITIONAL ANALYSIS PER SERVING: Calories 70; Protein 2g; Carbohydrate 8g (3%DV); Fat, total 3g (5%DV); Fat, saturated 0g; Fat, trans 0g; Cholesterol 0mg; Fibre 2g (8%DV); Sodium 100mg (4%DV).

Southwestern-Spiced Nuts

Lightly whisked egg whites act as a neutral-flavoured binding agent for the spices in this recipe. This not-so-secret ingredient can be used to coat almost any baked snack and will also stick lightweight coatings onto fish and chicken.

Prep time: 5 minutes
Cook time: 15 minutes
Makes 2 cups (2 tbsp per serving)

½ tsp each dried, ground chipotle chili powder (or chili powder)
  and ground coriander
½ tsp ground cumin
Pinch cayenne pepper
1 tbsp packed brown sugar
¼ tsp salt
1 egg white
2 cups raw, mixed, shelled, unsalted nuts

Preheat oven to 350°F.

In a bowl, combine chili powder, coriander, cumin, cayenne, sugar and salt. Set aside.

In another bowl, whisk egg white to foam-like consistency.

Gently stir spice mixture into egg white until combined; stir in nuts until well coated.

Arrange nuts in single layer on a parchment paper–lined baking sheet. Bake in centre of preheated oven until golden, about 15 minutes. Let cool completely; break apart to serve. (Nuts can be stored in an airtight container at room temperature for up to 3 months.)

NUTRITIONAL ANALYSIS PER SERVING: Calories 170; Protein 6g; Carbohydrate 8g (3%DV); Fat, total 14g (22%DV); Fat, saturated 2g (10%DV); Fat, trans 0g; Cholesterol 0mg; Fibre 2g (8%DV); Sodium 60mg (3%DV).

❦ Health Savvy: Nuts 101

Selection and Storage

The optimal time to buy nuts is in the late fall, when most types, such as walnuts, pecans and hazelnuts, are freshly harvested.

Buy nuts that look plump, meaty and crisp. Go for heft; all nuts should feel heavy for their size. If buying in bulk, buy from a store with a high turnover and buy only what you need. And don't be afraid, if you can, to taste one. If the nuts have a bitter, stale flavour, then they've gone rancid.

The high fat content of nuts makes them especially prone to rancidity. Nuts still in the shell will keep the longest. Unshelled nuts should be stored in an airtight container in the freezer. They should never be stored in tin or metal containers because the metal hastens their deterioration. Nuts will keep for 9 to 12 months if stored properly in the freezer. Frozen nuts will thaw very quickly at room temperature.

Toasting

Toasting nuts prior to using them means, in most cases, that your final dish will be sweeter, richer and more intensely flavoured than otherwise. Toasting can be done in a dry skillet over medium heat for 5 to 8 minutes or in a 350°F oven for about 5 minutes. The exceptions to this rule are pine nuts and macadamia nuts. When used in baking recipes, they usually toast enough during the baking process to make pre-toasting unnecessary. However, if you're sprinkling a salad or pasta with pine nuts, toasting will help round out their flavour. Pine nuts and macadamia nuts burn quickly, so always keep an eye on them.

Types

Almonds are a powerhouse of nutrients! They contain fibre, unsaturated fatty acids and phytochemicals, which may help in the prevention of chronic diseases such as cancer and heart disease. Almonds have less saturated fat than any other tree nut. One ounce equals about 23 almonds. Imagine that this handful of almonds contains only 160 calories, most of which come from heart-healthy polyunsaturated (20%) and monounsaturated (51%) fats. It will also provide you with 3 grams of fibre and 6 grams of protein! That same handful of almonds will give you 35% of your daily recommended allowance of vitamin E as well as hefty doses of phosphorus, calcium, iron and folate.

It's easy to add almonds to your daily diet. Throw some into your morning granola or yogurt. Sprinkle some on a salad. Use finely chopped almonds along with bread crumbs to coat fish or poultry.

Almonds come in two main types: sweet and bitter. Sweet almonds are delicately flavoured and slightly sweet. Bitter almonds have more of an intense flavour and contain traces of prussic acid. The toxicity of this acid can make them lethal when ingested and they are therefore illegal in North America.

Walnuts are pretty unique when compared with other nuts. They have the highest amount of plant-based omega-3 essential fatty acids required by the human body. This puts them right next to salmon as a source of omega-3 fatty acids. Eating ¼ cup of walnuts five times a week may reduce the risk of heart disease by as much as 35%. Comprised primarily of polyunsaturated fats, they also contain zinc, iron, folate, calcium, and vitamins A, E and C. Beware, however: although most of the fat is the heart-healthy unsaturated type, walnuts are high in overall fat and calories. One ounce (the equivalent of 14 walnut halves) provides approximately 185 calories and 18.5 grams of fat.

Pecans are a rich source of nutrients including vitamins A and E, folate, calcium, magnesium and phosphorus. They also have the dubious distinction of being the highest-fat nut—they contain more than 70% fat! However, pecans contain unsaturated fat, the type that's linked to heart health. In fact, it has been determined that eating pecans can help lower blood cholesterol and reduce the risk of heart disease. Pecans have an especially high antioxidant content, helpful in protecting our cells against oxidative damage. Choose plump deep-coloured pecans. And, as with almonds and walnuts, add them to a variety of daily dishes to boost your nutrient intake.

Hazelnuts are characterized by a robust, deep flavour and are a good source of protein, fibre, and a variety of vitamins and minerals. As with consuming most nuts, eating a handful of hazelnuts a day—about 1.5 ounces (about 20 hazelnuts)—may help reduce the risk of heart disease. Perhaps most notable is hazelnut's high monounsaturated fat content—the same type of fat found in olive oil. A ¼-cup serving of hazelnuts contains 18 grams of total fat, and 15 of those are heart-healthy monounsaturated fat.

Hazelnuts are best lightly toasted and skinned before using, and complement fresh fruits and chocolate exceptionally well.

Pine nuts are rich in unsaturated fats and an excellent source of vitamin E. They are also an excellent source of the B-complex group of vitamins such as thiamine, riboflavin, niacin, pantothenic acid, vitamin B_6 and folate. Furthermore, pine nuts contain healthy amounts of essential minerals such as manganese, potassium, calcium, iron, magnesium, zinc and selenium.

Pistachios have the fewest calories per ounce relative to other nuts (¼ cup has 178 calories). Additionally, they are a rich source of the antioxidants lutein, beta carotene and vitamin E. They are also rich in heart-healthy monounsaturated fats and have a fair amount of vitamin B_6, potassium and magnesium. Studies have shown that consumption of pistachios helps lower LDL ("bad") cholesterol.

When purchasing pistachios, opt for nuts that have a hard shell and an intact kernel. In general, the greener the kernel, the fresher the nut. Make sure to choose pistachios that have their shell open at one end. A closed shell is a sign that the nut was picked prematurely. A good whiff of the nuts will help determine their freshness—if they smell off, they've likely gone rancid (this happens quickly due to their high fat content). Avoid any nuts that have visible mould on them.

Cashews provide good amounts of protein and fibre, and contain plenty of B vitamins along with iron, magnesium, vitamin E, folate and some calcium. However, they have long been identified as the nut with a high fat content. This tarnished reputation comes from the fact that while cashews are lower overall in fat than other nuts, they have more of the unhealthy saturated fat than other nuts. For example, ¼ cup almonds contains 18.2 grams of total fat, compared to 15.9 grams in the same amount of cashews. But—and it's a big but—that ¼ cup of almonds contains 1.4 grams of saturated fat, compared to 3.1 grams in cashews.

Cashews are always sold shelled and roasted since the outer shell contains a toxic oil and the nuts must be roasted or bleached to remove any residue. Raw cashews tend to have little flavour, but when roasted they have a buttery, smooth, meaty flavour that makes them ideal not only for snacking but a favourite in Latin American cuisine.

Macadamia nuts are probably one of the most expensive nuts. Native to Australia, they typically come from Hawaii these days. Although their creamy, buttery texture belies it, they contain no cholesterol. The natural oils in these nuts contain 78% monounsaturated fats, the highest of any oil, including olive oil. They are also a good source of protein, calcium and fibre, and are of course naturally low in sodium.

Peanuts Although not a true nut—the peanut is actually a legume—peanuts share the heart-healthy monounsaturated fat common to pecans, walnuts and macadamia nuts. A source of protein, they also provide many vitamins and minerals such as folate, vitamin E, copper, selenium, magnesium and zinc. Peanuts also supply some dietary fibre. Be mindful, however, that peanuts are relatively high in fat so, despite their nutritional properties, should be consumed sparingly.

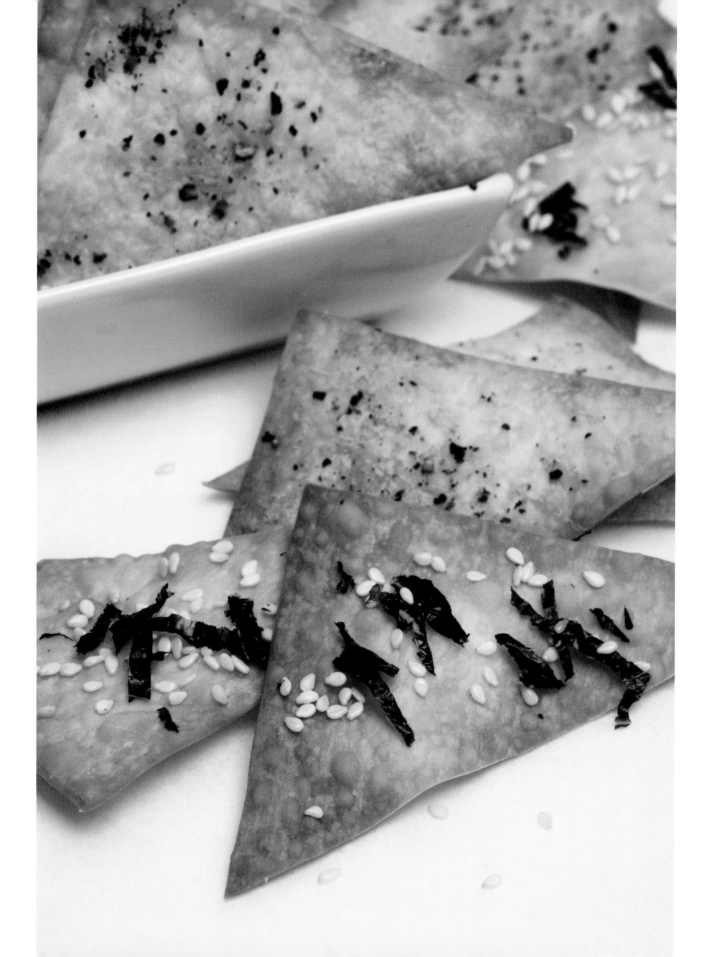

Seaweed and Sesame Wonton Crackers

Want chips without all the salt and oil? Use small amounts of naturally salty ingredients (such as cheese or seaweed) and seasonings that provide a flavourful punch (such as pepper or sesame seeds). Wonton wrappers provide crunch with minimal oil and act as a great substitute for deep-fried potatoes. So you can satisfy your craving without a trip to the vending machine!

Prep time: 5 minutes
Cook time: 10 minutes
Makes 50 crackers

25 wonton wrappers, halved diagonally (for 2 triangles) or vertically
    (for 2 narrow strips)
1½ tbsp olive oil
1 tbsp sesame seeds
½ sheet toasted nori seaweed, crumbled to flakes or finely sliced

Preheat oven to 350°F.

Arrange wonton wrappers on two parchment paper–lined baking sheets; brush lightly with oil. Sprinkle wontons with sesame seeds and nori.

Bake, one tray at a time, in centre of preheated oven until golden, 8 to 10 minutes. If you prefer, you can bake both trays at once in the upper and middle third of the oven, transferring pans from bottom to top halfway through baking.

Cool before serving. (Crackers can be stored in an airtight container at room temperature for up to 5 days.)

NUTRITIONAL ANALYSIS PER CRACKER: Calories 15; Protein 0g; Carbohydrate 2g (1%DV); Fat, total 0.5g (1%DV); Fat, saturated 0g; Fat, trans 0g; Cholesterol 0mg; Fibre 0g; Sodium 25mg (1%DV).

Parmesan and Pepper Wonton Crackers

Another delicious, low-fat cracker, this time with a cheesy kick!

Prep time: 5 minutes
Cook time: 10 minutes
Makes 50 crackers

25 wonton wrappers, halved diagonally (for 2 triangles) or vertically
    (for 2 narrow strips)
1½ tbsp olive oil
1 piece (1 x 1 inch) Parmesan cheese
½ tsp freshly ground black pepper

Preheat oven to 350°F.

Arrange wonton wrappers on two parchment paper–lined baking sheets; brush lightly with oil.

Using a microplane or hand grater, grate Parmesan directly onto wontons so that each is sprinkled but not covered with cheese. Sprinkle pepper over wontons.

Bake, one tray at a time, in centre of preheated oven until golden, 8 to 10 minutes. Or, if you prefer, you can bake both trays at once in the upper and middle third of the oven, transferring pans from bottom to top halfway through baking.

Cool before serving. (Crackers can be stored in an airtight container at room temperature for up to 5 days.)

NUTRITIONAL ANALYSIS PER CRACKER: Calories 15; Protein 0g; Carbohydrate 2g (1%DV); Fat, total 0.5g (1%DV); Fat, saturated 0g; Fat, trans 0g; Cholesterol 0mg; Fibre 0g; Sodium 25mg (1%DV).

❧ Health Savvy: Seeds 101

Seeds, no matter what variety, tend to be high in natural oils and thus prone to rancidity. Store all seeds in airtight containers in the freezer. There's no need to thaw them if either baking or cooking with them. Toasting seeds, as with nuts, will enhance their natural flavours. Always smell seeds before you use them. If they smell even a bit musty or rancid, discard them.

Flaxseeds Flaxseeds have a mild nutty flavour and are typically tiny, glossy, oval and brown. But don't let their size fool you—flaxseeds pack a whopper of a nutritional punch. Just 2 tablespoons of ground flaxseeds provide 2 to 3 grams of ALA, a type of omega-3 fatty acid that can help fight against heart disease and stroke. Flaxseeds also contain more lignans (a type of phytoestrogen) than any other food source. Some research has shown that lignans may help protect against cancers that are sensitive to hormones, including breast, ovarian and prostate cancer. Flaxseeds are also a good source of fibre and magnesium.

Thanks to a hard shell that can pass through the body undigested, ground flaxseeds offer more healthful benefits than eating the whole seed. Two tablespoons of ground flaxseed have less than 80 calories and contain 4 grams of fibre.

Two types of flaxseeds are readily available: golden yellow and reddish brown. According to the Flax Council of Canada, golden and brown flaxseeds are nutritionally very similar and are both a healthy choice.

Poppy seeds If you can imagine, it takes about 900,000 of these miniscule, black-grey seeds to equal 1 pound. They have a slightly bitter taste, sweet and nutty at the same time, and are much enhanced by toasting. The seeds are an excellent source of B-complex vitamins such as thiamine, pantothenic acid, vitamin B_6, riboflavin, niacin and folic acid. They also contain good levels of minerals such as iron, calcium and potassium. The outer coat is rich in dietary fibre.

Pumpkin seeds (pepitas) Although rich in calories, these sweet and nutty seeds boast a wealth of nutritional benefits. While somewhat high in saturated fat (60%), they are especially rich in ALA, an omega-3 fatty acid that has been shown to lower LDL, the "bad cholesterol," and raise HDL, the "good cholesterol." They are a good source of protein and a very good source of vitamin E. Popular in Mexican and South American cuisine, they also contain very good levels of essential minerals including copper, manganese, potassium, calcium, iron, magnesium, zinc and selenium.

Sesame seeds Brought to this continent by African slaves, sesame seeds originally flourished in Southern cooking, where they were known as benne seeds. Sesame seeds contain a multitude of nutritional benefits. They contain ALA, are a source of protein and are a very good source of B-complex vitamins such as niacin, folic acid, thiamine, vitamin B_6 and riboflavin. They are especially high in folic acid and niacin. Sesame seeds are available in both white and black varieties.

Sunflower seeds These teardrop-shaped seeds are native to North America. With a mild nutty flavour, sunflower seeds are a rich source of vitamin E, have a healthy fat profile and can provide a hefty dose of folic acid. They are a very good source of B-complex vitamins such as niacin, thiamine and riboflavin. Calcium, iron, manganese, zinc, magnesium, selenium and copper are especially concentrated in sunflower seeds.

✎ Kitchen Savvy: Snack-Time Swaps

Satisfy your cravings for run-of-the-mill snacks, which are loaded with fat, sugar and salt, with these tasty options!

- High-salt potato chips: Replace with **Kale Chips** (below), pretzels or **Wonton Crackers** (pages 133 and 134).

- High-fat cookies (e.g., chocolate chip cookies): Replace with **Fennel-Spiced Asiago Biscotti** (page 123) or **Cranberry Pumpkin Seed Crunchy Snack** (page 124).

- High-fat peanuts or cashews: Replace with **Indian-Spiced Chickpeas** (page 127).

- High-fat crackers: Replace with **Wonton Crackers** (pages 133 and 134).

- Chocolate bars: Replace with dried fruit or **Chili Chocolate Bark with Cherries and Pistachios** (page 125).

- High-fat ice cream: Replace with frozen yogurt or frozen fruit smoothies.

Easy Kale Chips

Rather than munching on potato chips or butter-laden popcorn, try our new version of a healthy snack. Kale chips are a delicious alternative and are surprisingly easy to make!

Simply whisk together 2 tbsp canola oil, 1 tbsp sherry vinegar, 1 tsp sesame oil and a pinch of cayenne pepper. Toss in 1 bunch of kale, stems removed and torn into pieces. Arrange on two parchment paper–lined baking sheets and bake, one sheet at a time, in a preheated 350°F oven until crispy, about 22 minutes. (Chips can be stored in an airtight container for up to 4 days.)

NUTRITIONAL ANALYSIS PER 1/2 CUP SERVING: Calories 35; Protein 1g; Carbohydrate 3g (1%DV); Fat, total 2.5g (4%DV); Fat, saturated 0g; Fat, trans 0g; Cholesterol 0mg; Fibre 1g (4%DV); Sodium 15mg (1%DV).

Roasted Edamame Bean Dip

This beautiful pale green dip is infused with the flavours of sushi. Edamame (soybeans) and tofu are the main ingredients, making it a great way to get all the healthful properties of soy in your afternoon snack.

Prep time: 15 minutes, plus 20 minutes to shell the edamame beans if necessary
Cook time: 20 minutes
Makes 1½ cups (1 tbsp per serving)

1 lb edamame, frozen if fresh not available
1 tsp + 2 tbsp canola oil
¾ cup soft tofu
3 tbsp water
¾ tsp wasabi paste (increase to 1 tsp if you prefer a little more heat)
2 tbsp coarsely chopped pickled (sushi) ginger
1 tbsp white miso paste
½ tsp each salt and black pepper

Preheat oven to 375°F.

If using fresh edamame, shell, discarding shells. If using frozen, unshelled edamame, bring 8 cups salted water to full boil over high heat in a large pot. Add frozen edamame; cook until shells are defrosted and soft, about 2 minutes. Drain under cold water. Remove edamame beans from shell. This should yield between 1 and 1⅓ cups of beans. Frozen shelled edamame beans can be used directly.

In a bowl, toss beans with 1 tsp oil; transfer to a parchment paper–lined baking sheet. Bake in centre of preheated oven for 20 minutes. Remove from oven; let cool.

Place beans, tofu, 2 tbsp water, wasabi paste, pickled ginger, miso paste, salt, pepper and remaining 2 tbsp oil in the bowl of a food processor. Process at high speed until a creamy paste is obtained. Add additional water to achieve desired consistency.

NUTRITIONAL ANALYSIS PER SERVING: Calories 35; Protein 2g; Carbohydrate 3g (1%DV); Fat, total 2.5g (4%DV); Fat, saturated 0g; Fat, trans 0g; Cholesterol 0mg; Fibre 1g (4%DV); Sodium 90mg (4%DV).

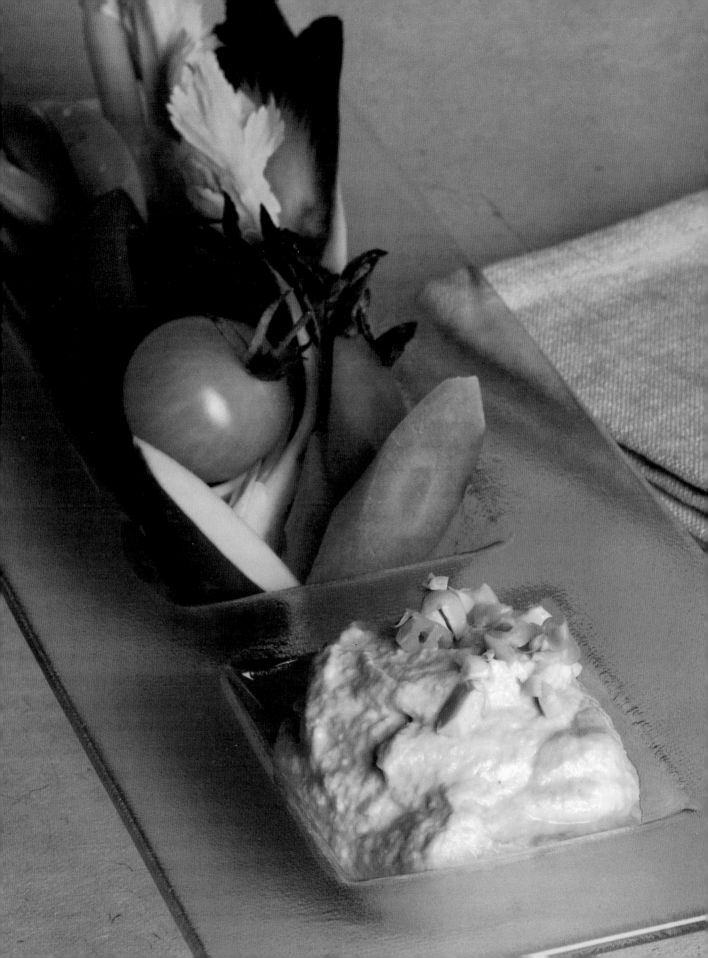

Thai-Inspired Almond and Peanut Dipping Sauce

This dipping sauce also works well using almonds only. If you need to avoid peanuts, simply replace the peanut butter with additional almond butter.

Prep time: 10 minutes
Cook time: 10 minutes
Makes 1½ cups (1 tbsp per serving)

2 tbsp canola oil
2 tbsp sesame oil
½ cup chopped onion
6 large cloves garlic, chopped
2 tbsp chopped fresh ginger
½ green chili, seeded and coarsely chopped (use the whole chili if you prefer a hotter dipping sauce)
½ cup water
2 tbsp red wine vinegar
2 tbsp ketchup
2 tbsp creamy almond butter
2 tbsp creamy peanut butter
2 tbsp low-sodium soy sauce
1 tbsp lime juice
¼ cup coarsely chopped fresh coriander leaves
1½ tbsp granulated sugar
¼ cup coarsely chopped fresh basil leaves, preferably Thai basil

Heat canola and sesame oils in a pot set over medium heat. Add onion, garlic, fresh ginger and green chili; cook for 5 minutes, stirring occasionally. Do not allow to brown.

Add water, vinegar, ketchup, almond and peanut butters, soy sauce, lime juice, coriander, and sugar. Bring to a boil. Reduce heat; simmer for 5 minutes. Remove from heat; cool to room temperature.

Transfer mixture to a blender or the bowl of a food processor and add basil; process until smooth. (Mixture can be refrigerated in an airtight container for up to 2 weeks.)

NUTRITIONAL ANALYSIS PER SERVING: Calories 45; Protein 1g; Carbohydrate 3g (1%DV); Fat, total 3.5g (5%DV); Fat, saturated 0g; Fat, trans 0g; Cholesterol 0mg; Fibre 0g; Sodium 70mg (3%DV).

Bite-Size Nut Scones

These bite-size scones are a great pick-me-up in the afternoon. They can also double up as mini sandwiches enclosing slices of cold cuts and/or cheese. As a bonus, they freeze extremely well, meaning you'll always have something satisfying when the 3 o'clock slump descends.

Prep time: 10 minutes
Cook time: 15 minutes
Makes 24 scones

2 cups all-purpose flour
¼ cup packed light brown sugar
2 tsp baking powder
½ tsp salt
3 tbsp cold unsalted butter, cubed
¾ cup chopped toasted walnuts
¾ cup buttermilk

Preheat oven to 425°F. Line a baking sheet with parchment paper.

In a bowl, combine flour, brown sugar, baking powder and salt. Using a pastry cutter or two knives, cut in butter until butter is broken down into very small pieces. Stir in walnuts.

Pour buttermilk over, stirring with a fork until mixture forms a cohesive, roughly shaped ball. Transfer mixture to a lightly floured work surface. With floured hands, pat into ½-inch thick circle.

Using a floured 1½-inch cookie cutter, cut out between 20 and 24 rounds. Transfer to prepared baking sheet.

Bake in centre of preheated oven until golden on top, 12 to 14 minutes. Transfer to rack and let cool for 5 minutes.

NUTRITIONAL ANALYSIS PER SCONE: Calories 90; Protein 2g; Carbohydrate 11g (4%DV); Fat, total 4g (6%DV); Fat, saturated 1g (5%DV); Fat, trans 0g; Cholesterol 5mg (2%DV); Fibre 1g (4%DV); Sodium 80mg (3%DV).

Appetizing Appetizers: Navigating the Witching Hour

We have all attended receptions in the late afternoon and early evening where we are tempted by high-fat, savoury treats offered by individuals with encouraging smiles. Well, overindulging in these treats is one more way we add extra pounds. We are also likely to sit down to a full dinner afterward. But you can be kind to yourself and your guests by avoiding high–saturated-fat treats and choosing—or serving—easy-to-prepare, healthy, low-fat alternatives instead.

Why We Gorge on Hors D'oeuvres

There's a term in science called "sensory-specific satiety." It refers to a phenomenon where our appetites decline with repeated consumption of the same taste and texture. However, our appetite picks up when we consume something new.

This phenomenon explains why many of us overeat at buffet-style meals with multiple choices. We constantly renew our appetite as we taste a new offering. The same thing can occur when multiple and varied tidbits are offered at receptions. Each new taste sensation can make us hungrier for more. Compound that with the fact that receptions often occur at a time of day when we are usually hungry and ready to sit down to dinner. So the best way to avoid this trap is to stick to one or two of the tidbits you are served. Or, if you are hosting the event, limit the number of offerings that you provide.

Role of High Fat

As we discussed in Chapter 1, protein is the most satiating nutrient that we can consume, followed by carbohydrates and then fat. If we consume a high-protein food just before a meal, we are likely to reduce our overall intake at the meal.

Contrast this with fat. When we eat high-fat snacks, we don't reduce our meal intake at all, resulting in excess consumption. Scientists study this by giving a test food to volunteers in close proximity to a meal and then determining how much an individual eats at the meal. These studies closely mimic the natural intake of hors d'oeuvres and foods offered before the meal.

To help promote satiety prior to a meal and discourage overeating, the recipes in this chapter are designed to be low in fat and high in protein. This combination should lead to satiety and naturally reduce your appetite when you sit down to a meal.

How to Use This Information

Keep in mind that eating or snacking just before a meal can lead to overconsumption, unless you consciously reduce your intake of calories at the meal. But foods that are naturally high in protein and low in fat are more likely to promote satiety and help you reduce your meal intake.

In addition, the more choices you have, the more likely you are to stimulate your appetite and overeat. So if you are preparing hors d'oeuvres and appetizers, choose foods that are naturally satiating and limit the number of choices that you offer. Many caterers will suggest that "three bites per person" is sufficient for a pre-meal event. With the low-fat recipes in this chapter, the calories in single bites range from 30 to 150 calories. Remember to take this into consideration and adjust your serving sizes for the actual meal.

Chapter 5

Appetizing Appetizers

Recipes

Salmon Tartare with Wasabi-Spiked Avocado "Mousse"   147

Thai Shrimp on Lemongrass Skewers   148

Summer Rolls with Thai Dipping Sauce   150

Sushi Stacks   153

Malaysian Fish Cakes with Easy Dipping Sauce   155

Whitefish "Tartare"   159

Persian Platter   160

Coconut Shrimp   161

Figs with Walnuts, Gorgonzola and Balsamic Drizzle   162

Cinnamon-Skewered Lamb Kebabs   164

Roasted Squash Soup with Roasted Pumpkin Seeds   166
by Chef Anne Desjardins

Fresh Fried and Roasted Almonds with Spicy Marinated Olives   168

Salmon Tartare with Wasabi-Spiked Avocado "Mousse"

This might sound fancy, but it's a cinch to make! There's a ton of flavour and texture in this one-bite dish, but the best part could be the crushed wasabi peas; adding a burst of heat and crunch, they are like Japanese Pop Rocks in a sophisticated starter.

Prep time: 15 minutes
Cook time: 7 minutes
Makes 20 canapés

CRACKERS
10 wonton wrappers, halved diagonally
1 tbsp canola oil
1 tsp raw sesame seeds

TARTARE
½ lb sushi-grade salmon
1 tbsp wasabi peas, coarsely crushed
1 tsp finely chopped fresh coriander leaves
1 tsp finely sliced green onion (white and light green parts only)

½ tsp each sesame oil and low-sodium soy sauce or tamari
1 tsp seasoned rice vinegar

MOUSSE
1 ripe avocado
¼ tsp wasabi paste
1 tbsp lime juice
½ tsp salt
1 tbsp sesame seeds

Preheat oven to 350°F.

Crackers: Arrange wonton wrappers on two parchment paper–lined baking sheets; brush lightly with oil. Sprinkle wrappers with sesame seeds. Bake in centre of pre-heated oven until golden, 6 to 7 minutes.

Tartare: Meanwhile, cut salmon against the grain into ½-inch thick slices. Stack slices; cut into strips, then cut across strips into cubes.

In a bowl, stir together salmon, wasabi peas, coriander, green onion, sesame oil, soy sauce and rice vinegar. Cover with plastic wrap and refrigerate until ready to use or for up to 1 day.

Mousse: In a separate bowl, smash avocado with fork; stir rigorously until smooth and creamy. Stir in wasabi paste, lime juice and salt.

Assembly: Top each wonton cracker with 1 scant tbsp tartare and 1 tsp avocado mousse. Sprinkle with sesame seeds for garnish.

NUTRITIONAL ANALYSIS PER CANAPÉ: Calories 30; Protein 2g; Carbohydrate 2g (1%DV); Fat, total 1.5g (2%DV); Fat, saturated 0g; Fat, trans 0g; Cholesterol 5mg (2%DV); Fibre 0g; Sodium 60mg (3%DV)

Thai Shrimp on Lemongrass Skewers

The spicy citrus flavour of the lemongrass skewer gives these shrimp a little extra zing from the inside out! Adventuring away from the typical toothpick or bamboo skewer is a great method to add unexpected flavour and an element of surprise to your cocktail nibbles. Shrimp can be swapped out for any firm whitefish, such as halibut, sea bass or swordfish.

Prep time: 15 minutes plus 20 minutes marinating time
Cook time: 10 minutes
Makes 12 skewers

2 small fresh red hot chili peppers, seeded
½ cup loosely packed fresh coriander, leaves and stems
1 lime, zested and juiced
1 tbsp canola oil
1 can (14 oz/398 mL) light coconut milk
1 clove garlic
1 piece fresh ginger (about 1 inch)
2 tsp low-sodium soy sauce or tamari
Pinch each salt and black pepper
12 black tiger shrimp, peeled and deveined (about 14 oz total)
12 stalks lemongrass (each 3 to 4 inches long)

In a blender, purée peppers, coriander, lime zest and juice, oil, coconut milk, garlic, ginger, soy sauce, salt and pepper until smooth. Pour mixture into a bowl. Add shrimp; marinate at room temperature for 20 minutes.

Preheat oven to 375°F.

Shake excess marinade off shrimp and discard marinade. Skewer 1 shrimp onto each lemongrass stalk. Arrange skewers in single layer on a parchment paper–lined baking sheet. Bake in centre of preheated oven until shrimp are pink, about 10 minutes.

NUTRITIONAL ANALYSIS PER SKEWER: Calories 70; Protein 8g; Carbohydrate 1g; Fat, total 3g (5%DV); Fat, saturated 2g (5%DV); Fat, trans 0g; Cholesterol 75mg (25%DV); Fibre 0g; Sodium 210mg (9%DV).

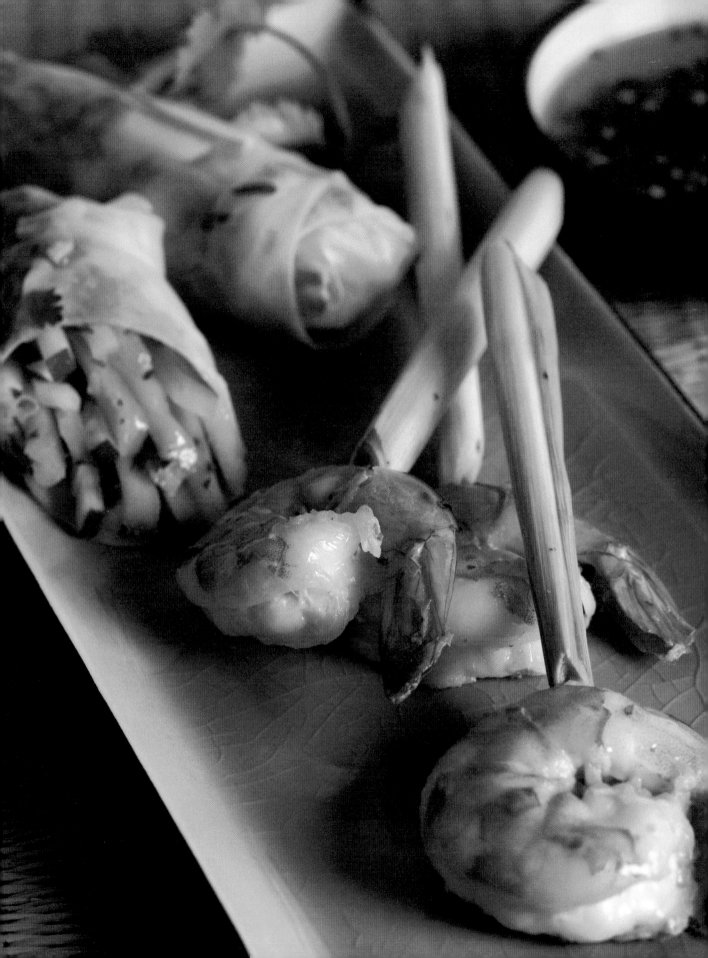

Summer Rolls with Thai Dipping Sauce

The fresh herbs in this vegetable bundle explode in your mouth. What could be better than a flavourful, no-fat, vegetable-packed roll? Even the dipping sauce is fat-free!

Prep time: 20 minutes
Makes 6 rolls

1 mango, julienned (about 1 cup)
½ English cucumber, julienned (about 1 cup)
¼ cup julienned radishes
¼ cup chopped peanuts
¼ cup finely chopped fresh coriander leaves
1 tbsp finely chopped fresh mint leaves
1 tsp lime juice
6 medium-sized rice paper wrappers
4 cups boiling water

In a bowl, combine mango, cucumber, radishes, peanuts, coriander, mint and lime juice.

Place two deep-set plates, large enough to accommodate rice paper wrappers, on work surface. Carefully pour ½ cup boiling water into one plate; immediately submerge one wrapper in boiling water, until softened and pliable, about 5 seconds. Transfer wrapper to the dry plate.

Spoon about ½ cup filling onto centre of wrapper, leaving 2 inches uncovered over and under and 3 inches uncovered on either side. Mould filling into narrow log.

Fold top and bottom of wrapper over filling. Gently fold one side over the filling, then roll up until wrapper has sealed around the stuffing. Cut each roll in half on an angle. Repeat process with each wrapper.

Serve with Thai Dipping Sauce (page 151).

NUTRITIONAL ANALYSIS PER ROLL: Calories 120; Protein 4g; Carbohydrate 18g (6%DV); Fat, total 4.5g (7%DV); Fat, saturated 0.5g (3%DV); Fat, trans 0g; Cholesterol 0mg; Fibre 2g (8%DV); Sodium 20mg (1%DV).

Thai Dipping Sauce

Prep time: 5 minutes
Cook time: 25 minutes
Makes ½ cup (1 tsp per serving)

1 cup white vinegar
½ cup granulated sugar
1 tsp salt
¾ tsp dried red pepper flakes (increase to 1 tsp if you prefer a spicier dipping sauce)
3 cloves garlic, minced

In a small pot set over medium heat, combine vinegar and sugar. Cook until sugar has dissolved. Add salt, red pepper flakes and garlic. Bring to a boil; reduce heat to low and simmer, stirring occasionally, until volume is reduced by half, about 20 minutes.

Cool; serve at room temperature. (Sauce can be refrigerated in an airtight container for up to 3 weeks.)

NUTRITIONAL ANALYSIS PER SERVING: Calories 20; Protein 0g; Carbohydrate 5g (2%DV);
Fat, total 0g; Fat, saturated 0g; Fat, trans 0g; Cholesterol 0mg; Fibre 0g; Sodium 100mg (4%DV).

TIP—Mangoes Out of Season?

If fresh mangoes are unavailable, feel free to combine the same amount of julienned cucumbers, half a sweet red pepper (halved, seeded and thinly sliced), 1 carrot (peeled and julienned) with 1 bunch each finely chopped fresh coriander, mint and basil leaves, along with the other ingredients.

✿ Health Savvy: Flavour without Fat

Chefs often promote fat as flavour, but in reality fat is a nutrient we should limit in our diet. Butter, lard and certain oils can be high, concentrated sources of trans and saturated fats; if consumed too often, these ingredients increase the risk of dementia and other health-degenerative conditions. Thankfully, flavour is not a one-trick pony! Explore new options for injecting full-bodied taste into your cooking without harmful fat. You might be surprised at how many flavourful ingredients have been hiding in your pantry.

Vinegars add a bright, tangy, sour yet spicy kick to dishes. Similar to citrus juices, vinegars contribute a light flavour to rich and hearty recipes. Sherry, apple cider, malt, rice, balsamic and wine vinegars are fantastic additions to your pantry and daily cooking.

Citrus fruits add a tart zing with light sweetness to dishes. Each citrus fruit varies in sugar content, but all provide essential well-rounded flavour. Lemons, limes, grapefruit, oranges and pomelos will brighten up any dish.

Aromatic vegetables are humble ingredients, often underappreciated for their contribution to complex flavour profiles. Usually sautéed as the base for proteins and sauces, or simmered for long hours for soups and stews to absorb their flavours, aromatics are never the star of the show. But without them, there would be no earthy notes or mellow sweetness. This family of flavour is vast, and each member tickles a different part of the tongue. Mix and match your favourites to create a flavour base for almost any dish: onions, garlic, ginger, mushrooms, carrots, celery/celeriac, leeks, peppers, parsnips and turnips.

Chili peppers add a burst of fresh, spicy flavour that wakes up a dish. Too much can overpower a recipe and prevent you from tasting anything but its hot spice, so use with caution. Chilies are available fresh, dried and in a wide variety of sauces. Jalapeño, serrano, ancho/poblano, cayenne and paprika are easily found.

Fresh herbs liven up a plate when sprinkled or stirred in just before serving; think of them as giving a tall drink of water to a very thirsty dish! Fresh herbs—such as dill, parsley, cilantro/coriander, basil, tarragon, oregano, chives and mint—have a way of refreshing long-simmered ingredients and making each one pop.

Tea, coffee and cocoa add a rich, earthy and sometimes smoky undertone to dishes. They can be used as a complementary seasoning for meat and fish. Stick with neutral varieties when first experimenting with these, as those blended with floral and potent ingredients may interfere with the desired flavour profile of a dish.

Sushi Stacks

All the sushi with none of the rolling work! If you are buying fish at the supermarket, be sure to ask the fishmonger if it is sushi grade. Alternatively, stop in at your local sushi restaurant, where chefs are usually happy to sell you a portion of their day's delivery. If you're a bit squeamish about using raw fish, this dish is equally delicious made with smoked salmon.

Prep time: 20 minutes plus 1½ hours waiting time
Cook time: 20 minutes
Makes 16 squares

SUSHI
1 cup sushi rice
2 cups water
2 tbsp seasoned rice vinegar
3 tbsp toasted white or black sesame seeds
1 square sheet nori
½ lb sushi-grade tuna or salmon
½ English cucumber, peeled
1 large avocado (or 2 small avocados)
1 tbsp lime juice
2 tbsp low-sodium soy sauce or tamari

GARNISH
1 tbsp sesame seeds
1 green onion (white and light green parts only), finely sliced

In a deep pot, bring rice and water to a boil over medium-high heat. Stir; reduce heat to low. Cook, leaving lid slightly ajar, until liquid is absorbed and rice is cooked, 20 to 22 minutes. Stir in rice vinegar and sesame seeds until evenly distributed.

Line an 8-inch square baking pan with plastic wrap. Trim nori to evenly fit bottom of pan. Top with warm rice. Using a wooden spoon or palette knife, spread rice to form an even layer. Refrigerate to cool slightly.

Meanwhile, thinly slice tuna. Arrange in a single layer to cover rice. Cover with plastic wrap; refrigerate for at least 1 hour or for up to 24 hours.

Remove pan from refrigerator; unwrap and cut into 16 even squares. Arrange on platter. Just before serving, cut cucumber in half lengthwise; discard seeds and cut cucumber into thin strips. Cut across strips to make small cubes. Place in a bowl. Halve avocado; discard pit. Run large spoon under skin to remove avocado half in one piece. Repeat for other half. Cut avocado into thin strips; cut across strips to make small cubes. Sprinkle avocado with lime juice. Add to bowl and stir gently to combine with cucumber. Spoon about 1 tsp cucumber mixture onto each sushi square. Drizzle with soy sauce. Sprinkle each stack with sesame seeds and green onion. Serve immediately.

NUTRITIONAL ANALYSIS PER SQUARE: Calories 130; Protein 9g; Carbohydrate 15g (5%DV); Fat, total 4.5g (7%DV); Fat, saturated 1g (5%DV); Fat, trans 0g; Cholesterol 10mg (3%DV); Fibre 1g (4%DV); Sodium 160mg (7%DV).

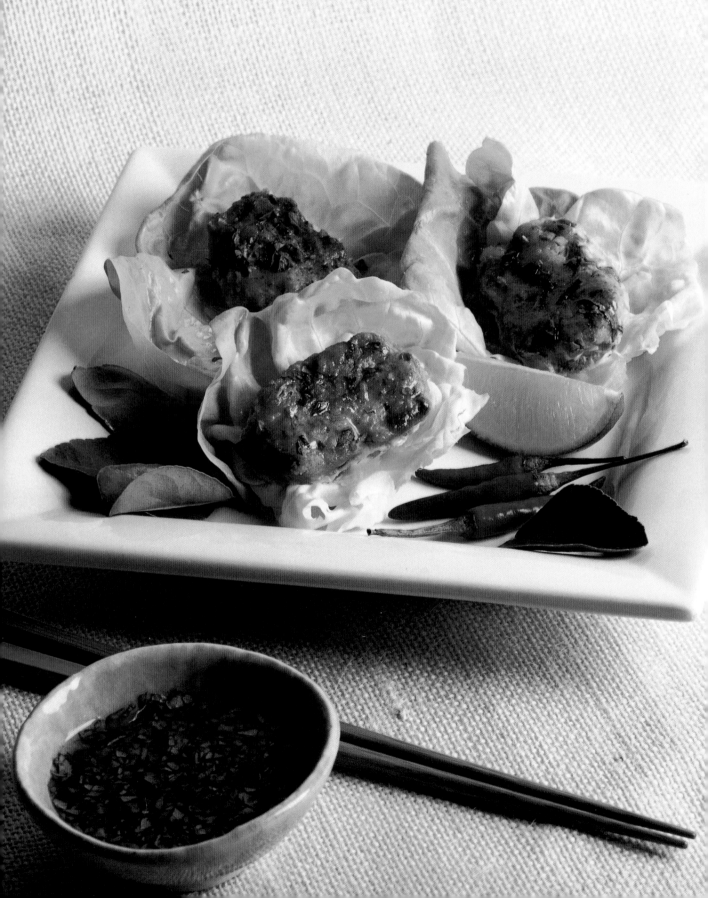

Malaysian Fish Cakes with Easy Dipping Sauce

Common on the streets of Thailand and surrounding countries, these fish cakes are flavour-packed with a hot, spicy finish. They are usually deep-fried, but the calorie count of these cakes has been dramatically reduced by having you bake them instead. This has the added advantage of freeing up your time so you can mingle with family and guests. To up the heat, feel free to use the entire chili.

Prep time: 20 minutes plus 20 minutes resting time
Cook time: 12 minutes
Makes 16 cakes

1 lb cod or tilapia
2 tbsp unsweetened shredded dried coconut
2 tsp Thai red curry paste
2 tsp fish sauce
½ green chili, seeded and coarsely chopped
3 kaffir lime leaves, finely sliced (or ½ tsp grated lime zest)
1 tbsp lime juice
¼ tsp salt
1 egg
2 tbsp cornstarch
⅓ cup chopped fresh coriander leaves
2 green onions (white and light green parts only), finely chopped
6 fresh green beans, cut into very thin slices
2 tbsp (approx) panko bread crumbs
16 soft lettuce leaves, such as Bibb lettuce, torn into 2 x 4-inch pieces (approx)

Preheat oven to 400°F.

Using paper towels, pat fish as dry as possible. If using previously frozen fish, squeeze the fish to remove as much excess moisture as possible—the fish must be very dry for this recipe to work. Cut fish into large chunks. Place in the bowl of a food processor; process until fish is in very small pieces and paste begins to appear.

Add coconut, curry paste, fish sauce, chili, lime leaves, lime juice, salt, egg and cornstarch; process until mixture is consistency of paste. Transfer to a bowl; stir in coriander, onions, beans and panko. If paste is too runny to form cakes, add 1 to 2 tbsp more panko. Set aside for 20 minutes before proceeding, to allow bread crumbs to absorb any excess moisture.

Shape heaping tablespoon of fish paste into oblong cake ¼ inch thick and 1 inch wide; place on a well-oiled or -sprayed parchment paper–lined baking sheet. Spray tops of fish cakes with baking spray. (Fish cakes can be covered with plastic wrap and refrigerated for up to 6 hours.)

Bake in centre of preheated oven until bottoms of cakes are well browned, about 6 minutes. Flip; bake 5 minutes. Let cool slightly. Serve warm, with lettuce leaf and Easy Dipping Sauce (recipe follows).

NUTRITIONAL ANALYSIS PER CAKE: Calories 45; Protein 5g; Carbohydrate 3g (1%DV); Fat, total 1g (2%DV); Fat, saturated 0.5g (3%DV); Fat, trans 0g; Cholesterol 20mg (7%DV); Fibre 1g (4%DV); Sodium 120mg (5%DV).

Easy Dipping Sauce

Prep time: 5 minutes
Makes ½ cup (1 tsp per serving)

¼ cup lime juice
2 tbsp fish sauce
2 tsp liquid honey
2 tbsp each finely chopped fresh coriander, mint and basil leaves (preferably Thai basil)

In a bowl, mix together all ingredients.

NUTRITIONAL ANALYSIS PER SERVING: Calories 5; Protein 0g; Carbohydrate 0g; Fat, total 0g; Fat, saturated 0g; Fat, trans 0g; Cholesterol 0mg; Fibre 0g; Sodium 115mg (5%DV).

✹Brain Savvy: Fats—The Good, the Bad and the Ugly

When we use the word "fat," we are referring to a specific component called "fatty acids." Fatty acids are long chains of carbon, linked together by chemical bonds.

Saturated fatty acids only have single bonds; monounsaturated fatty acids have one double bond in addition to the single bonds; and polyunsaturated fatty acids have two or more double bonds. Why is this important? Because the types of bonds in fats influence their physical characteristics. For example, animal-based fats, which are high in saturated fatty acids, are solid at room temperature. Fats high in monounsaturated fatty acids, such as olive oil, are liquid at room temperature but become thick and sludge-like in the refrigerator. Fats high in polyunsaturated fatty acids, like most vegetable oils, are liquid at both room temperature and in the refrigerator.

Now, imagine how these fats behave inside your body and cell membranes. The more fluid a membrane is, the easier it is for it to carry out its work. The type of fatty acids incorporated into our cell membranes depends, in part, on the types of fatty acids we consume. One advantage of eating monounsaturated or polyunsaturated fatty acids over saturated fatty acids is that it helps us keep our cell membranes fluid. We also know that monounsaturated fatty acids help lower the "bad" LDL cholesterol in our bodies.

So the first rule of thumb in selecting fat is that it should be vegetable, not animal, based. Both monounsaturated and polyunsaturated fatty acids are healthy if not consumed in excess. Select a fat based on the flavour requirements for the food being prepared. Olive oil will bring a fruity, nutty flavour to a dish whereas canola or soybean oils are reasonably tasteless.

Also keep in mind that some foods are inherently high in fat. Avocados, peanut butter, and many nuts and seeds are high in fat—but this fat is monounsaturated. As a result, these higher-fat foods are consistent with both a heart-healthy and brain-healthy diet.

Omega-3 and omega-6 fatty acids

What about the omega-3 fats you've heard so much about? *Omega-3* and *omega-6* are scientific terms that refer to where the first double bond is located in the fatty acid chain. Mammals, including humans, are unable to make omega-3 and omega-6 fatty acids naturally, so we must consume them in our diet, primarily from plant oils and fish. Both of these fatty acids play essential roles in cell-to-cell communication, maintaining the health of our blood vessels and reducing inflammation. Unfortunately, the typical North American diet contains too much omega-6 fat and too little omega-3 fat, so the balance or ratio of these two fatty acids is often less than optimal.

We need to eat more foods that are high in omega-3 fatty acids to improve this balance. We can do that by using canola or soybean oil, which are naturally higher in omega-3 fatty acids. Flax is particularly high in omega-3 fatty acids. However, it is easier to absorb flaxseed oil if we consume ground flax rather than the whole seed, which tends to exit the body intact. Other good choices for healthy oils include fatty fish, walnuts and soybeans.

Fish versus other foods as a source of omega-3 fatty acids

Fish contain two omega-3 fatty acids that are particularly important: eicosapentaenoic acid or EPA, and docosahexaenoic acid or DHA. These are longer-chain fatty acids than those found in plant foods. While our bodies can convert the shorter omega-3s in plants into this longer form, we are very inefficient at doing so. What's more, many of the biological processes supported by omega-3 fatty acids require these longer-chain versions. So it's simply more efficient to get them from fish.

Your brain, relative to other organs, is particularly high in DHA. The DHA in your brain supports nerve cell communication and protects the brain from inflammation, which can damage cells and leads to cell death. Indeed, many studies demonstrate that people who routinely eat fish (usually 2 to 3 servings per week) have better cognitive retention with aging.

Safety of eating fish

You have no doubt seen reports in the last few years questioning the safety of eating fish due to potential mercury contamination and other toxins. Fish accumulate mercury directly from the water in which they live (if polluted) and by eating other fish that may also contain mercury.

You can limit your exposure to mercury by choosing certain types of fish, according to Health Canada. Fish that are both high in healthy EPA and DHA but are also low in mercury include anchovies, capelin, char, hake, herring, Atlantic mackerel, mullet, pollock (Boston bluefish), salmon, smelt, rainbow trout, lake whitefish, blue crab, shrimp, clams, mussels and oysters. In contrast, larger, predatory fish tend to contain higher levels of mercury and consequently should be avoided or consumed in limited amounts. These larger fish include fresh or frozen tuna, shark, swordfish, marlin, orange roughy and escolar.

What about tuna, one of the more popular types of fish? The fish used in canned tuna products are generally younger and smaller and have significantly less mercury than fresh or frozen tuna, according to Health Canada. This is particularly true for flaked white or dark meat tuna. However, you may want to avoid albacore tuna, which has the potential for higher levels of mercury.

Farmed versus wild salmon

There have been reports raising concerns about the levels of toxins, PCBs and other contaminants in farmed fish, including salmon. Levels of contaminants in the food supply are routinely monitored by the Canadian Food Inspection Agency and compared with Health Canada–established standards for safe levels. Health Canada's current risk assessment says that consuming farmed salmon does not pose a health risk. This suggests that you can safely choose wild or farmed fish based on price and taste preference and not worry that you are risking your health if you consume fish two to three times per week.

Whitefish "Tartare"

Where's the beef? This "tartare," our riff on a fantastic Bonnie Stern recipe, is full of all the ingredients in a traditional beef tartare, but mixed into a base of flaked smoked fish. Carrying a wallop of flavour, these easy-to-make hors d'oeuvres embrace the healthfulness of fish.

Prep time: 15 minutes
Cook time: 10 minutes
Makes 16 croûtes

1 lb smoked whitefish, skinned, boned and torn into large flakes
3 tbsp finely chopped fresh dill
2 green onions, minced
½ tsp finely grated lemon zest
2 tbsp drained capers
2 tbsp lemon juice
1 tbsp (approx) olive oil
¼ tsp hot sauce such as Tabasco (optional)
1 baguette

In a bowl, gently toss together fish, dill, green onions, lemon zest, capers, lemon juice, oil and hot sauce (if using). If mixture seems dry, add an additional tablespoon of oil. Transfer to a bowl.

Preheat oven to 350°F.

Cut baguette into 16 ½-inch thick slices. Place on ungreased cookie sheets in a single layer. Bake in centre of preheated oven until lightly browned, about 10 minutes.

Cool and serve topped with 2 tbsp tartare.

NUTRITIONAL ANALYSIS PER CROÛTE: Calories 70; Protein 5g; Carbohydrate 7g (2%DV); Fat, total 1.5g (2%DV); Fat, saturated 0g; Fat, trans 0g; Cholesterol 5mg (2%DV); Fibre 0g; Sodium 300mg (13%DV).

Persian Platter

Revamp your typical cheese platter with this Iranian-inspired spread. Salty cheese is wrapped up with walnuts and cherries in layers of fresh herbs—an unexpectedly perfect marriage of flavours in just one bite. The assembly here should be DIY, but it's a good idea to have one or two bites prepared on the side of the plate, so guests get the idea. Pita isn't really necessary, but is a great base for those who wish to include it. Otherwise, leave your basil leaves whole and wrap the other flavours in the leaf.

Prep time: 10 minutes plus 2 hours resting time
Serves 8

1 cup low-fat or light feta cheese (about 4 oz)
4 tsp low-fat ricotta cheese
1 bunch fresh basil leaves
1 bunch fresh tarragon leaves
1 bunch fresh mint leaves
½ cup halved walnuts
¼ cup preserved sour cherries
1 tbsp olive oil
4 whole-wheat pitas

Using a fork or food processor, mix feta and ricotta cheeses until well combined. Line a small flat-bottomed container, measuring about 3 inches wide, with plastic wrap. Transfer cheese into container and press down, using container as a mould. Flatten top so that it is smooth. Cover with plastic wrap and refrigerate for at least 2 hours or up to 3 days.

When ready to serve, unmould cheese. Place on platter surrounded by delicate piles of whole fresh basil, tarragon and mint leaves, one small bowl of walnuts and one small bowl of cherries.

Heat a grill or grill pan set over medium-low heat; brush with oil. Grill pita until warmed through with light grill marks, about 2 minutes per side.

Stack grilled pita on platter for guests to tear from; encourage diners to spread their pita pieces with cheese mixture and layer herbs, cherries and nuts for a delicious bite!

NUTRITIONAL ANALYSIS PER EACH OF 8 SERVINGS: Calories 150; Protein 6g; Carbohydrate 12g (4%DV); Fat, total 9g (14%DV); Fat, saturated 2.5g (13%DV); Fat, trans 0g; Cholesterol 5mg (2%DV); Fibre 2g (8%DV); Sodium 300mg (13%DV).

Coconut Shrimp

Most recipes for coconut shrimp have you deep-fry the shrimp, turning a healthy food into a high-fat appetizer. Baking the shrimp not only turns this into a lower-fat version but also allows the flavour of the toasted coconut to sing.

Prep time: 15 minutes
Cook time: 10 minutes
Makes 20 shrimp

2 cups unsweetened shredded dried coconut
1 cup panko bread crumbs
2 tsp curry powder
½ tsp salt
4 egg whites
1 lb large shrimp (about 20), peeled but leaving the last section and tails intact
Cooking spray

Preheat oven to 350°F.

Line a baking sheet with coconut; toast in centre of preheated oven, stirring once or twice, until lightly browned, 5 to 8 minutes. Let cool.

On a plate, mix together toasted coconut, panko, curry powder and salt.

In a bowl, lightly beat egg whites until frothy. Add shrimp to bowl; gently toss until well coated.

Place shrimp, one or two at a time, in coconut mixture, gently pressing so that coconut adheres to shrimp. Place on parchment paper–lined baking sheet. Repeat until all shrimp are coated. Lightly spray shrimp with cooking spray. (Shrimp can be covered with plastic wrap and refrigerated for up to 3 hours.)

Increase oven temperature to 400°F. Bake shrimp in centre of oven until cooked through, about 10 minutes. Serve while still warm, allowing guests to use shrimp tails as handles.

NUTRITIONAL ANALYSIS PER SHRIMP: Calories 76; Protein 8g; Carbohydrate 4g (1%DV); Fat, total 3g (4%DV); Fat, saturated 2g (9%DV); Fat, trans 0g; Cholesterol 44mg (15%DV); Fibre 1g (3%DV); Sodium 124mg (5%DV).

Figs with Walnuts, Gorgonzola and Balsamic Drizzle

Figs are extremely perishable, so buy them close to use. Calimyrna figs from California, with their white flesh and green exterior, are particularly good with this recipe. Also look for Mission figs, with their characteristic purple-black skin, which are available from June through mid-September.

Prep time: 10 minutes
Cook time: 10 minutes
Makes 8 figs

½ cup balsamic vinegar
2 tbsp packed light brown sugar
8 fresh figs
½ cup crumbled Gorgonzola cheese
⅓ cup toasted chopped walnuts

In a small pot set over medium-high heat, stir together vinegar and brown sugar. Bring to a boil; boil gently, without stirring, until reduced by half, about 8 minutes. Set aside to cool. (Vinegar can be covered with plastic wrap and kept at room temperature for up to 3 days.)

Starting at stem end but without cutting all the way through, cut each fig into quarters. Transfer to a serving platter. Gently press figs open, as if creating a flower with four petals.

In a bowl, gently stir together cheese and walnuts. Spoon mixture evenly into centre of each fig. Drizzle with balsamic glaze.

NUTRITIONAL ANALYSIS PER FIG: Calories 100; Protein 3g; Carbohydrate 12g (4%DV); Fat, total 5g (8%DV); Fat, saturated 1.5g (8%DV); Fat, trans 0g; Cholesterol 5mg (2%DV); Fibre 2g (8%DV); Sodium 100mg (4%DV).

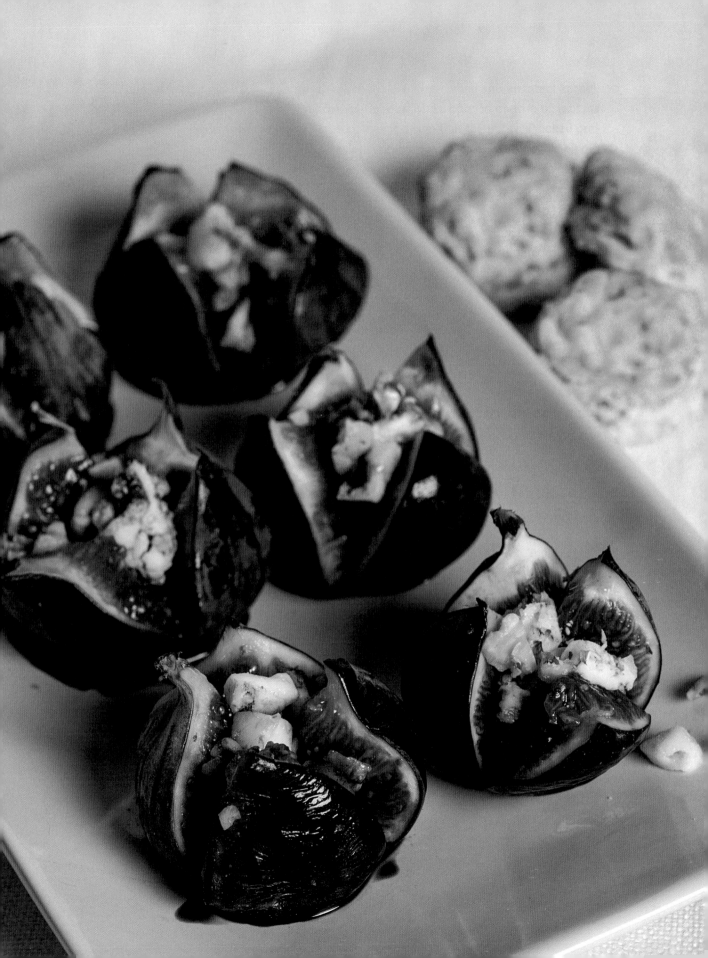

Cinnamon-Skewered Lamb Kebabs

Using cinnamon as the skewer instead of bamboo or steel is a great way to season kebabs while cooking. The same technique can be applied with any skewer-sturdy aromatic, such as rosemary or lemongrass (as used in **Thai Shrimp on Lemongrass Skewers** on page 148). Be sure to leave space on the sticks for guests to grab hold! However, these are equally scrumptious on metal or bamboo skewers.

Prep time: 15 minutes
Cook time: 10 minutes
Makes 15 kebabs

¾ lb ground lamb or beef
2 tsp finely chopped fresh mint leaves
1 tsp minced or grated shallot
1 clove garlic, minced or grated
2 tbsp red wine
½ tsp ground ginger
½ tsp ground coriander
¼ tsp ground cinnamon
½ tsp salt
¼ tsp black pepper
15 cinnamon sticks (each about 3 inches long)
1 tbsp olive oil

Preheat broiler to 500°F or to high. Position rack in top third of oven.

In a bowl, mix together lamb, mint, shallots, garlic, wine, ginger, coriander, cinnamon, salt and pepper.

Divide mixture into 15 equal portions; form each into log. Push cinnamon stick into each log, leaving enough of the cinnamon stick exposed to use as a handle. Cover handle with aluminum foil to prevent cinnamon stick from burning.

Arrange kebabs on an aluminum foil–lined baking sheet; brush lightly with oil. Broil, flipping halfway through cooking time, until no longer pink inside, about 10 minutes. Remove foil from cinnamon sticks.

NUTRITIONAL ANALYSIS PER KEBAB: Calories 80; Protein 6g; Carbohydrate 0g; Fat, total 5g (8%DV); Fat, saturated 2g (10%DV); Fat, trans 0g; Cholesterol 25mg (8%DV); Fibre 0g; Sodium 95mg (4%DV).

✏ Kitchen Savvy: Small Plates, Big Meal

"Small plates" is a fairly new craze that's hitting North America in a huge way. Rather than sitting down to individual blue-plate entrées, food enthusiasts are opting to share scaled-down portions of various dishes that are served over multiple courses. This dining experience is already common in the Mediterranean: Greece and Turkey have dubbed this meal of many plates "mezze," the Spanish refer to it as "tapas," while the Italians offer it as "antipasti." All showcase the olives, seafood, meats and dairy proudly produced in their regions. This practice can also be found in Asian cultures—"dim sum," the traditional brunch in China, consists of various steamed and fried dumplings, served four to six at a time for families to share. Similarly, Japanese pubs, called "izikayas," cater to the after-work crowd with an endless offering of miniature morsels to accompany their sake. If you'd like to plan a small-plate meal with big impact, here are three suggested menus with recipes from this chapter:

Mezze-Inspired Menu

Fresh Fried and Roasted Almonds with Spicy Marinated Olives (page 168)
Persian Platter (page 160)
Cinnamon-Skewered Lamb Kebabs (page 164)
Figs with Walnuts, Gorgonzola and Balsamic Drizzle (page 162)

Flavours of the Far East

Summer Rolls with Thai Dipping Sauce (page 150)
Thai Shrimp on Lemongrass Skewers (page 148)
Coconut Shrimp (page 161)
Salmon Tartare with Wasabi-Spiked Avocado "Mousse" (page 147)
Malaysian Fish Cakes with Easy Dipping Sauce (page 155)

A Winter Night In

Fresh Fried and Roasted Almonds with Spicy Marinated Olives (page 168)
Roasted Squash Soup with Roasted Pumpkin Seeds (page 166)
Figs with Walnuts, Gorgonzola and Balsamic Drizzle (page 162)

Roasted Squash Soup with Roasted Pumpkin Seeds

By Chef Anne Desjardins

Anne Desjardins is the brilliant chef and owner of the restaurant l'Eau à la Bouche, tucked away in the postcard-worthy village of Sainte-Adèle in Quebec.

A perfect autumn starter in a pretty little teacup!

Prep time: 10 minutes
Cook time: 1 hour
Serves 8 (¾ cup per serving)

1 butternut squash (about 3 lb)
1 onion, peeled and halved
2 cloves garlic, unpeeled
2 tbsp olive oil
2 cups (approx) chicken broth, preferably low-sodium
½ tsp salt
½ tsp cider vinegar
Dash hot pepper sauce such as Tabasco
3 tbsp 2% plain yogurt
2 tbsp pumpkin seed oil
2 tbsp roasted unsalted pumpkin seeds

Preheat oven to 425°F.

Cut squash in half lengthwise; scoop out seeds. Place squash on an aluminum foil–lined baking sheet along with onion and garlic. Brush oil all over vegetables.

Roast in centre of preheated oven, turning onion and garlic a couple of times, until golden brown and softened, 40 to 50 minutes. Let cool slightly. Peel garlic.

Using a spoon, scoop out cooked squash; transfer to a blender or the bowl of a food processor along with onion and garlic. Pour in 1 cup broth. Purée until completely smooth. Return mixture to pot, adding remaining 1½ cups broth. Whisk in salt, vinegar and hot pepper sauce. If soup is too thick, whisk in ½ cup more stock. Heat over medium heat until steaming.

Pour ¾ cup soup into each of eight teacups. Top each with 1 tsp yogurt. Drizzle with 1 tsp oil and sprinkle with 1 tsp pumpkin seeds.

NUTRITIONAL ANALYSIS PER SERVING: Calories 130; Protein 3g; Carbohydrate 14g (5%DV); Fat, total 8g (12%DV); Fat, saturated 1.5g (8%DV); Fat, trans 0g; Cholesterol 0mg; Fibre 2g (8%DV); Sodium 170mg (7%DV).

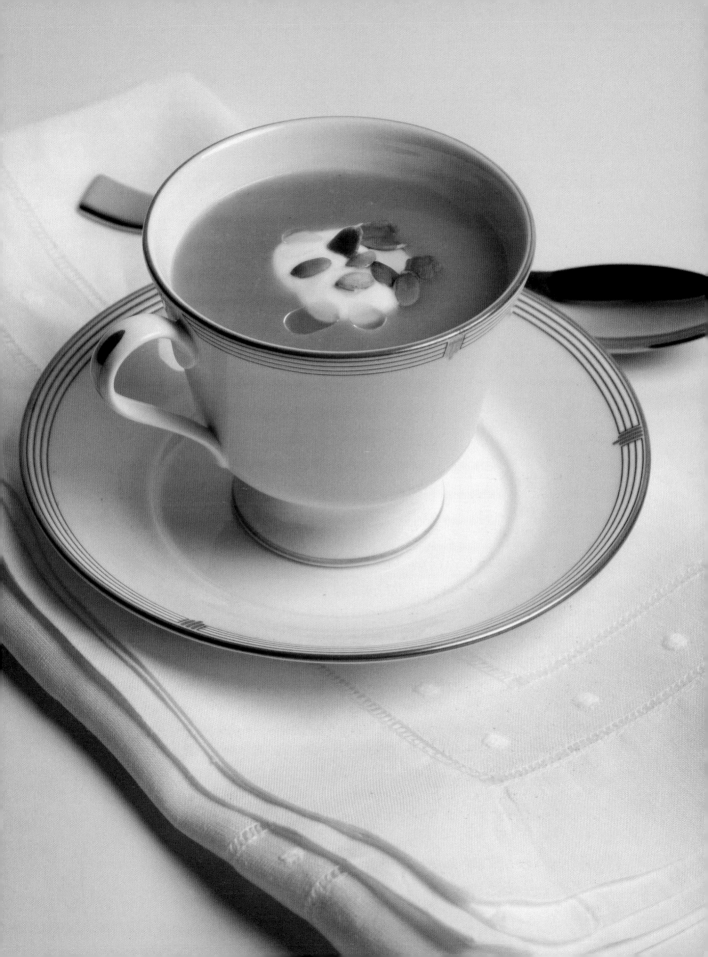

Fresh Fried and Roasted Almonds with Spicy Marinated Olives

Spain is well known for both its almonds and olives, so it's not surprising that small dishes offering these delicacies are common. Try roasting your own almonds to draw on the flavour of freshly roasted nuts, and pair this with olives you have purchased or, even better, olives that you have personalized with a homemade marinade, like the **Spicy Marinated Olives** that follow. For a boost of flavour, add some freshly chopped rosemary when stir-frying the almonds.

Prep time: 10 minutes
Cook time: 10 minutes
Makes 2 cups (2 tbsp each)

1 tbsp olive oil
2 cups blanched whole almonds

1 tsp salt, preferably sea salt

Preheat oven to 350°F.

In a large non-stick skillet, heat oil over medium heat. Add almonds and salt; cook, stirring frequently, until nuts are deep golden and crisp, 8 to 10 minutes. Spread almonds in a single layer on a parchment paper–lined baking sheet.

Bake in centre of preheated oven, stirring every 2 to 3 minutes, until almonds are just starting to brown, about 10 minutes. Remove from oven. Cool in pan. Serve at room temperature.

Spicy Marinated Olives

Prep time: 10 minutes plus 3 to 4 hours, or up to overnight, to marinate
Makes 2 cups

1 lemon
2 cups large brine-cured green olives, drained
2 tsp finely chopped fresh rosemary

2 cloves garlic, finely sliced
3 tbsp olive oil
½ tsp crushed red pepper flakes (optional)

Using a sharp knife or vegetable peeler, remove long slices of lemon zest, leaving behind as much white pith as possible. Squeeze lemon, reserving 2 tbsp juice.

In a large bowl, toss together lemon zest and reserved juice, olives, rosemary, garlic, olive oil and red pepper flakes (if using). Place olives in an airtight container; let stand for several hours or overnight before serving. Olives will keep in the refrigerator for several weeks.

NUTRITIONAL ANALYSIS PER 2 TBSP MIXED ALMONDS AND OLIVES: Calories 105; Protein 2g; Carbohydrate 4g (1%DV); Fat, total 10g (15%DV); Fat, saturated 1g (4%DV); Fat, trans 0g; Cholesterol 0mg; Fibre 1g (4%DV); Sodium 385mg (16%DV).

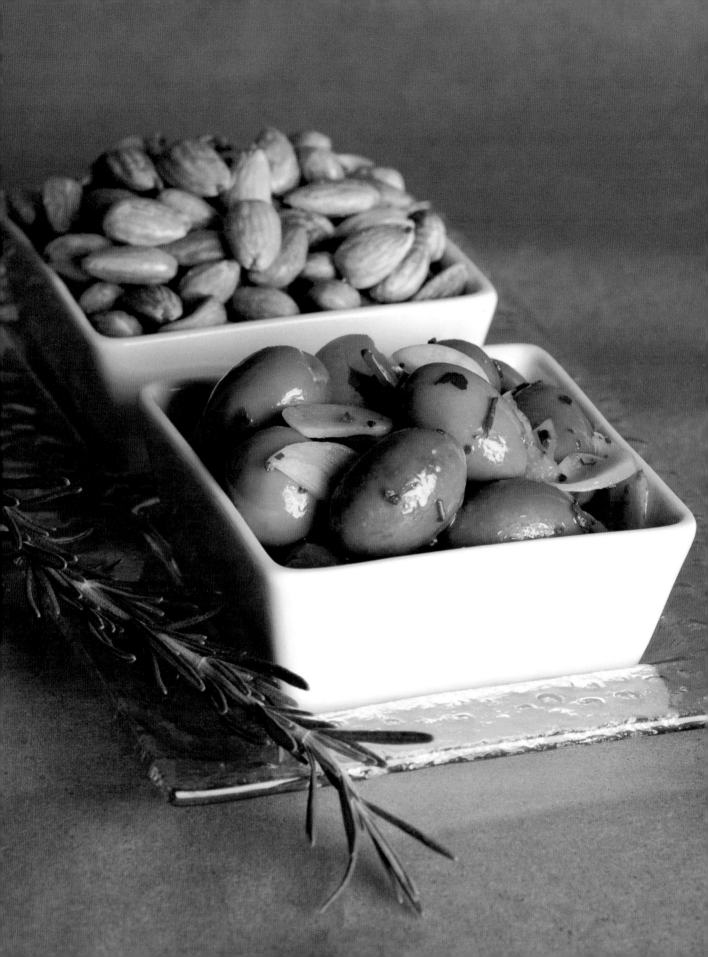

The Dinner Plate: Colour, Crunch and a Whole Lot of Versatility

Think of sitting down to a colourful plate full of all the goodness of fruits and vegetables. What a great way to end the day in a brain-healthy way! So be environmentally friendly and "green up" your plate. Try to view your plate as a painter's palate with a vast array of fruits and vegetables and create your picture of health. Here are some fundamental principles that you can follow.

Meet Your Fruit and Vegetable Needs

Canada's Food Guide recommends that all adults over 50 years of age consume at least 7 servings of fruits and vegetables per day. Younger adult women (19 to 50 years old) should consume 7 to 8 servings per day and younger adult men should consume 8 to 10 servings per day. The best way to meet this target is by consuming fruits and vegetables in a variety of forms—juices, soups, salads, ingredients in mixed dishes and on their own. Unfortunately, most Canadians consume well below this recommendation and as a consequence are not benefitting from the brain-healthy nutrients in these foods.

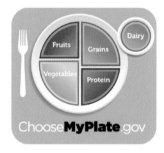

Trying to count the number of servings of fruits and vegetables is a bit tricky. What makes "a serving" is not always clear. So recently, the United States Department of Agriculture developed a new icon called "MyPlate" as a way to help consumers understand how to meet their fruit and vegetable needs. They recommend that at least half of your plate be fruits and vegetables. Try to focus on variety when it comes to these vegetables and whole fruits.

These recommendations are consistent with a brain-healthy diet. As we mentioned previously (see page 23), there is no evidence that super foods exist, so you should eat as wide a variety as possible. Choosing highly coloured fruits and vegetables ensures that you are eating foods rich in antioxidants and other healthful components.

The recipes in this chapter have all been developed to help you achieve a plate that is 50% fruit and vegetables. How?

- By coupling a protein with a suggested vegetable, e.g., **Haddock Wraps with Crunchy Southwestern Salad** (page 179), **Halibut with Two Tomato and Avocado Salsa** (page 184), **Marinated Tofu over Wilted Napa Cabbage and Vegetables** (page 193), and **Tandoori-Spiced Lamb with Roasted Cauliflower Purée** (page 225)

- By including a vegetable as a core ingredient in the dish, e.g., **Ribollita** (page 197) and **Lamb Stew with Root Vegetables** (page 229)

- By using fruit as part of the main dish itself, e.g., **Roasted Fruit and Vegetable Stuffed Chicken** (page 206) and **Farfalle with Walnuts, Goat Cheese, Arugula and Caramelized Apples** (page 230)

In addition, you'll find a bunch of ways to create fruit-laden sweet treats to help you meet your fruit recommendations in the next chapter.

Choose Healthy Protein Sources

MyPlate recommends that you choose lean proteins. In addition, research into brain health suggests that you should minimize your intake of red meat and processed meats (e.g., salami, ham, hot dogs). Focus on fish, poultry, and meat alternatives.

This does not mean you have to abstain from red meat altogether, but you should select lean cuts of beef, e.g., flank steak, such as in **Flank Steak with Pine Nut, Herb and Currant Stuffing** (page 224), or tenderloin in **Thyme-Roasted Beef Tenderloin with Three-Mushroom Ragout** (page 221). Also, trim the fat from chops and stew meat in the lamb recipes, and choose red meat only occasionally.

Fish is probably one of the most powerful foods when it comes to brain health. As mentioned previously, your brain needs high levels of omega-3 fats, especially those found in fish. Try to eat fish two to three times a week by drawing on the recipes in both the lunch and dinner sections (see the section on fish safety on page 158).

Also, be certain to select fatty fish—e.g., salmon, as in **Asian Salmon Burgers** (page 187)—to obtain the highest levels of omega-3 fats. The leaner fish used throughout this chapter (halibut, tilapia, basa, trout) will also contain healthy omega-3 fats.

Also try some meat alternatives once in a while. Meat alternatives are generally lower in fat and bring other healthy food components, like the fibre in beans and nuts, as in **Black Bean Soup** (page 198), **Ribollita** (page 197) and **South African Peanut Stew** (page 233), and the phytoestrogens in tofu, as in **Miso-Glazed Tofu with Toasted Sesame Green Beans** (page 188) and **Marinated Tofu over Wilted Napa Cabbage and Vegetables** (page 193).

Select High-Quality Grains

MyPlate recommends that you eat whole grains with at least half of your meals. This helps to ensure that you are eating a low-glycemic index carbohydrate. You will also benefit from the other nutrients found in less-processed grains.

Again, this recommendation is consistent with brain-health literature. You can easily draw upon whole grains by using recipes such as **Peruvian-Spiced Grilled Chicken** (page 212) with **Cracked Wheat and Chayote or Zucchini Pilaf** (page 213) or **Moroccan Chicken Stew with Couscous and Homemade Harissa** (page 203). Also, remember that both white and whole-grain pastas are reasonably low on the glycemic index. Finally, try to replace your white potatoes with sweet potatoes to draw upon the extra nutrients found in sweet potatoes. Try **Turkey Shepherd's Pie with Mushrooms, Spinach, Cranberries and Sweet Potatoes** (page 209) or **Lamb Stew with Root Vegetables** (page 229).

Include Milk Products in Your Meal

Most Canadians are not consuming enough dairy products to meet their calcium and vitamin D needs. We do not know the impact of this on brain function. However, the evidence suggests that people who are severely vitamin D deficient are at higher risk for cognitive impairment and dementia, relative to those with good vitamin D status. We don't yet understand whether individuals with poor cognitive function simply consume fewer dairy products, or whether poor intake of dairy, and consequently vitamin D, increases risk of cognitive decline. So it simply makes sense at this point to make sure you are consuming dairy products to help meet your vitamin D needs. However, it is equally important to understand that these data address individuals with vitamin D deficiency—this does not support an argument that consuming vitamin D in high doses, over and above vitamin D requirements, will be any better than simply ensuring that you are meeting your needs.

While drinking a glass of low-fat milk is one way to increase your dairy intake, try other low-fat dairy foods, too, as a source of protein in your diet. Some helpful recipes in this chapter include **Farfalle with Walnuts, Goat Cheese, Arugula and Caramelized Apples** (page 230) and **Squash, Spinach and Onion Lasagna** (page 234). If you choose to use milk alternatives, such as soy or rice milk, be certain to select milks that have added calcium and vitamin D. Also remember that coconut milk contains very little calcium and, unless you are choosing a low-fat or light alternative, is extremely high in fat, especially saturated fat; it is also considered a highly inflammatory food. This is something you may want to avoid to help maintain brain health.

Chapter 6
The Dinner Plate

Recipes

Haddock Wraps with Crunchy Southwestern Salad   179

Herbed Fish Stew   181

Basa and Asparagus Steamed in White Wine   183

Halibut with Two Tomato and Avocado Salsa   184

Poached Coconut Fish   186

Asian Salmon Burgers   187
By Chef Michael Smith

Miso-Glazed Tofu with Toasted Sesame Green Beans   188

Marinated Tofu over Wilted Napa Cabbage and Vegetables   193

Hot and Sour Soup   195

Ribollita   197

Black Bean Soup   198

Iberian Chickpea Soup   199

Lemon Thyme Turkey with Spicy Smoky Succotash   200

Moroccan Chicken Stew with Couscous and Homemade Harissa   203

Roasted Fruit and Vegetable Stuffed Chicken   206

Grilled Chicken with Pomegranate Vinaigrette   207
By Chef Brad Smoliak

Turkey Shepherd's Pie with Mushrooms, Spinach,
Cranberries and Sweet Potatoes   209

Peruvian-Spiced Grilled Chicken   212

Cracked Wheat and Chayote or Zucchini Pilaf   213

Provençal-Style Rabbit with Polenta   214

Spicy Honeyed Chicken Thighs with Peanut Coleslaw   218

Thyme-Roasted Beef Tenderloin with Three-Mushroom Ragout   221

Flank Steak with Pine Nut, Herb and Currant Stuffing   224

Tandoori-Spiced Lamb with Roasted Cauliflower Purée   225

Warm Quinoa Salad over Bitter Greens   227

Lamb Stew with Root Vegetables   229

Farfalle with Walnuts, Goat Cheese, Arugula and
Caramelized Apples   230

South African Peanut Stew   233

Squash, Spinach and Onion Lasagna   234

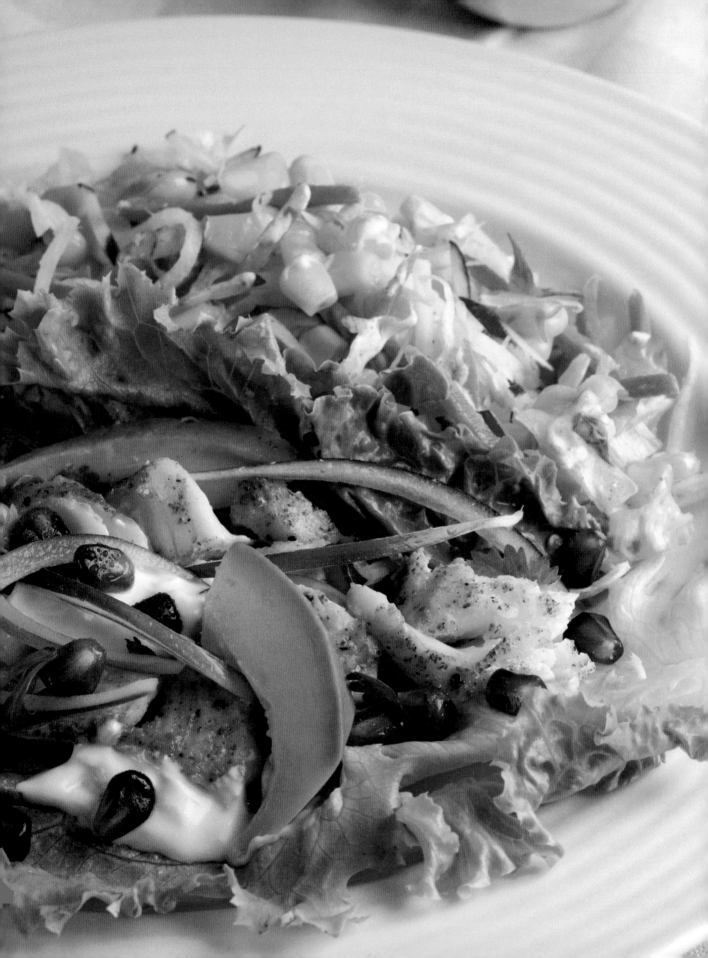

Haddock Wraps with Crunchy Southwestern Salad

Pomegranate seeds add both colour and a surprising tart burst to this dish—a refreshing antidote to the spiciness of the marinade's jalapeño pepper and the hot sauce in the Crunchy Southwestern Salad.

Prep time: 15 minutes plus 15 minutes marinating time
Cook time: 8 minutes
Serves 6

FISH
¼ cup canola oil
1 lime, juiced
1 jalapeño, seeded and thinly sliced
2 cloves garlic, thinly sliced
¼ cup fresh coriander, leaves and stems
1½ tsp chipotle/ancho chili powder or chili powder
1 tsp ground cumin
¼ tsp each salt and black pepper
4 skinless haddock fillets (24 oz total)

TACOS
6 lettuce leaves or whole-wheat tortillas
¼ red onion, thinly sliced
½ cup low-fat plain yogurt or light sour cream
¼ cup loosely packed fresh coriander leaves
1 large avocado, sliced
½ cup pomegranate seeds
½ lime

Preheat broiler to 500°F. Position rack in top third of oven.

In a bowl, combine oil, lime juice, jalapeño, garlic, coriander, chili powder, cumin, salt and pepper. Add fish to bowl, gently stirring until well coated; marinate for 15 minutes.

Transfer fish to an aluminum foil–lined baking sheet; discard marinade. Broil until fish turns opaque, 6 to 8 minutes. Using 2 forks, flake fish.

Place lettuce leaves on work surface. Layer each with fish, onion, yogurt, coriander, avocado and pomegranate seeds. (For tips on extracting pomegranate seeds, see page 49.) Squeeze lime juice overtop. Roll up lettuce. Serve with Crunchy Southwestern Salad, below).

NUTRITIONAL ANALYSIS PER SERVING: Calories 200; Protein 22g; Carbohydrate 7g (2%DV); Fat, total 9g (14%DV); Fat, saturated 1g (5%DV); Fat, trans 0g; Cholesterol 65mg (22%DV); Fibre 3g (12%DV); Sodium 140mg (6%DV).

Crunchy Southwestern Salad

This crunchy salad is a snap to make, especially if you buy pre-julienned carrots, available at many grocery stores. Jicama, often referred to as the Mexican potato, is a large bulbous-looking root vegetable known for its crunch and sweet, juicy flesh. Peel only what you need and keep the rest well wrapped in the refrigerator for up to 5 days—it's great as a snack, dipped in hummus, mustard or sun-dried tomato pesto.

Prep time: 20 minutes
Serves 6 (1⅓ cups each)

SALAD
2 cups julienned jicama (or celery or fennel)
2 cups julienned radish
1½ cups cooked corn kernels
1 cup julienned carrots
2 cups finely shredded lettuce

DRESSING
½ cup low-fat plain yogurt
⅓ cup chopped fresh coriander leaves
2 tbsp lime juice
½ tsp each granulated sugar and chili powder
¼ tsp ground cumin
¼ tsp each salt and black pepper
¼ tsp hot sauce such as Tabasco

Salad: In a large bowl, toss together jicama, radishes, corn, carrots and lettuce.

Dressing: In a separate bowl, whisk together yogurt, coriander, lime juice, sugar, chili powder, cumin, salt, pepper and hot sauce. Pour over salad, tossing gently until well coated.

NUTRITIONAL ANALYSIS PER SERVING: Calories 90; Protein 3g; Carbohydrate 19g (6%DV); Fat, total 1g (2%DV); Fat, saturated 0g; Fat, trans 0g; Cholesterol 0mg; Fibre 5g (20%DV); Sodium 150mg (6%DV).

Herbed Fish Stew

Lycopene is the antioxidant compound that makes fruits and vegetables vibrantly red. Tomatoes have the highest concentration of lycopene over all other food sources, and lycopene is better absorbed by the body if the tomatoes are cooked. This tomato-based stew is a great way to draw on the antioxidant properties of tomatoes.

Prep time: 10 minutes
Cook time: 35 minutes
Serves 6 (1⅓ cups each)

2 tbsp olive oil
1 fennel, finely chopped, reserving fronds for garnish
1 leek (white and light green parts only), sliced into half-moons
1 onion, finely chopped
3 cloves garlic, minced
2 tsp dried basil
1 tsp dried oregano
¼ tsp dried rosemary
1 tsp grated lemon zest
1 tbsp tomato paste
1 can (19 oz/540 mL) white kidney beans, drained and rinsed
½ tsp each salt and black pepper
½ cup dry white wine
½ cup vegetable stock, preferably low-sodium
1 can (28 oz/796 mL) diced tomatoes
2 halibut fillets, or any firm white-fleshed fish (6 oz each)
¼ cup olive oil
6 lemon wedges

Heat oil in a large deep skillet set over medium heat. Add fennel, leek and onion; cook, stirring, until softened, about 4 minutes. Stir in garlic, basil, oregano, rosemary, lemon zest and tomato paste until paste melts into vegetables, about 2 minutes. Stir in beans, salt and pepper until well combined.

Add wine; cook until reduced by one-third, about 5 minutes. Add stock and tomatoes. Reduce heat to low; simmer, covered, for 15 minutes.

Cut fish into bite-size pieces. Add to stew; cook until fish is opaque, about 5 minutes. Garnish with drizzle of oil, lemon wedges to squeeze over and fennel fronds.

NUTRITIONAL ANALYSIS PER SERVING: Calories 370; Protein 26g; Carbohydrate 27g (9%DV); Fat, total 16g (25%DV); Fat, saturated 2g (10%DV); Fat, trans 0g; Cholesterol 30mg (10%DV); Fibre 8g (32%DV); Sodium 290mg (12%DV).

❧ Health Savvy: Beans 101

Just call them legumes, if you please! Dried beans, chickpeas, lentils and split peas are all part of the all-star team called legumes. They are little treasures filled with vitamins (especially those of the vitamin B variety), minerals (we're talking magnesium), nutrients (think potassium, calcium, iron, copper, zinc and manganese), fibre, protein and antioxidants. Additionally, they have the distinct perk of falling low on the glycemic index rating, helping to steady blood glucose and insulin levels.

In general, the larger the beans, the longer they need to soak—and the longer you soak beans, the faster they cook. Soaking allows the dried beans to absorb water, which begins to dissolve the starches that cause intestinal discomfort. While beans are soaking, they will double to triple in size.

Most beans need to be soaked in three times their volume in cold water, for a maximum of 6 hours. But beware of soaking for too long: If allowed to soak overnight, they may ferment, which can affect their flavour and make them more difficult to digest. The optimal method is to put them in cold water and bring them gently to a boil, then take the saucepan off the heat, allowing them to remain in the water for 1 to 2 hours only.

Remember to discard the water in which the beans have been soaked. There's no need to add any other ingredients or flavourings to the soaking water—let your recipe do that trick for you.

Split peas and lentils don't need to be soaked. They take about 30 minutes to cook. Dried beans will keep indefinitely if stored in a cool, dry place, but as time passes, their flavour degrades and their nutritive value declines.

Of course, canned, already-cooked beans are a convenient way to add nutrients to your diet. Just make sure to rinse them well before using. Rinsing helps lower the high levels of sodium found in most canned beans. Also, choose low-salt canned varieties whenever available.

Types
- Black beans
- Split peas
- Black-eyed peas
- White kidney beans
- Chickpeas
- Red kidney beans
- Lentils
- Pinto beans

Basa and Asparagus Steamed in White Wine

Sometimes labelled bocourti, basa is a lesser-known flaky white fish belonging to the catfish family. Native to Southeast Asia, this delicate fillet is a great replacement for sea bass or halibut.

Prep time: 10 minutes
Cook time: 20 minutes
Serves 2

2 tbsp olive oil
¼ tsp dried red pepper flakes (optional)
1 leek (white and light green parts only), finely chopped
½ fennel bulb, finely chopped
½ bunch asparagus (roughly 8 to 12 stalks), cut into bite-size pieces
2 cloves garlic, thinly sliced
1 lemon, zested
3 sprigs fresh thyme
½ cup dry white wine
¼ cup vegetable stock, preferably low-sodium
¼ tsp each salt and black pepper
2 Basa or sole fillets (6 oz/180 g each)

Heat oil in a deep-set pan set over medium heat. Add red pepper flakes (if using); cook for 1 minute. Stir in leek, fennel, asparagus and garlic until coated with oil. Add lemon zest and thyme; cook until vegetables have softened slightly, about 2 minutes.

Add white wine, stock and half of salt and pepper. Push vegetables into centre of pan to form bed for fish. Place fish on top of vegetables; sprinkle with remaining salt and pepper. Cover pan; steam until fish turns opaque, 8 to 10 minutes.

Transfer fish to a plate and keep warm. Bring mixture in pan to a boil; boil until sauce is slightly thickened, about 3 minutes. Remove thyme sprigs.

Serve fish topped with vegetable medley.

NUTRITIONAL ANALYSIS PER SERVING: Calories 450; Protein 48g; Carbohydrate 17g (6%DV); Fat, total 17g (26%DV); Fat, saturated 2.5g (13%DV); Fat, trans 0g; Cholesterol 120mg (40%DV); Fibre 6g (24%DV); Sodium 570mg (24%DV).

Halibut with Two Tomato and Avocado Salsa

Whether served over fish, as it is here, or over grilled boneless skinless chicken breasts, this salsa makes each bite resonate with the acid tones of the sherry vinegar, the piquancy of the capers, the earthiness of the fresh thyme and the juiciness of the tomatoes. It's like an explosion in the mouth! The salsa performs best if its flavours are allowed to mingle for a couple of hours before serving. For it to be at its optimum, be sure to serve it at room temperature.

Prep time: 20 minutes plus at least 2 hours marinating time
Cook time: 10 minutes
Serves 6

SALSA
1 lb mixed yellow and red cherry tomatoes, halved
½ cup julienned oil-packed sun-dried tomatoes, drained
1 large ripe avocado, diced
3 tbsp drained capers
3 tbsp sherry vinegar
3 large cloves garlic, minced
2 tbsp chopped fresh thyme leaves
1 tsp Dijon mustard
¼ tsp each salt and black pepper
⅓ cup olive oil

FISH
2 tbsp chopped fresh thyme leaves
½ tsp each salt and black pepper
2 tbsp olive oil
6 halibut fillets (6 oz/180 g each)

Salsa: In a large bowl, combine cherry and sun-dried tomatoes, avocado and capers. In a separate bowl, whisk together vinegar, garlic, thyme, mustard, salt and pepper. Gradually whisk in oil until emulsified. Pour over tomato mixture, tossing gently until well coated. Marinate at room temperature for at least 2 hours and for up to 8 hours.

Fish: Preheat broiler; place oven rack approximately 6 inches from heat source. In a small bowl, stir together thyme, salt, pepper and oil. Brush over halibut fillets; place on broiler pan, skin-side down. Broil for 5 minutes. Flip fish so that it is skin-side up. Broil until fish flakes easily with a fork, about 5 more minutes for 1-inch thick fillets. Broiling time should be adjusted depending upon thickness of fillet so that total cooking time is 10 minutes per inch.

Serve topped with heaping mound of salsa.

NUTRITIONAL ANALYSIS PER SERVING: Calories 490; Protein 50g; Carbohydrate 10g (3%DV); Fat, total 28g (43%DV); Fat, saturated 4g (20%DV); Fat, trans 0g; Cholesterol 75mg (25%DV); Fibre 4g (16%DV); Sodium 600mg (25%DV).

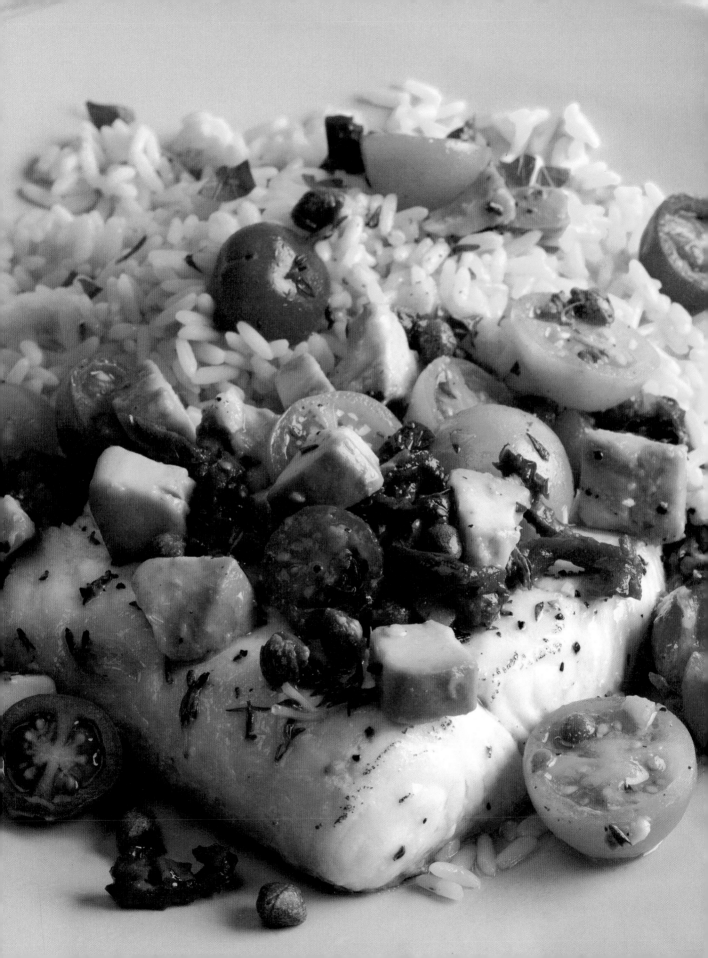

Poached Coconut Fish

Reducing the poaching liquid into a sauce is a great technique. The reduction concentrates all of the flavours and thickens it without having to add any rich ingredient such as butter or cream. Serve this over a steaming bed of rice.

Prep time: 10 minutes
Cook time: 25 minutes
Serves 4

2 tbsp canola oil
1 red hot chili pepper, seeded and finely sliced
3 cloves garlic, minced
10 shiitake mushrooms, stemmed and sliced
2 stalks lemongrass (or 2 tbsp grated lemon zest)
1 can (14 oz/398 mL) light coconut milk
2 tbsp low-sodium soy sauce or tamari

2 tsp grated lime zest
1 piece fresh ginger (about 1 inch), finely grated
4 salmon or snapper fillets (6 oz/180 g each)
1 cup frozen peas
¼ cup loosely packed fresh coriander leaves
4 lime wedges

Heat oil in a deep-set pan set over medium heat. Add chili, garlic and mushrooms; cook for 2 minutes.

Using the back of a knife, lightly dent lemongrass stalk. Add lemongrass to pan; cook until fragrant, about 1 minute.

Stir coconut milk, soy sauce, lime zest and fresh ginger into pan until well combined. Bring to a slight boil; reduce heat to medium-low. Lay salmon in pan (at least three-quarters of the salmon should be submerged in coconut milk). Cover; poach until salmon turns opaque, 10 to 12 minutes. Transfer salmon to a plate; keep warm. Bring sauce to a boil; boil until thickened, about 5 minutes. Add peas; cook for 1 minute. Remove lemongrass from pan. Divide salmon among 4 plates. Pour sauce evenly overtop.

Garnish with coriander and lime wedges.

NUTRITIONAL ANALYSIS PER SERVING: Calories 420; Protein 51g; Carbohydrate 15g (5%DV); Fat, total 17g (26%DV); Fat, saturated 7g (35%DV); Fat, trans 0g; Cholesterol 85mg (28%DV); Fibre 4g (16%DV); Sodium 390mg (16%DV).

TIP—How to "Bruise" Lemongrass

Using the back (dull edge) of a chef's knife, dent the lemongrass so that the surface layers crack slightly. This will allow the natural oils and aroma of the lemongrass to permeate the dish while cooking.

Asian Salmon Burgers

By Chef Michael Smith

Michael Smith is a bestselling cookbook author, the winner of a James Beard media award and the host of Food Network's Chef at Home, Chef at Large *and* Chef Abroad.

You can fill your grill with more than just beefy burgers! Try a batch of these salmon burgers: they're super simple to make, full of Asian-influenced flavour and taste great.

Prep time: 5 minutes
Cook time: 10 minutes
Serves 2

½ lb salmon fillet, skin removed, cubed
1 tbsp grated fresh ginger
1 tsp low-sodium soy sauce
2 tbsp minced red onion or sliced green onion (white and green parts)
1 handful fresh coriander leaves
2 tsp canola oil
2 whole-wheat burger buns

Preheat grill or barbecue to highest setting.

In the bowl of a food processor, combine salmon, ginger, soy sauce, onion and coriander; pulse until coarse mixture is formed. Do not over-process—a rough chop is all that's needed. Form into two large burgers or four smaller ones. The mixture will seem wet and loose, but it will firm up as it cooks.

Lightly brush each burger with oil. Carefully place on the grill and sear until cooked through, about 5 minutes per side. Serve on bun.

NUTRITIONAL ANALYSIS PER SERVING: Calories 400; Protein 29g; Carbohydrate 24g (8%DV); Fat, total 21g (32%DV); Fat, saturated 3.5g (18%DV); Fat, trans 0g; Cholesterol 70mg (23%DV); Fibre 4g (16%DV); Sodium 270mg (11%DV).

Miso-Glazed Tofu with Toasted Sesame Green Beans

Miso, fermented soybean paste, is used as a seasoning in Japanese cooking. There are a couple varieties of miso, which intensify in colour and flavour depending on the volume of ingredients used and length of fermentation. We recommend using shiromiso, "white miso," for this recipe, as it is the mildest of the varieties.

Prep time: 10 minutes plus 10 minutes marinating time
Cook time: 20 minutes
Serves 2

1 package (450 g) firm tofu, drained
1½ tbsp miso paste
¼ cup rice vinegar
¼ cup water
3 tbsp liquid honey or agave nectar
2 tbsp canola oil

1 tbsp sesame oil
1 tbsp low-sodium soy sauce or tamari
Dash hot sauce such as sriracha or Tabasco (optional)
2 green onions (white and green parts), thinly sliced

Wrap tofu in a double thickness of paper towel. Place on a plate. Place a heavy weight, such as a skillet, on top. Let stand until excess liquid has been released, 5 to 10 minutes.

Meanwhile, in a large bowl, whisk together miso, vinegar, water, honey, canola and sesame oils, soy sauce and hot sauce (if using).

Position oven rack in top third of oven. Preheat broiler to highest setting.

Transfer tofu to cutting board; discard paper towel and any excess liquid. Cut tofu into 1-inch cubes (about 18 cubes); toss with miso sauce. Marinate for 10 minutes.

Spread tofu on an aluminum foil–lined baking sheet, reserving as much of the marinade as possible in the bowl. (If you'd like to take the extra step, use your fingers to gently brush excess marinade off the cubes as you transfer them to the baking sheet.)

Broil for 10 minutes. Remove from oven; transfer tofu cubes to reserved marinade, tossing quickly to coat. Redistribute on baking tray (don't worry about saving sauce this time). Broil until tofu is lightly charred around the edges, about 10 minutes more.

Sprinkle with green onions and serve with Toasted Sesame Green Beans (page 189) and rice.

NUTRITIONAL ANALYSIS PER EACH OF 2 SERVINGS: Calories 250; Protein 21g; Carbohydrate 12g (4%DV); Fat, total 16g (25%DV); Fat, saturated 1g (5%DV); Fat, trans 0g; Cholesterol 0mg; Fibre 1g (4%DV); Sodium 310mg (13%DV).

Toasted Sesame Green Beans

Prep time: 5 minutes
Cook time: 15 minutes
Serves 2

10 oz green beans (about 2 large handfuls)
1 tbsp raw sesame seeds
1 tbsp sesame oil
2 tbsp water
1 tbsp liquid honey or agave nectar
¼ tsp each salt and black pepper

Discard stem ends of green beans; cut beans in half crosswise.

In a non-stick skillet over medium heat, lightly toast sesame seeds until fragrant and golden, about 5 minutes. Remove to a plate.

Add oil to skillet; heat for 1 minute. Add beans; gently toss until lightly coated in oil. Add water. Cook, tossing occasionally, until beans are warmed through and turn a bright emerald green, about 6 minutes.

Drizzle beans with honey; season lightly with salt and pepper. Cook, tossing gently, for 3 minutes. Serve sprinkled with reserved sesame seeds.

NUTRITIONAL ANALYSIS PER EACH OF 2 SERVINGS: Calories 160; Protein 3g; Carbohydrate 16g (5%DV); Fat, total 9g (14%DV); Fat, saturated 1g (5%DV); Fat, trans 0g; Cholesterol 0mg; Fibre 4g (16%DV); Sodium 300mg (13%DV).

✸Brain Savvy: Midlife Mindfullness— Menopause and Soy

Some women view menopause as marking their entry into "Freedom 55"; others mourn the loss of their reproductive years. The gradual decrease in estrogen and progesterone levels that occur with menopause is commonly accompanied by heart pounding or racing, hot flashes, night sweats, skin flushing and sleeping problems.

In addition, some women experience decreased interest in sex, forgetfulness, headaches, mood swings, urine leakage, vaginal dryness and infection, and joint pain. The severity and frequency of these symptoms differ among women.

Some women decide to use hormone replacement therapy (HRT) in consultation with their family physician as a means of reducing menopausal symptoms. Other women turn to soy products, since soy contains compounds called isoflavones that are a type of phytoestrogen and have weak estrogen-like activity in the body.

Estrogen and Memory

The brain is an estrogen-responsive organ. Estrogen aids in nerve cell communication in the hippocampus—an area of the brain involved in memory. That could be why menopausal women with declining estrogen levels often report memory problems. As a result, scientists studied HRT in the 1990s as a way of helping women retain their memory function and possibly reverse early age-related memory loss. Unfortunately, many of these trials were cancelled when women reported adverse effects from HRT.

There are many conflicts and controversies when it comes to HRT. Some studies began HRT in women who were 65 years of age or older. Re-introducing estrogen to postmenopausal women who have been estrogen-free for over a decade can be harmful. Results from newer studies, where HRT has been initiated at menopause, are inconsistent. Many of these studies were conducted using hormones made from horse urine rather than the "bio-identical" hormones that have become more popular today.

Nevertheless, the National Institutes of Health in the USA has concluded that "randomized trials of estrogen have not shown any preventive effects on cognitive decline, and conjugated equine estrogen plus methylprogesterone may worsen cognitive outcome." It was, however, recognized that many of the studies had limitations and that these findings may not extend to women who have undergone early surgical removal of their ovaries.

Soy and Menopausal Symptoms

Scientists have also explored the relationship between soy consumption and memory loss with aging. The results have been equally inconclusive. Some studies in Japan and

Indonesia report that high intake of tofu can be associated with poorer memories and greater brain atrophy (shrinkage), although consumption of tempeh (a fermented soy product) was associated with better memory.

Given the relatively low intake of soy products in North America, it is unlikely that tofu consumption would be associated with harm. It is also unlikely that consuming soy is an effective means, in and of itself, to delay memory loss in older adults.

Despite these discouraging results, the North American Menopause Society recently reviewed two studies reporting that consumption of soy and soy isoflavones (80 to 110 milligrams isoflavones per day) may have some cognitive benefit in women younger than 65 years of age. Women participating in these studies were predominantly in their 50s and in their early postmenopausal years. While these two studies provide insufficient evidence to support any recommendations, particularly in light of the National Institutes of Health statement with regards to HRT, the data are consistent with the potential for modest benefits of soy isoflavone consumption on brain health.

Can soy help with menopause symptoms? Some studies have focused on hot flashes and other vasomotor symptoms. This originated from the fact that only 10 to 20% of Asian women report hot flashes compared to 70 to 80% of North American women. Scientists wondered if a higher intake of soy products, and consequently isoflavones, confers some degree of protection.

In a recent review of the scientific literature, the North American Menopause Society concluded that "soy-based isoflavones are modestly effective in relieving menopausal symptoms and that the minimal dose at which benefit can be seen is 50 mg of total isoflavones/day." While many of these studies were conducted using isoflavone supplements, this dose of isoflavones can be achieved through the consumption of soy foods. If you are consuming soy foods, or using isoflavone supplements, be certain to mention this to your family physician, especially if you are considering HRT.

Isoflavone Content of Soy Foods

The isoflavone content of soy foods varies tremendously based on growing conditions and the types of processing of the soybean. Many processing conditions result in the loss of isoflavones. In general, the closer the soybean is to its original form, the higher the isoflavone content (see table on page 192). Isoflavones are fairly stable and are not destroyed with normal cooking methods. Please note that soy oil, soy butter, soy-based margarines, and soy sauce do not contain isoflavones. Also, note that different brands of soy foods vary in their isoflavone content. Check the label or check with the manufacturer for the exact isoflavone content.

Typical Isoflavone Content in Some Soy Foods

FOOD	SERVING SIZE	ISOFLAVONE (mg/serving)
Mature soybean, uncooked	½ cup	176
Green soybean, uncooked (edamame)	½ cup	70
Soy flour	¼ cup	44
Tofu, uncooked	3 oz	29
Soy beverage (milk)	1 cup	20
Soy yogurt	100 g	16
Soy hot dog	1 soy hot dog; 38 g	6
Soy cheese, mozzarella	1 oz	2

See www.ars.usda.gov/Services/docs.htm?docid=6382 for the isoflavone content of additional foods.

Marinated Tofu over Wilted Napa Cabbage and Vegetables

High in protein and containing no cholesterol, tofu is a versatile ingredient to say the least. Soft tofu is perfect for smoothies and making into desserts. It can be frozen easily and thawed in 10 minutes by covering it with boiling water. Be sure to use firm tofu for this recipe or the pieces will end up sticking to your wok and turning mushy. Napa cabbage is easily found in the produce section of your supermarket and is a great addition to salads and coleslaws.

Prep time: 15 minutes plus 30 minutes resting time
Cook time: 15 minutes
Serves 6 (1⅓ cups each)

1½ lb firm tofu
2 tbsp (approx) canola oil
4 green onions (white and green parts), sliced
2 cloves garlic, minced
1 tbsp minced fresh ginger
½ tsp dried red pepper flakes
2 tbsp water
1 cup sliced carrots
3 cups shredded napa cabbage
1½ cups snow peas, trimmed
1 cup sliced water chestnuts
½ sweet red pepper, cored and cut into thin strips

SAUCE
⅔ cup water
⅓ cup ketchup
¼ cup granulated sugar
3 tbsp rice vinegar
2 tsp low-sodium soy sauce
1 tsp sesame oil
1 tbsp cornstarch

Wrap tofu in a double thickness of paper towel. Place on a plate. Place a heavy weight, such as a skillet, on top. Let stand for 30 minutes or until excess liquid has been released. Cut tofu into ½-inch thick slices and then crosswise into 2-inch squares. Set aside.

Sauce: Meanwhile, prepare sauce. In a bowl, whisk together water, ketchup, sugar, vinegar, soy sauce, sesame oil and cornstarch; set aside.

Heat oil in a large skillet or wok set over medium-high heat. In batches, stir-fry tofu cubes, adding more oil if necessary, until golden brown on all sides. Remove to a plate. Add green onions, garlic, fresh ginger, red pepper flakes and water; stir-fry for 20 seconds, stirring to scrape up any browned bits from the bottom of the pan. Add carrots; stir-fry for 1 minute. Stir in cabbage, snow peas, water chestnuts and red pepper until well combined. Pour in half of sauce. Stir-fry for 2 minutes. Add tofu cubes and remainder of sauce. Stir until sauce has thickened and vegetables are tender, 2 to 3 minutes.

NUTRITIONAL ANALYSIS PER SERVING: Calories 300; Protein 20g; Carbohydrate 25g (8%DV); Fat, total 15g (23%DV); Fat, saturated 1g (5%DV); Fat, trans 0g; Cholesterol 0mg; Fibre 3g (12%DV); Sodium 360mg (15%DV).

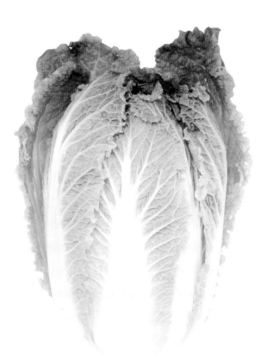

Hot and Sour Soup

Unlike most hot and sour soups, this one is not thickened with cornstarch, giving it a lighter consistency. But don't be fooled: a bowl of this will fill you up quickly!

Prep time: 20 minutes
Cook time: 15 minutes
Serves 6 (1⅓ cups each)

1 tbsp vegetable oil
2 tbsp sesame oil
2½ cups sliced mushrooms (enoki, shiitake, cremini, oyster)
2 cups finely shredded napa cabbage
2 cups finely shredded or julienned carrots
1 package (250 g) medium or soft tofu, cut into bite-size pieces
3 pieces fresh ginger (each about 1-inch thick), unpeeled
¼ cup rice vinegar
1 tbsp low-sodium soy sauce
1 tsp granulated sugar
½ tsp black pepper
1 tsp Asian chili paste
5 cups chicken or vegetable stock, preferably low-sodium
½ cup frozen peas, defrosted
2 green onions (white and green parts), thinly sliced

Heat vegetable oil and 1 tsp sesame oil in a large pot set over medium-high heat. Add mushrooms; cook, stirring, for 5 minutes. Stir in cabbage, carrots, tofu and ginger. Pour in rice vinegar, soy sauce, sugar, pepper and chili paste, stirring just until vegetables are coated. Pour in stock. Bring to a boil. Reduce heat to low; simmer, uncovered, for 5 minutes.

Remove pot from heat. Stir in peas, remaining sesame oil and green onions. Remove ginger and discard. Serve in warmed bowls.

NUTRITIONAL ANALYSIS PER SERVING: Calories 210; Protein 11g; Carbohydrate 19g (6%DV); Fat, total 10g (16%DV); Fat, saturated 2g (10%DV); Fat, trans 0g; Cholesterol 0mg; Fibre 4g (16%DV); Sodium 510mg (21%DV).

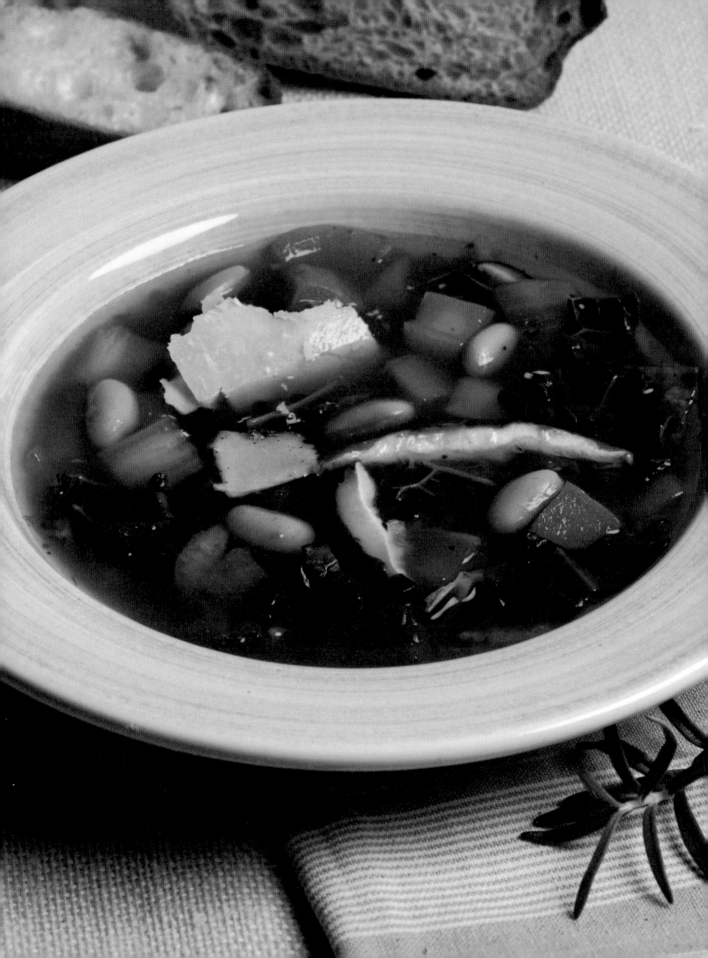

Ribollita

Ribollita hails from Tuscany, Italy, where it has the proud heritage of meaning "reboiled." With peasant origins, it was originally made by reheating or reboiling the leftover vegetable soup (minestrone) from the previous day. Traditionally, its main ingredients include beans, inexpensive vegetables such as carrots, celery and cabbage, and leftover bread. Although we've omitted the bread and upped the ante slightly by calling for shiitake mushrooms, we proudly salute this time-honoured potage. For an extra flourish, top soup with pieces of shaved Parmesan.

Prep time: 15 minutes
Cook time: 40 minutes
Serves 10 (1 cup each)

2 tbsp olive oil
1 onion, chopped
4 cloves garlic, minced
2 large carrots, diced
1 stalk celery, diced
1 tsp dried thyme
½ tsp each salt and black pepper
¼ tsp each crumbled dried rosemary and rubbed sage
1½ cups chopped cabbage
1½ cups sliced shiitake mushrooms, stems removed
4½ cups vegetable stock, preferably low-sodium
1 can (28 oz/796 mL) whole tomatoes, drained and chopped
2 tbsp sherry vinegar
1 can (19 oz/540 mL) white kidney beans, drained and rinsed
4 cups chopped spinach
½ cup grated Parmesan cheese

Heat oil in a large heavy saucepan set over medium heat. Add onion, garlic, carrots, celery, thyme, salt, pepper, rosemary and sage. Cook, stirring, for 5 minutes. Add cabbage and mushrooms; cook, stirring, for 3 minutes.

Stir in stock, tomatoes and vinegar. Bring to a boil. Reduce heat; cover and simmer for 20 minutes. Stir in beans and spinach. Cook, uncovered, until spinach is wilted and beans are warmed through, about 5 minutes.

Ladle soup into bowls; sprinkle with Parmesan.

NUTRITIONAL ANALYSIS PER SERVING: Calories 140; Protein 7g; Carbohydrate 20g (7%DV); Fat, total 4.5g (7%DV); Fat, saturated 1.5g (8%DV); Fat, trans 0g; Cholesterol 5mg (2%DV); Fibre 6g (24%DV); Sodium 370mg (15%DV).

Black Bean Soup

This soup eats like a meal and is a tasty way to include more black beans in your diet. Black beans are particularly rich in fibre, omega-3 fat and antioxidants, making it a perfect choice for a brain-healthy soup.

Prep time: 15 minutes
Cook time: 35 minutes
Serves 6 (1 cup each)

1 tbsp canola oil
½ cup finely chopped plum tomatoes
1 onion, chopped
2 large cloves garlic, finely chopped
1 jalapeño pepper, seeded and finely chopped
2 cans (19 oz/540 mL each) black beans, drained and rinsed
2 cups water
1 bay leaf
1 tbsp ground cumin
1 tbsp dried oregano
1 tsp dried thyme
½ tsp salt
¼ tsp cayenne pepper
1½ oz (6 tbsp) grated farmer's cheese or Monterey Jack cheese
¼ cup low-fat or no-fat sour cream

Heat oil in a pot set over medium heat. Add tomato, onion, garlic and jalapeño; cook, stirring, until onion is softened, about 5 minutes.

Place black beans and ¼ cup water in the bowl of a food processor; purée, adding a little more water as necessary to purée smoothly.

Add black bean mixture and remaining water to pot along with bay leaf, cumin, oregano, thyme, salt and cayenne. Bring to a boil. Reduce heat to medium-low; simmer, uncovered, for 30 minutes, adding more water if mixture becomes too thick. Remove and discard bay leaf.

Place a spoonful of grated cheese in bottom of each soup bowl. Cover with soup; garnish with a dollop of sour cream.

NUTRITIONAL ANALYSIS PER SERVING: Calories 160; Protein 8g; Carbohydrate 13g (4%DV); Fat, total 9g (14%DV); Fat, saturated 4g (20%DV); Fat, trans 0g; Cholesterol 20mg (7%DV); Fibre 4g (16%DV); Sodium 350mg (15%DV).

Iberian Chickpea Soup

Iberian cuisine is shaped by its rich history, with strong undertones of Moorish and Christian traditions. The yellow colours in this soup, contributed by the saffron and chickpeas, are a reflection of the Moorish influences. Chorizo sausage contributes a lovely smokiness to this dish. When available, choose low-fat sausage, and before cooking always prick sausages with a fork to release as much of the fat as possible. If you prefer to retain the nutrients in the potato skin, simply scrub the potatoes well, and cube the potatoes with skins on.

Prep time: 20 minutes
Cook time: 1 hour
Makes 10 servings (1½ cups each)

Pinch saffron (about 8 small threads)
2 tbsp hot water
2 chorizo sausages
1 can (19 oz/540 mL) chickpeas, drained and rinsed
10 cups chicken stock, preferably low-sodium
2 bay leaves
4 large cloves garlic, minced
2 onions, chopped
3 cups chopped cabbage
2 cups peeled and cubed potatoes
¼ tsp salt
½ tsp black pepper

In a small bowl, crush saffron and add water. Set aside.

Grill sausages for 10 minutes or cook in a frying pan over medium heat. Pierce sausages several times during cooking to help release the fat. Cut into ½-inch coins. The sausage does not need to be cooked through at this stage and may still be slightly pink in the centre.

Meanwhile, combine chickpeas, chicken stock, bay leaves, garlic, onions, cabbage and potatoes in a large pot. Bring to a boil over high heat. Add the saffron and sausage. Reduce heat to low and simmer, covered, for 1 hour.

Add salt and pepper. Remove and discard bay leaves. Taste and adjust seasonings as needed.

NUTRITIONAL ANALYSIS PER SERVING: Calories 209; Protein 14g; Carbohydrate 22g (7%DV); Fat, total 5.0g (8%DV); Fat, saturated 1.5g (7%DV); Fat, trans 0g; Cholesterol 18mg (6%DV); Fibre 3g (12%DV); Sodium 403mg (18%DV).

Lemon Thyme Turkey with Spicy Smoky Succotash

It's easy to make your own scaloppine at home. Buy a skinless boneless turkey breast and slice very thinly, following the grain. For best health purposes and to make cooking easier, make sure that each slice weighs roughly about the same, namely 5 to 6 ounces. If using frozen turkey, it's not necessary to fully thaw it before slicing. Defrost it halfway and then slice—it's much easier this way.

Prep time: 5 minutes
Cook time: 12 minutes
Serves 6 (⅔ cup each)

¾ cup fresh bread crumbs or panko bread crumbs
2 tbsp finely grated lemon zest
1 tbsp grated Parmesan cheese
1½ tsp each dried thyme and dry mustard
¼ tsp each salt and black pepper
1 egg
6 pieces turkey scaloppine (each about 5 oz)
3 tbsp olive oil
12 lemon wedges for garnish

In a large flat bowl, combine bread crumbs, lemon zest, Parmesan, thyme, mustard, salt and pepper.

In a separate bowl, beat egg until broken up.

One piece at a time, coat turkey scaloppine in egg. Then coat each side with bread crumbs, pressing so coating adheres well.

Heat 2 tbsp oil in a large non-stick skillet set over medium-high heat. Add 3 pieces of breaded scaloppine. Cook, turning once, until no longer pink inside, about 6 minutes. Remove to a plate. Repeat with 3 remaining scaloppine, adding remaining oil if necessary.

Serve with lemon wedges and Spicy Smoky Succotash (page 202).

NUTRITIONAL ANALYSIS PER SERVING: Calories 270; Protein 35g; Carbohydrate 11g (4%DV); Fat, total 10g (15%DV); Fat, saturated 1.5g (8%DV); Fat, trans 0g; Cholesterol 85mg (28%DV); Fibre 1g (4%DV); Sodium 340mg (14%DV).

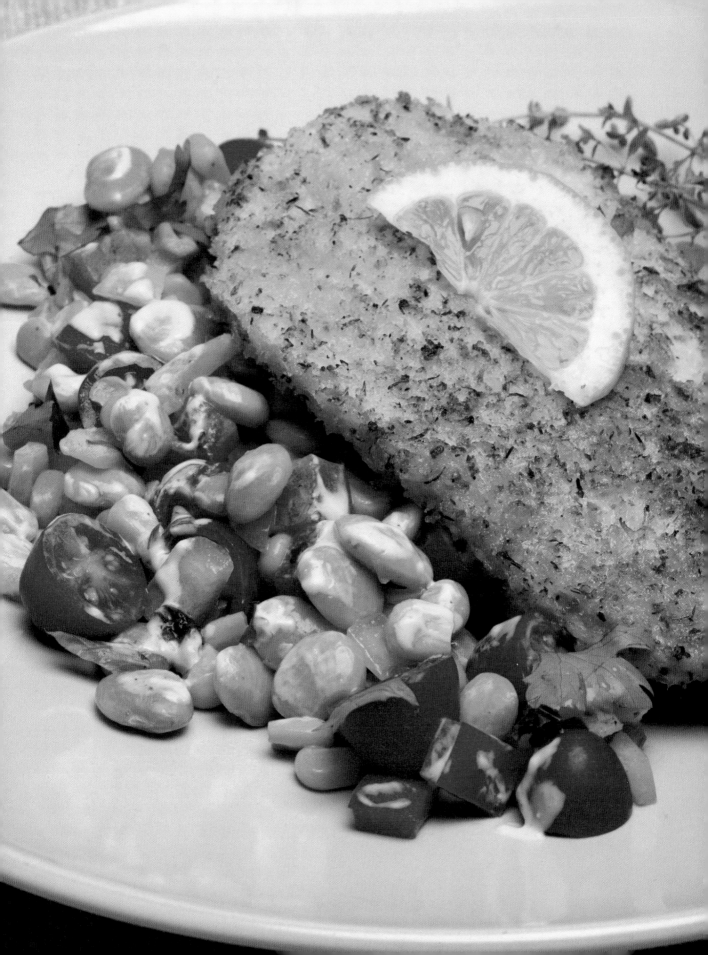

Spicy Smoky Succotash

Prep time: 15 minutes
Cook time: 15 minutes
Serves 6 (⅔ cup each)

2 tbsp olive oil
1 onion, chopped
2 cloves garlic, minced
2 cups cooked corn kernels, fresh or frozen
2 cups cherry tomatoes, halved
2 cups cooked lima or fava beans, fresh or frozen (or green beans, halved crosswise)
1 sweet red pepper, cored and chopped
½ tsp each salt and black pepper
2 tbsp light sour cream
2 tbsp lime juice
2 tsp chopped chipotles in adobe sauce
¼ cup chopped fresh coriander leaves

Heat oil in a large skillet set over medium heat. Add onion and garlic; cook, stirring, for 3 minutes. Add corn, tomatoes, lima beans, red pepper, salt and pepper. Cook, stirring, until vegetables are tender and juices have been released, 5 to 7 minutes. Stir in sour cream, lime juice and chipotles for 3 minutes. Stir in coriander.

NUTRITIONAL ANALYSIS PER SERVING: Calories 190; Protein 7g; Carbohydrate 30g (10%DV); Fat, total 6g (9%DV); Fat, saturated 1g (5%DV); Fat, trans 0g; Cholesterol 0mg; Fibre 5g (20%DV); Sodium 240mg (10%DV).

Moroccan Chicken Stew with Couscous and Homemade Harissa

This chicken recipe, based on one by Martha Stewart, is reasonably mild in flavour. So for those who prefer a spicier version, simply add a bit of harissa to your plate. But be cautious at first—this paste packs a lot of heat!

Prep time: 10 minutes
Cook time: 35 minutes
Serves 8

STEW
4 skinless chicken breasts, halved crosswise
3 carrots, cut into 1½-inch chunks
3 onions, thinly sliced
1 can (14 oz/398 mL) whole tomatoes
1 can (15 oz/443 mL) chickpeas, drained and rinsed
1 can (10 oz/284 mL) chicken stock, preferably low-sodium, undiluted
1 cup water
1 tsp salt
½ tsp ground ginger
¼ tsp each ground turmeric and ground cinnamon
Pinch each chili powder and black pepper
2 zucchini (about 1 lb), halved crosswise and quartered lengthwise

COUSCOUS
2 cups whole-grain couscous
½ tsp each salt and black pepper
2 tbsp olive oil

In a Dutch oven, stir together chicken, carrots, onions, tomatoes, chickpeas, stock, water, salt, ginger, turmeric, cinnamon, chili powder and pepper; stir, breaking up tomatoes with the back of a spoon.

Bring to a simmer over medium heat. Cook, covered, for 15 minutes. Stir in zucchini; simmer until chicken is cooked through, about 15 minutes.

Meanwhile, prepare couscous. Place couscous, salt and pepper in a large bowl. Stir in oil until evenly coated.

Bring 2½ cups water to a boil; stir one-third into couscous. Cover remaining water to keep it hot.

Press couscous gently with the back of a fork. Cover with plastic wrap; let stand for 3 minutes. Repeat with remaining water in 2 additions, letting couscous stand for 3 minutes in between additions. Break up any clumps with a fork or your fingers.

Divide couscous equally among 8 bowls. Spoon chicken, vegetables and broth overtop.

Pass the Harissa (see recipe below) and allow individuals to spice as desired.

NUTRITIONAL ANALYSIS PER EACH OF 8 SERVINGS: Calories 350; Protein 33g; Carbohydrate 41g (14%DV); Fat, total 6g (9%DV); Fat, saturated 1g (5%DV); Fat, trans 0g; Cholesterol 65mg (22%DV); Fibre 5g (20%DV); Sodium 530mg (22%DV).

Harissa

Prep time: 10 minutes plus 30 minutes soaking time
Makes ⅓ cup (1 tsp per serving)

12 whole dried chilies
2 tbsp coriander seeds
1 tbsp caraway seeds
½ tsp cumin seeds
Pinch salt
5 cloves garlic, coarsely chopped
¼ cup olive oil

Cover dried chilies with hot water; set aside to soften, 20 to 30 minutes. Drain, discarding most of the seeds and membranes.

Grind coriander, caraway and cumin seeds in a spice grinder until finely ground before proceeding.

Place chilies, ground coriander, caraway and cumin seeds, salt, garlic, and oil in a small electric blender/chopper; blend until you get a smooth paste. Taste and adjust seasonings. Sauce should be very thick but easy to spread. (Harissa can be stored in an airtight container, with olive oil on top to act as a sealant, and refrigerated for up to 3 weeks.)

NUTRITIONAL ANALYSIS PER SERVING: Calories 40; Protein 0g; Carbohydrate 1g (0%DV);
Fat, total 3.5g (6%DV); Fat, saturated 0.5g (2%DV); Fat, trans 0g; Cholesterol 0mg; Fibre 0.5g (2%DV);
Sodium 12mg (0.5%DV).

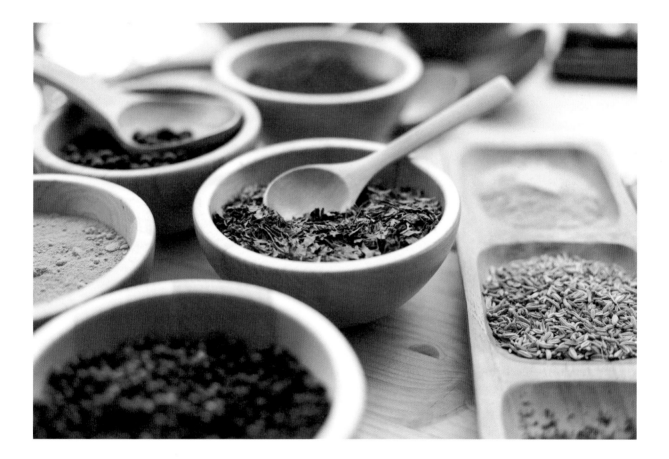

Roasted Fruit and Vegetable Stuffed Chicken

Stuffing meat or poultry is a clever way to get more fruits and vegetables onto your dinner plate. This chicken dish, for example, is replete with zucchini and sweet red peppers as well as chopped peaches, all wrapped up in one neat bundle. It's super easy to assemble, and the tasty mix of fruit and vegetables adds levels of flavour and interest to the protein.

Prep time: 15 minutes
Cook time: 35 minutes
Serves 6

1 zucchini, trimmed and cut lengthwise into strips
1 sweet red pepper, cored and quartered
1 peach, quartered and pitted
3 tbsp olive oil
3 cloves garlic, minced
1 onion, chopped

⅓ cup shredded smoked Gouda cheese
1 tbsp each chopped fresh basil and mint leaves
¾ tsp salt
½ tsp black pepper
6 boneless chicken breasts, with skin
Basil and mint leaves, for garnish

Preheat grill to medium-high.

Place zucchini, red pepper and peach in a large bowl. Toss with 2 tbsp oil until evenly coated. Transfer to a lightly greased grill and cook, turning often, for about 10 minutes or until vegetables and peach quarters are softened but still intact. Coarsely chop and return to bowl.

Heat remaining oil in a non-stick skillet set over medium heat; cook garlic and onion until softened, about 3 minutes. Remove from heat. Stir into vegetable/fruit mixture along with cheese, basil, mint, ½ tsp salt and ¼ tsp pepper.

Pry skin away from thick end of chicken breasts to form pocket, leaving skin attached at the edges. Stuff about ⅓ cup vegetable/fruit mixture into each pocket. Close opening at edges with toothpicks. Sprinkle skin of chicken with remaining salt and pepper.

Place chicken on lightly greased grill set over medium heat. Grill, turning once, until chicken is no longer pink inside, 15 to 20 minutes. Remove toothpicks. Garnish with basil and mint leaves.

NUTRITIONAL ANALYSIS PER SERVING: Calories 480; Protein 55g; Carbohydrate 10g (3%DV); Fat, total 24g (37%DV); Fat, saturated 7g (35%DV); Fat, trans 0g; Cholesterol 175mg (58%DV); Fibre 2g (8%DV); Sodium 280mg (12%DV).

Grilled Chicken with Pomegranate Vinaigrette

By Chef Brad Smoliak

Brad's career includes cooking at the Hardware Grill and helping to organize Alberta's official food contributions at the Vancouver Olympics. He is now cooking at Kitchen in Edmonton and also does product development, teaching and catering.

We always think that vinaigrettes are for salads, but they are also a great way to add flavour to grilled items. This particular dressing is wonderful with any meat. Try it with leg of lamb sprinkled with some crushed pistachios.

Prep time: 30 minutes plus 30 minutes resting time
Cook time: 20 minutes
Serves 4

CHICKEN
4 boneless skinless chicken breasts
1 tbsp canola oil
½ tsp each salt and black pepper

POMEGRANATE VINAIGRETTE
4 tsp pomegranate juice
2 tsp pomegranate molasses
2 tsp red wine vinegar
1 tsp Dijon mustard
1 tsp liquid honey
Pinch each salt and black pepper
¼ cup olive oil

Rub chicken breasts with canola oil; sprinkle with salt and pepper. Transfer to a plate; cover with plastic wrap. Refrigerate for 30 minutes or up to 6 hours.

Meanwhile, in a bowl, mix together pomegranate juice and molasses, vinegar, Dijon mustard, honey, salt and pepper until well combined. Gradually whisk in oil until well emulsified. (Dressing can be stored in an airtight container in the refrigerator for up to 2 weeks.)

Place chicken breasts on a lightly greased grill set over medium-high heat. Grill until juices run clear, about 20 minutes.

To serve, slice each chicken breast on the bias, into two or three pieces. Drizzle with vinaigrette.

NUTRITIONAL ANALYSIS PER SERVING: Calories 390; Protein 47g; Carbohydrate 5g (2%DV); Fat, total 19g (29%DV); Fat, saturated 3g (15%DV); Fat, trans 0g; Cholesterol 120mg (40%DV); Fibre 0g; Sodium 500mg (21%DV).

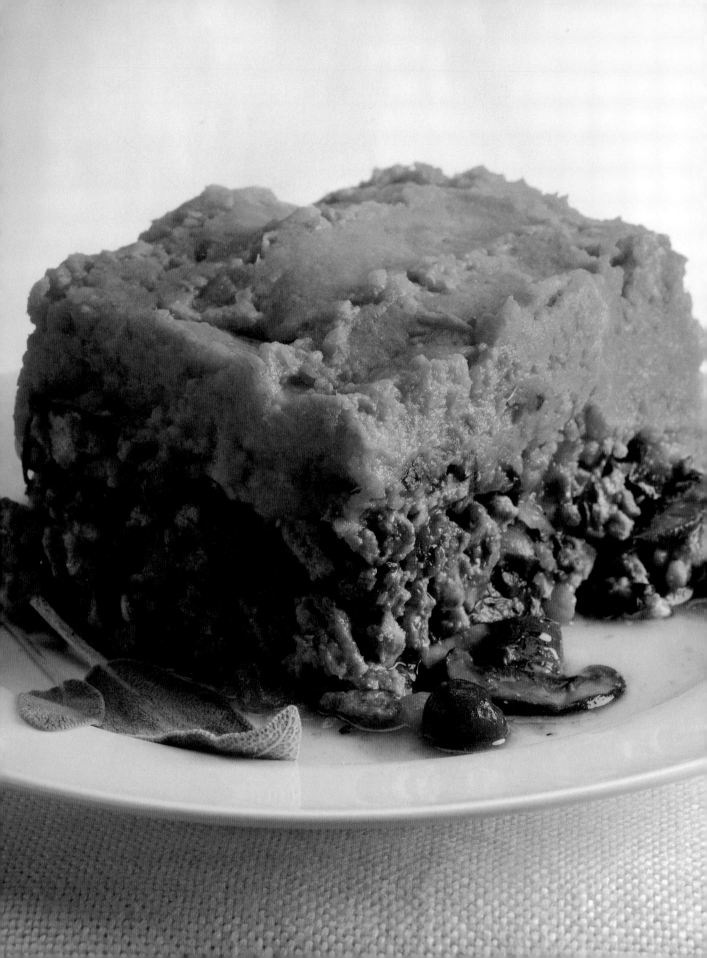

Turkey Shepherd's Pie with Mushrooms, Spinach, Cranberries and Sweet Potatoes

It's Thanksgiving in a pan! Traditional shepherd's pie gets a lean, vitamin-packed makeover in this recipe, so you won't feel guilty reaching for seconds … or thirds.

Prep time: 15 minutes
Cook time: 1½ hours
Serves 8

6 large sweet potatoes
6 cups packed fresh baby spinach
2 tbsp canola oil
2 lb lean ground turkey
½ tsp each salt and black pepper
1 large onion, finely chopped
2 tbsp finely chopped fresh sage
6 cups sliced cremini mushrooms
10 cloves garlic, grated
½ cup frozen whole cranberries
3 tbsp all-purpose flour
½ cup chicken or vegetable stock, preferably low-sodium
½ tsp ground cinnamon

Preheat oven to 450°F.

Prick each potato all over with a fork so that skin is peppered with small holes (this will allow steam to escape while cooking). Wrap each potato in aluminum foil. Bake in centre of preheated oven for 50 minutes.

Meanwhile, working in batches, neatly pile spinach leaves and role like a cigar. Slice spinach "cigar" into thin ribbons. Repeat until you have worked through the entire amount.

Heat oil in a large pot set over medium-high heat. Add turkey and half of salt and pepper; cook, breaking up meat with a wooden spoon, until lightly browned, 6 to 8 minutes. Remove meat from pan; reserve.

Reduce heat to medium; add onion and sage. Cook until onion softens and turns translucent, about 2 minutes. Add mushrooms; cook until mushrooms brown and soften, about 8 minutes. Add spinach and garlic; cook until all the spinach has wilted, about 1 minute. Stir in remaining salt and pepper.

Transfer turkey and any accumulated juices to pot with vegetables and add cranberries; stir until well combined.

Sprinkle flour into pot. Cook, stirring until contents stick together, about 3 minutes. Stir in stock. Bring to a boil. Reduce heat to medium-low; simmer until mixture reaches a stew-like consistency.

Remove potatoes from oven. Reduce oven temperature to 350°F. Cut an "X" across top of potato skins. Using the back of a knife, peel skin, working from centre of "X" outward (skin should release easily from flesh). Discard skin; place potato flesh in a bowl. Using a ricer, potato masher or fork, mash potatoes. Season with more salt and pepper, if desired; stir in cinnamon.

Transfer turkey and vegetables to a 9 x 9-inch square baking pan. Evenly spread mashed sweet potatoes overtop.

Bake in centre of preheated oven until heated through, about 20 minutes.

NUTRITIONAL ANALYSIS PER EACH OF 8 SERVINGS: Calories 410; Protein 26g; Carbohydrate 51g (17%DV); Fat, total 12g (18%DV); Fat, saturated 2.5g (13%DV); Fat, trans 0g; Cholesterol 75mg (25%DV); Fibre 7g (28%DV); Sodium 290mg (12%DV).

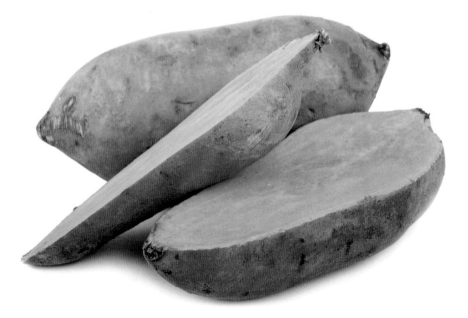

❧Health Savvy: Is Fresh Better?

We all know we have to eat more fruits and vegetables. But what about during the winter months, when local produce is scarce and what is available costs a small ransom?

First of all, remember that just because it's fresh doesn't mean it's the best option. In the dead of winter, fresh produce often has to travel thousands of miles to reach you. This means that raspberries or leafy greens are harvested before they're ripe, affording them less time to develop the full spectrum of their nutrient potential. Outwardly, they may appear ripe, but these vegetables will never have the same nutritive value as if they had been allowed to fully ripen on their own. In addition, their journey to your local grocery store exposes them to lots of heat and light, which can degrade some of the more delicate nutrients such as vitamins C and B.

Frozen fruits and vegetables, on the other hand, are often harvested at their peak, generally when they're most nutrient-packed, and prepared for freezing within hours of being picked. Canned vegetables, although still a viable option, tend to lose nutrients during the preservation process and can have high levels of sodium.

While the first step of freezing vegetables—blanching them in hot water or steam to kill bacteria and arrest the action of food-degrading enzymes—causes some water-soluble nutrients such as vitamins C and B to break down or leach out, the subsequent flash-freeze locks the vegetables in a relatively nutrient-rich state.

The bottom line is, when fruits and vegetables are in season, buy them fresh and ripe. Frozen produce is the next best option, while canned varieties fall at the bottom. If you are buying frozen, however, it's best not to keep them in your freezer for too long. Over many months, nutrients in frozen vegetables do inevitably degrade.

Peruvian-Spiced Grilled Chicken

Peruvian cooking blends local ingredients with influences from immigration—particularly from Spain, China, Italy, West Africa and Japan—creating a unique and flavourful cuisine.

Prep time: 10 minutes plus 6 to 8 hours resting time
Cook time: 20 minutes
Serves 8

10 cloves garlic
½ cup low-sodium soy sauce
¼ cup lime juice
4 tsp ground cumin
2 tsp paprika
1 tsp dried oregano
2 tbsp canola oil
8 small boneless skinless chicken breasts or 16 boneless skinless chicken thighs

Using a food processor, chop garlic until finely minced. Add soy sauce, lime juice, cumin, paprika, oregano and oil; process until well mixed.

Place chicken in a resealable bag; add half of marinade. Refrigerate for 6 to 8 hours or overnight.

Preheat grill to medium heat.

In a pot set over medium heat, boil remaining marinade until reduced by half; reserve.

Remove chicken from marinade; discard marinade. Grill chicken until juices run clear, about 8 minutes per side; alternatively, broil chicken, approximately 6 inches from the heat, until juices run clear, 8 to 10 minutes per side.

Drizzle each piece of chicken with 1 tsp reduced marinade. Pass any remaining marinade at the table. Serve with Cracked Wheat and Chayote or Zucchini Pilaf (page 213).

NUTRITIONAL ANALYSIS PER SERVING: Calories 290; Protein 56g; Carbohydrate 2g (1%DV); Fat, total 5g (8%DV); Fat, saturated 1g (5%DV); Fat, trans 0g; Cholesterol 150mg (50%DV); Fibre 0g; Sodium 360mg (15%DV).

Cracked Wheat and Chayote or Zucchini Pilaf

Chayote is a pear-sized squash with light green wrinkly skin. It is common in Central and South American cuisine and has a very mild cucumber-like flavour. Low in calories and high in vitamin C, this squash does not have to be peeled before cooking and is easily cut, even when raw. If unavailable, zucchini can be substituted—unlike chayote, it doesn't need to be precooked (see instructions below).

Prep time: 20 minutes
Cook time: 30 minutes
Serves 8 (1 cup each)

2 chayote squash, halved and seeds removed, or 2 medium zucchini, unpeeled and chopped
1 tbsp canola oil
1 onion, chopped
2 cloves garlic, minced
1 cup chopped tomato
¼ cup golden raisins
1 tsp dried oregano

¾ tsp chipotle chili powder (or ½ tsp each ground cumin and paprika)
½ tsp salt
¼ tsp black pepper
2½ cups chicken stock, preferably low-sodium
1 cup medium bulgur (cracked wheat)
¾ cup chopped pecans

Preheat oven to 350°F.

In a pot of lightly salted boiling water, cook chayote until fork-tender, 10 to 15 minutes (if using zucchini, skip this step). Remove from water; set aside to cool.

Heat canola oil in a large non-stick skillet set over medium heat. Add onion and garlic; cook until onion is translucent but has not yet begun to brown, 3 to 5 minutes. Peel chayote; chop into ½-inch cubes. Add chayote (or zucchini, if using), tomato, raisins, oregano, chipotle powder, salt, pepper and stock to skillet. Bring to a light boil. Add bulgur and pecans; cook for 5 minutes, stirring occasionally (if using zucchini, increase cooking time to 10 minutes).

Lightly spray an 8-cup casserole dish with cooking spray. Add bulgur mixture; cover with lid or aluminum foil. (Pilaf can be made in advance and refrigerated for up to 8 hours. Remove from refrigerator an hour before cooking to return to room temperature, and increase cooking time to 40 minutes.)

Bake in centre of preheated oven until broth has been absorbed by bulgur and pilaf is warm throughout, about 30 minutes.

NUTRITIONAL ANALYSIS PER SERVING: Calories 240; Protein 7g; Carbohydrate 33g (11%DV); Fat, total 11g (17%DV); Fat, saturated 1g (5%DV); Fat, trans 0g; Cholesterol 0mg; Fibre 6g (24%DV); Sodium 180mg (8%DV).

Provençal-Style Rabbit with Polenta

While popular in Europe, rabbit is an underappreciated lean meat in North America. Its mild flavour is similar to chicken. Indeed, chicken (bone-in legs, thighs or breasts) can easily be substituted—just be certain to purchase skinless chicken or remove the skin yourself before cooking. This dish is based on a recipe by David Rosengarten featured in *The Dean & Deluca Cookbook*.

Prep time: 25 minutes
Cook time: 2 hours
Serves 4

1 rabbit (about 2¼ lb), cut into 6 to 8 pieces
   (have your butcher do this for you, if possible)
¼ cup all-purpose flour
¼ cup Dijon mustard
2 tbsp olive oil
1 cup chopped onion
¼ cup chopped carrots
2 cloves garlic, minced
½ cup white wine
1 sprig fresh thyme
1 bay leaf
1 tbsp tomato paste
3 cups (approx) chicken stock, preferably low-sodium
½ tsp salt
½ lb tomatoes
⅓ cup brine-cured green olives
⅓ cup capers
2 cups bite-size pieces fresh green beans

GREMOLATA
2 tbsp finely minced fresh parsley leaves
1 clove garlic, finely minced
1 tsp finely grated lemon zest

Preheat oven to 375°F.

Remove any organs from rabbit and discard. Place flour in a flat dish. Brush rabbit pieces with mustard; dip into flour, shaking off excess. Heat oil in a large ovenproof pan set over high heat. The pan should be large enough to hold the rabbit pieces in one layer. Sear rabbit until golden brown on both sides; remove from pan and set aside.

Reduce heat to medium; add onion, carrots and garlic to pan. Cook until onion is slightly browned, about 3 minutes, adding a little more oil if needed. Sprinkle leftover flour over onions; cook, stirring until well blended, 1 minute. Increase heat to high;

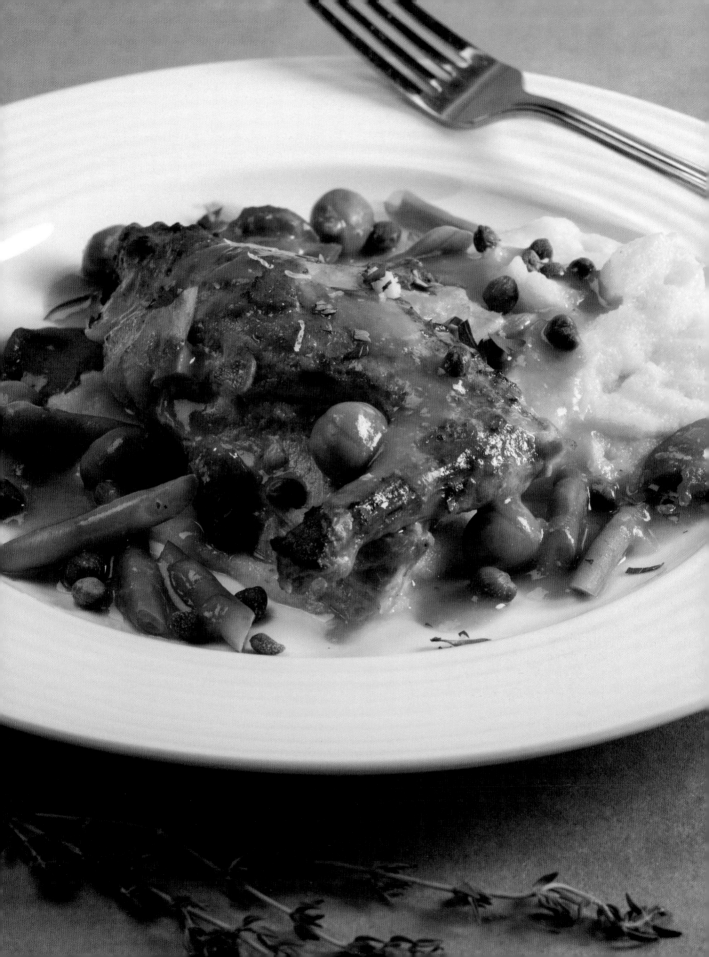

stir in wine, stirring to scrape up any browned bits from bottom of pan. Add thyme, bay leaf and tomato paste, mixing well.

Return rabbit to pan. Add stock, making sure to cover meat by ½ inch. Bring to a boil; stir in salt. Cover; cook in centre of preheated oven until the meat is just starting to fall off the bone, about 1½ hours.

Meanwhile, bring a pot of water to a boil. Cut a small and shallow "X" into the bottom of each tomato. Transfer to boiling water for 30 seconds. Immediately refresh under cold running water. Peel skin, cut in half and remove seeds. Coarsely chop. Rinse olives and capers in cold water; set aside.

Prepare gremolata. Stir together parsley, garlic and zest in a bowl. Season with salt and pepper, if desired.

Remove rabbit from pan; keep warm on plate. Strain sauce through a colander, discarding vegetables and herbs.

Return sauce to pan; bring to a boil over medium heat. Add tomatoes, green beans, olives and capers; gently boil until sauce is reduced by about half and green beans are tender, about 5 minutes. Adjust seasonings.

When sauce is ready, add rabbit back to pan to warm. Sprinkle with prepared gremolata.

Serve with Polenta (page 217), mashed potatoes or rice.

NUTRITIONAL ANALYSIS PER EACH OF 4 SERVINGS: Calories 430; Protein 55g; Carbohydrate 9g (3%DV); Fat, total 18g (28%DV); Fat, saturated 4.5g (23%DV); Fat, trans 0g; Cholesterol 145mg (48%DV); Fibre 2g (8%DV); Sodium 300mg (13%DV).

Polenta

Polenta is easy Italian fare that goes so well with winter stew or even served on its own topped with Gorgonzola cheese. It splatters when cooking, so make sure to use a large enough saucepan.

Cook time: 30 minutes
Serves 4 (1 cup each)

4 cups water
½ tsp salt
1 cup fine cornmeal
2 tbsp butter
½ cup grated Parmesan cheese

In a large saucepan set over medium-high heat, bring 2 cups water plus salt to a boil.

In a bowl, combine cornmeal and remaining 2 cups water; stir to combine. Let sit for 2 minutes; the cornmeal will absorb some of the water.

Slowly whisk cornmeal and water into boiling water. Continue to whisk until polenta begins to thicken, about 3 minutes.

Reduce heat to low; cook, stirring every few minutes, until polenta is no longer grainy and has a soft and creamy texture, 15 to 20 minutes.

Stir in butter and Parmesan until well combined. As polenta sits, it will begin to thicken. If it becomes thicker than desired, stir in a little milk or water.

NUTRITIONAL ANALYSIS PER SERVING: Calories 280; Protein 9g; Carbohydrate 40g (13%DV); Fat, total 10g (15%DV); Fat, saturated 6g (30%DV); Fat, trans 0g; Cholesterol 25mg (8%DV); Fibre 2g (8%DV); Sodium 270mg (11%DV).

Spicy Honeyed Chicken Thighs with Peanut Coleslaw

This chicken is an adaptation of a recipe featured in Suvir Saran's *American Masala*. Save leftovers for lunch because this recipe is also great as a sandwich, topped with coleslaw on a ciabatta bun.

Prep time: 5 minutes plus 1 hour to overnight marinating time
Cook time: 30 minutes
Serves 6 (2 thighs each)

2½ tbsp liquid honey
2 tbsp canola oil
1 tsp salt
1 tsp black pepper
½ tsp garam masala
1 tsp paprika
¼ tsp cayenne pepper
12 boneless skinless chicken thighs
1½ tbsp white wine vinegar

In a bowl, whisk together 1 tbsp honey plus oil, salt, pepper, garam masala, paprika and cayenne pepper. Add chicken thighs, mixing until thighs are coated with marinade. Place in a resealable bag; refrigerate for 1 hour or overnight.

Preheat oven to 400°F.

Line a baking sheet with aluminum foil or parchment paper; place wire rack on baking sheet. Remove chicken from marinade; discard marinade. Place chicken thighs on rack. Bake in centre of preheated oven for 20 minutes.

Mix together remaining honey and white wine vinegar. Remove chicken from oven; brush with honey/vinegar mixture. Return to oven; bake until chicken is cooked through, 5 to 10 minutes. Lightly sprinkle with salt, if desired; cool for 5 minutes.

For each serving, slice 2 chicken thighs into 4 or 5 diagonal slices. Arrange in a circle on each dinner plate. Top with Peanut Coleslaw (recipe follows).

NUTRITIONAL ANALYSIS PER SERVING: Calories 200; Protein 25g; Carbohydrate 5g (2%DV); Fat, total 8g (12%DV); Fat, saturated 2g (10%DV); Fat, trans 0g; Cholesterol 95mg (32%DV); Fibre 0g; Sodium 135mg (6%DV).

Peanut Coleslaw

Prep time: 15 minutes
Cook time: 10 minutes
Serves 6 (1⅔ cups each)

DRESSING
2 tbsp canola oil
¼ cup chopped onion
3 large cloves garlic, chopped
1 tbsp chopped fresh ginger
⅓ cup water
2 tbsp ketchup
3 tbsp creamy peanut butter
2 tbsp chopped fresh mint leaves
2 tbsp fresh lime juice
¼ tsp (approx) hot chili sauce

COLESLAW
7 cups finely sliced cabbage (about ½ small cabbage)
2 carrots, grated
2 green onions (white and light green parts only), thinly sliced
½ sweet red pepper, cored and julienned
1 cup bean sprouts
¼ cup chopped fresh mint leaves

Dressing: Heat oil in a small pan set over medium heat. Add onion, garlic and fresh ginger; cook, stirring occasionally, for 3 minutes. Add water, ketchup, peanut butter, mint, lime juice and chili sauce. Simmer for 5 minutes. Cool; place in a blender and process until smooth.

Coleslaw: Mix together cabbage, carrots, onions, red pepper and bean sprouts. Toss with peanut dressing. Sprinkle with mint and gently toss again.

NUTRITIONAL ANALYSIS PER SERVING: Calories 160; Protein 6g; Carbohydrate 18g (6%DV); Fat, total 9g (14%DV); Fat, saturated 1g (5%DV); Fat, trans 0g; Cholesterol 0mg; Fibre 4g (16%DV); Sodium 150mg (6%DV).

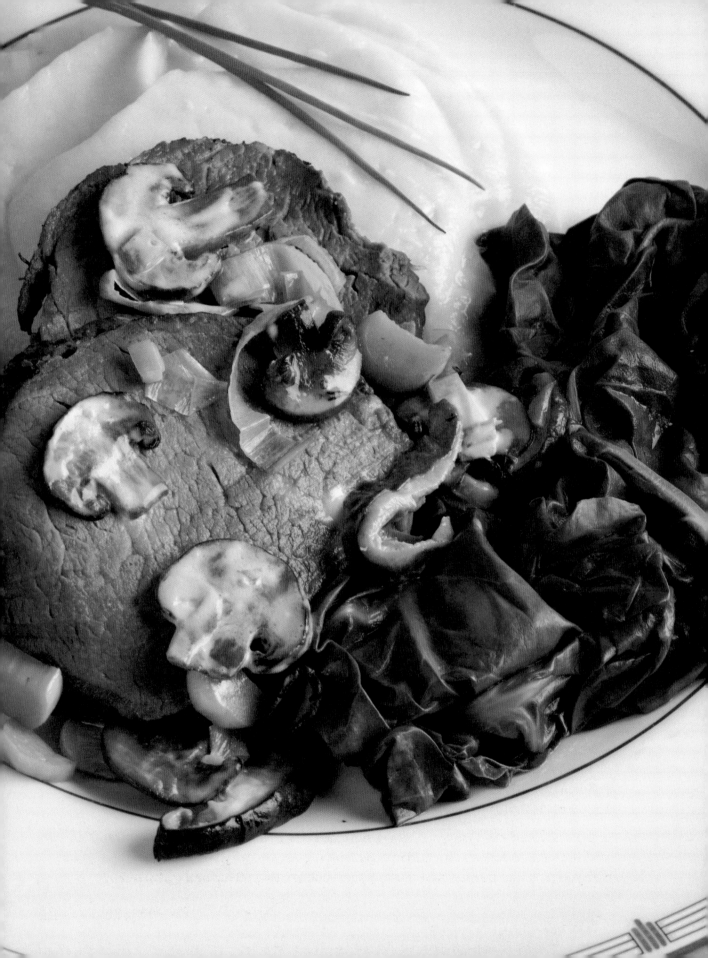

Thyme-Roasted Beef Tenderloin with Three-Mushroom Ragout

The path to brain health does not mean forsaking meals for special occasions. When choosing red meats, we suggest that you choose lean meats, and this tenderloin fits the bill quite beautifully. Although expensive, the tenderloin cut is so tender and special, it's well worth breaking the bank at certain times of year. Make sure that you cook it only to rare or its luscious tenderness will go to waste.

Prep time: 15 minutes
Cook time: 45 minutes
Serves 6

2 tsp olive oil
1 beef tenderloin (about 1½ lb)
1 tsp chopped fresh thyme leaves
½ tsp black pepper
¼ tsp salt

MUSHROOM RAGOUT
3 tbsp olive oil
1 leek, halved lengthwise and sliced thinly into half-moons
    (white and light green parts only)
2 cloves garlic, minced
1 tsp chopped fresh thyme leaves
½ tsp salt
¼ tsp black pepper
3 cups sliced cremini mushrooms
1½ cups sliced shiitake mushrooms
1 cup sliced oyster mushrooms
½ cup dry white wine
2 tbsp whipping cream (optional)
1 bunch Swiss chard, stemmed (about 12 oz)

Preheat oven to 400°F.

Rub oil all over top and sides of tenderloin. Sprinkle with thyme, pepper and salt. Place on rack in a roasting pan. Roast in centre of preheated oven for 35 to 40 minutes or until instant-read thermometer reads 120°F for rare or 125°F–130°F for medium-rare. Tent with aluminum foil and let stand for 10 minutes.

Meanwhile, halfway through roasting time, heat oil in a non-stick skillet set over medium heat. Add leek and garlic; cook, stirring occasionally, for 3 minutes. Stir in thyme, salt and pepper. Add mushrooms; cook, stirring often, until softened and starting to brown, about 8 minutes. Pour in wine and cream (if using). Bring to a boil; reduce heat and boil gently until reduced by two-thirds.

Place Swiss chard in colander; rinse well. Shake colander to remove most but not all of liquid. In a separate skillet set over medium heat, cook Swiss chard (with just the water that's clinging to the leaves) until wilted, 2 to 3 minutes.

Slice meat into 6 portions. Mound Swiss chard evenly among 6 plates. Top with meat and then mushroom ragout.

NUTRITIONAL ANALYSIS PER EACH OF 6 SERVINGS: Calories 330; Protein 33g; Carbohydrate 7g (2%DV); Fat, total 17g (26%DV); Fat, saturated 5g (25%DV); Fat, trans 0g; Cholesterol 70mg (23%DV); Fibre 2g (8%DV); Sodium 430mg (18%DV).

✹Health Savvy: Green as Gold

For optimal health and nutritional benefits, colour your palette green—dark green, to be exact. Dark green vegetables, such as kale, spinach, romaine lettuce, Swiss chard, rapini and kohlrabi, are high in nutrients and beneficial plant compounds that fight disease, making them heart- and brain-healthy. They are high in folic acid and a rich source of lutein. They also contain vitamin K and immune-enhancing vitamin C as well as beta carotene, potassium, magnesium, calcium and iron. These plants typically contain non-heme iron, which is not readily absorbed by the body. However, vitamin C, which these plants do carry in abundance, helps with the absorption of iron, making it all the more important to stock your grocery cart with these leafy greens.

⚛Brain Savvy: Is It Safe to Drink Alcohol?

Is it safe or beneficial to drink alcohol, especially red wine, as a means of retaining cognitive function with aging and reducing our dementia risk?

Since brain health is closely linked to the health of our heart and blood vessels, it would make sense that what is good for the heart is good for the brain. Many of the heart-health benefits of wine have been attributed to resveratrol—a polyphenol (plant-based) compound found in grapes. But please keep two things in mind. First, these heart-health benefits came from drinking moderate amounts of alcohol, a glass or two a day. And second, we have not uncovered any evidence that shows wine or alcohol consumption directly improves cognition function.

There is no doubt that excessive alcohol consumption damages the brain and can be associated with alcoholic dementia. Studies on low, moderate and excessive alcohol intake found no evidence that alcohol intake was associated with either an increase or a decrease in risk for developing cognitive impairment or Alzheimer's disease. A recent study, however, reported that women who engaged in light to moderate alcohol consumption at midlife were more likely to show better indicators of "successful aging" later in life. Furthermore, better adherence to a Mediterranean diet, including moderate alcohol consumption, for more than a decade was associated with higher overall cognitive performance in older women. Nevertheless, these positive indicators of potential brain benefits of alcohol need to be balanced with evidence that alcohol may increase your risk of breast cancer.

Clearly the evidence is confusing. Light to moderate red wine and/or alcohol consumption may be beneficial for heart health, and indirectly, brain health. It may also increase your risk of other diseases, including breast cancer.

What's your best path? Discuss the safety of alcohol consumption with your family physician, taking into account risks that you personally have. Also, if you currently do not drink, there's no need to begin in hope that it will protect future brain health. You could use grape juice as an alternate. If you do drink, limit yourself to one or two drinks a day, to a weekly maximum of 9 drinks for women and 14 for men.

Flank Steak with Pine Nut, Herb and Currant Stuffing

Usually braised, flank steak is also great grilled or broiled quickly—just go rare. Be sure to let it sit, so that its juices recede back into the meat, before slicing across the grain. For ease, toast the bread crumbs and pine nuts (separately) in a dry skillet set over medium heat, for about 5 minutes, shaking the pan frequently.

Prep time: 10 minutes plus 2 hours soaking time
Cook time: 10 minutes
Serves 6

½ cup orange juice
½ cup currants
½ cup toasted fresh whole-wheat bread crumbs
½ cup toasted pine nuts
½ cup chopped fresh mint leaves
⅓ cup chopped fresh parsley leaves
⅓ cup julienned packed-in-oil sun-dried tomatoes
2 tbsp olive oil
1 tbsp finely grated lemon zest
1 egg
1 flank steak (about 1 lb)
¼ tsp each salt and black pepper

In a bowl, pour orange juice over currants; let stand at room temperature for at least 2 hours or for up to 8 hours.

In a large bowl, combine bread crumbs, pine nuts, mint, parsley, sun-dried tomatoes, oil, lemon zest and egg. Drain currants; stir into pine nut mixture.

Place flank steak on a flat cutting board. Starting at long side of steak and holding long carving knife parallel to cutting board, cut in half almost but not all the way through; open up like a book. Spread stuffing over half of meat, leaving a ½-inch border on open side. Cover stuffing with other half of meat. Using toothpicks, secure open side so stuffing does not fall out. Sprinkle steak with salt and pepper. Transfer to a foil-lined baking sheet.

Broil steak, 4 to 6 inches from heat, for 5 minutes. Remove from oven and gently turn over. Broil for 4 minutes. Remove from oven; let stand, tented with foil, for 7 minutes. Remove toothpicks. Slice against the grain into thin slices.

NUTRITIONAL ANALYSIS PER EACH OF 6 SERVINGS: Calories 340; Protein 24g; Carbohydrate 18g (6%DV); Fat, total 20g (31%DV); Fat, saturated 4g (20%DV); Fat, trans 0g; Cholesterol 90mg (30%DV); Fibre 3g (12%DV); Sodium 190mg (8%DV).

Tandoori-Spiced Lamb with Roasted Cauliflower Purée

If you're an adventurous eater, by all means increase the cayenne pepper to ½ tsp. These chops work well on the barbecue—just cook over a hot grill. Cauliflower works particularly well with this Indian-inspired recipe. However, feel free to experiment. Puréed turnips, carrots or parsnips are equally as delicious.

Prep time: 15 minutes plus 4 hours marinating time
Cook time: 45 minutes
Serves 6

LAMB CHOPS
12 rib lamb chops, ¾ to 1 inch thick
4 cloves garlic, minced
1 piece fresh ginger (about 2 inches long), peeled and finely minced
3 tbsp Greek yogurt (see Tip on page 226)
1 tbsp lemon juice
1 tbsp white vinegar
2 tsp garam masala
1 tsp each ground coriander and ground cumin
1 tsp paprika
½ tsp salt
¼ tsp cayenne pepper

ROASTED CAULIFLOWER PURÉE
1 medium cauliflower, cut into florets
2 tbsp olive oil
½ tsp ground turmeric
¼ tsp salt
¼ tsp black pepper
1 cup (approx) low-fat or skim milk, or low-sodium chicken broth

Lamb chops: Trim lamb chops of excess fat. Using a fork, pierce each chop a couple of times to allow marinade to permeate meat.

In a bowl, combine garlic, ginger, yogurt, lemon juice, vinegar, garam masala, coriander, cumin, paprika, salt and cayenne pepper. Transfer mixture to a resealable bag; add lamb chops, massaging marinade into chops. Refrigerate for 4 hours or preferably overnight.

Roasted cauliflower purée: About 45 minutes before you plan to serve the meal, preheat oven to 400°F and start preparing the roasted cauliflower purée.

In a large bowl, toss together cauliflower, oil, turmeric, salt and pepper. Place on a large parchment paper–lined baking sheet. Roast in centre of preheated oven, turning once or twice, until lightly browned and very soft, about 30 minutes. In a microwave or pot set over medium heat, heat milk until warm. Transfer cauliflower and milk to the bowl of a food processor; purée, adding more liquid if necessary, to obtain the desired texture. The cauliflower will be slightly more rigid than mashed potatoes. Set aside, covered, to keep warm. (If necessary, the purée can be quickly reheated in the microwave if it becomes too cool.)

Switch oven to broil and preheat for 1 to 2 minutes. Broil lamb chops, 4 to 6 inches from heat, for 6 minutes per side. Allow to rest 3 to 5 minutes before serving.

NUTRITIONAL ANALYSIS PER SERVING: Calories 420; Protein 47g; Carbohydrate 10g (3%DV); Fat, total 21g (32%DV); Fat, saturated 6g (30%DV); Fat, trans 0g; Cholesterol 135mg (45%DV); Fibre 5g (20%DV); Sodium 460mg (19%DV).

TIP—How to Thicken Yogurt
If you don't have Greek yogurt, strain regular yogurt in cheesecloth for 2 hours.

Warm Quinoa Salad over Bitter Greens

Quinoa is a seed, native to South America, that has a fluffy, creamy, slightly crunchy texture once cooked. It is both rich in high-quality protein and a good source of dietary fibre. Not only is quinoa a good choice for brain-healthy eating, it is currently being considered a possible crop in NASA's Controlled Ecological Life Support System for long-duration human-occupied spaceflights. What's good for astronauts must be good for us!

Prep time: 10 minutes
Cook time: 30 minutes
Serves 4 (1½ cups each)

¼ cup quinoa
2 tbsp olive oil
½ sweet onion such as Vidalia, chopped
3 cloves garlic
2 cups cremini mushrooms, thinly sliced
2 cups fresh spinach, loosely packed
¼ tsp dried red pepper flakes, crushed
1 lemon, zested and juiced
¼ cup vegetable or chicken stock, preferably low-sodium

¼ cup dry white wine
3 cups bitter greens such as frisée (French curly endive) or arugula
1 can (10 oz/284 mL) artichoke hearts, well-rinsed and chopped into bite-sized pieces
Pinch black pepper
4 pieces shaved Parmesan cheese, each about ½ inch wide and 3 inches long (see Tip on page 93)
8 cherry tomatoes, halved

Rinse quinoa in a fine-mesh sieve; drain well. (If you skip this step, quinoa may have a slightly bitter taste.) Transfer to a dry skillet over medium-low heat and, stirring constantly, toast quinoa, about 5 minutes. Set aside.

Heat oil in a pot over medium heat. Add onion and garlic and cook until softened and translucent, about 5 minutes. Add mushrooms and cook until mushrooms have given off most of their liquid, about 5 minutes.

Meanwhile, chiffonade the spinach. Add prepared quinoa, spinach, red pepper flakes, and lemon zest to mushroom mixture; stir well. Stir in stock and wine. Increase heat to high and bring to a boil. Cover and reduce heat to low; simmer, undisturbed, until liquid has been absorbed and quinoa has puffed, about 14 minutes.

Meanwhile, tear frisée into large pieces and divide equally among 4 serving plates or large, shallow soup bowls.

Add artichoke hearts and 2 tsp lemon juice to quinoa mixture. Spoon equal amounts of quinoa mixture over frisée. Generously season with pepper and top with shaved Parmesan. Garnish with tomato and serve warm.

NUTRITIONAL ANALYSIS PER SERVING: Calories 220; Protein 8g; Carbohydrate 27g (9%DV); Fat, total 10g (15%DV); Fat, saturated 2.5g (13%DV); Fat, trans 0g; Cholesterol 5mg (2%DV); Fibre 9g (36%DV); Sodium 200mg (8%DV).

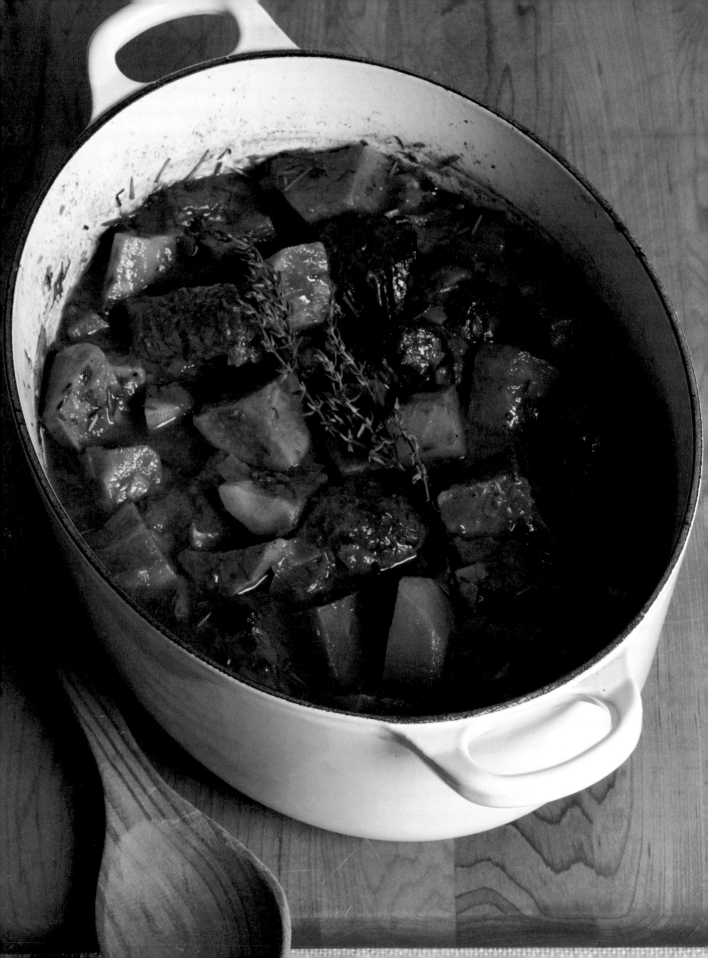

Lamb Stew with Root Vegetables

Parsnips, sweet potatoes *and* rutabagas—talk about a wallop of good-for-you! This stew is a bombshell of nutrients, with potassium, folate, beta carotene and fibre, all swathed in a luxurious French-inspired stew. So add some red wine, dim a few lights and enjoy, bistro-style!

Prep time: 20 minutes
Cook time: 1 hour 45 minutes
Serves 6 (1⅓ cups each)

2½ lb stewing lamb, cut into 1½-inch pieces, trimmed of visible fat
¼ cup all-purpose flour
3 tbsp canola oil
2 leeks (white part only), chopped
3 cloves garlic, minced
1½ tsp dried rosemary, crushed
1 tsp dried thyme
1 tbsp grated lemon zest
½ tsp each salt and black pepper
⅓ cup water
2¾ cups beef stock, preferably low-sodium
2 tbsp tomato paste
3 cups cubed peeled sweet potato
2 cups cubed peeled rutabaga
1½ cups cubed peeled parsnip
⅓ cup chopped fresh parsley leaves

Toss lamb with flour, reserving any excess flour. Heat 2 tbsp oil in a heavy saucepan or Dutch oven set over medium-high heat. In batches, brown lamb pieces on all sides, adding remaining oil as necessary to prevent sticking. Transfer browned meat to a plate after each batch.

Add leeks, garlic, rosemary, thyme, lemon zest, salt, pepper and water to pan. Cook, stirring, until leeks have softened, about 3 minutes. Stir in 1 tbsp reserved flour for 1 minute. Add stock and tomato paste. Bring to a boil over high heat, scraping up any browned bits from bottom of pan.

Return lamb to pot. Reduce heat to medium-low; cover and simmer for about 1 hour, until meat is tender. Stir in sweet potatoes, rutabaga and parsnips. Cover; cook for 20 minutes. Uncover and cook for 15 to 20 minutes, until vegetables are tender and sauce is thickened slightly. Serve sprinkled with parsley.

NUTRITIONAL ANALYSIS PER SERVING: Calories 530; Protein 49g; Carbohydrate 41g (14%DV); Fat, total 19g (29%DV); Fat, saturated 5g (25%DV); Fat, trans 0g; Cholesterol 135mg (45%DV); Fibre 7g (28%DV); Sodium 410mg (17%DV).

Farfalle with Walnuts, Goat Cheese, Arugula and Caramelized Apples

Pasta is always a good carbohydrate choice for a brain-healthy meal, as it has a reasonably low glycemic index. Where possible, purchase whole-grain pasta to increase your fibre intake and be certain to cook it only to the al dente stage—this will help keep the glycemic index of your pasta low.

Prep time: 15 minutes
Cook time: 25 minutes
Serves 4

2 tsp unsalted butter
1 apple, cored and cut into ½-inch cubes
1 tbsp granulated sugar
3 tsp finely grated lemon zest
½ lb farfalle or bow-tie pasta (whole-wheat, if available)
½ cup chopped walnuts
2 tbsp olive oil
3 large cloves garlic, minced
½ large sweet onion, such as Vidalia or Spanish, halved and cut into thin slices
1 cup white wine
4 oz fat-reduced soft goat cheese
½ tsp black pepper
2 cups baby arugula leaves, torn into bite-size pieces

In a large skillet set over medium heat, melt butter. Add apples to pan; sprinkle with 1 tsp sugar. Cook, stirring often, until apples just start to turn tender, about 5 minutes. Sprinkle remaining sugar and 1 tsp lemon zest over apples. Toss mixture gently; cook until sugar begins to caramelize and apples are crisp-tender, 4 to 5 minutes. Transfer to a bowl.

In a large pot of boiling salted water, cook farfalle until tender but firm, 8 to 10 minutes. Reserving 1 cup cooking liquid, drain pasta well.

Meanwhile, in the same skillet that was used for the apples, toast walnuts over medium heat until fragrant and beginning to brown, 4 to 5 minutes. Set aside. Reduce heat to low; add olive oil, garlic and onion. Cook until garlic is just starting to brown, 4 to 5 minutes. Pour in wine; cook until reduced to about ½ cup, about 4 minutes.

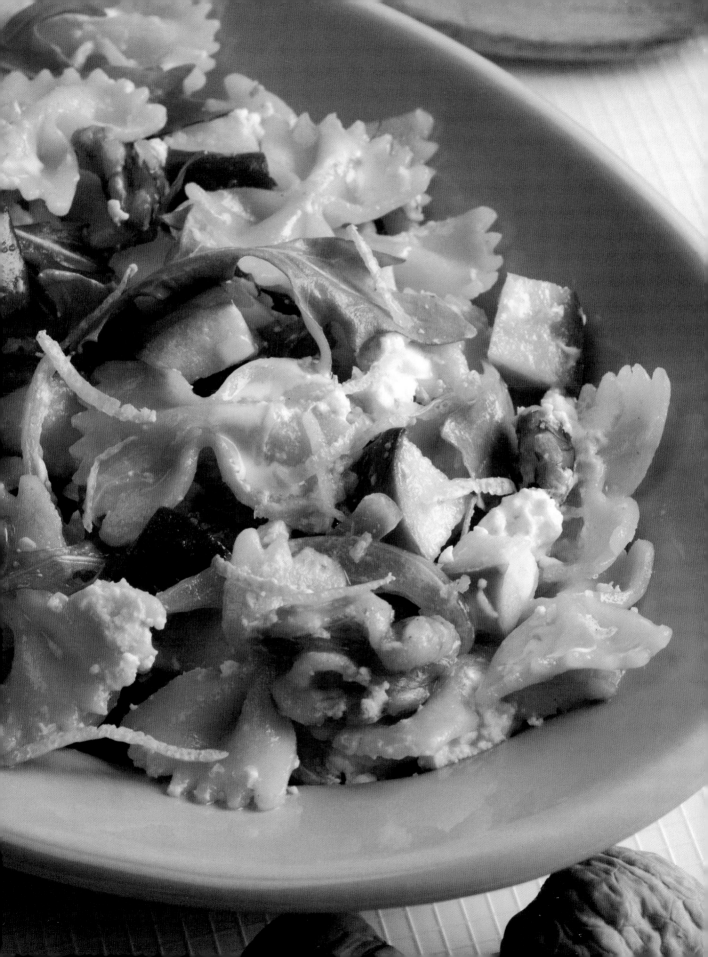

Transfer drained pasta and walnuts to skillet. Crumble goat cheese over pasta; stir until cheese begins to melt. Stir in pepper and remaining lemon zest. If pasta is too dry, add pasta water ½ cup at a time until a slight amount of liquid remains in pan. Stir in arugula just until leaves begin to wilt. Gently add caramelized apples. Season to taste with salt and pepper.

NUTRITIONAL ANALYSIS PER EACH OF 4 SERVINGS: Calories 430; Protein 15g; Carbohydrate 47g (16%DV); Fat, total 20g (31%DV); Fat, saturated 6g (30%DV); Fat, trans 0g; Cholesterol 15mg (5%DV); Fibre 5g (20%DV); Sodium 105mg (4%DV).

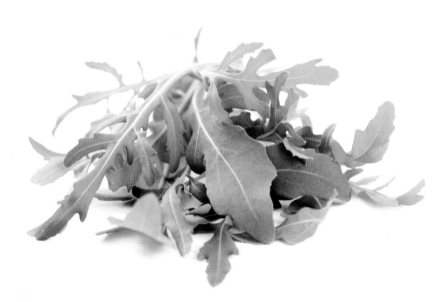

South African Peanut Stew

Serve on basmati rice, with a fruity chutney on the side. This vegetarian stew, generously donated by Carol's South African friend, Lourenza Fourie, is also fantastic served alongside simply prepared roast chicken breast slices. The stew can be frozen, but you may want to sprinkle fresh, coarsely chopped peanuts overtop before serving.

Prep time: 20 minutes
Cook time: 35 minutes
Serves 6 (1 cup each)

1½ tsp curry powder or garam masala
½ tsp coriander seeds
½ tsp black peppercorns
¼ tsp cumin seeds
¼ tsp dried red pepper flakes
1½ cups peanuts, roasted and lightly salted
2 tbsp olive oil
1 onion, chopped
1 tbsp grated fresh ginger (or ½ tsp ground ginger)
1 carrot, finely chopped
1 stalk celery, finely chopped
3 tbsp finely chopped garlic
3 cups chicken or vegetable stock, preferably low-sodium
1 large sweet potato, cut into chunks
1 cup chopped okra (or 1 cup shredded cabbage) (optional)
2 cups shredded baby spinach leaves

In a small spice grinder or mortar and pestle, grind together curry powder, coriander seeds, peppercorns, cumin seeds and red pepper flakes. Set aside.

In a large skillet set over medium heat, toast peanuts until just starting to turn golden and fragrant, about 3 minutes. Add half of oil plus onion, fresh ginger and prepared spice mixture; cook, stirring, until onion starts to brown, about 3 minutes. Add carrot and celery; cook, stirring, for 3 minutes. Add remaining oil and garlic; cook, stirring, for 2 minutes.

Add stock and sweet potato; cook, stirring occasionally, until vegetables are tender, about 20 minutes.

Add okra, if using; cook until just tender, about 5 minutes. Stir in spinach just until wilted.

NUTRITIONAL ANALYSIS PER SERVING: Calories 370; Protein 11g; Carbohydrate 29g (10%DV); Fat, total 24g (37%DV); Fat, saturated 3g (15%DV); Fat, trans 0g; Cholesterol 0mg; Fibre 7g (28%DV); Sodium 420mg (18%DV).

Squash, Spinach and Onion Lasagna

We have replaced the rich and fattening béchamel (white sauce) traditionally used in lasagnas with a lighter squash-based filling. If you don't have time to make your own squash purée, look for canned varieties with as little sodium as possible. Although this recipe takes time, you can do it in stages if you like—and the effort is well worth it.

Prep time: 20 minutes
Cook time: 30 minutes for onions plus 45 minutes for lasagna
Serves 8

2 tbsp olive oil
5 onions, sliced
2 bunches spinach, trimmed and washed well
¼ cup unsalted butter
½ cup all-purpose flour
4 cups 2% milk
⅓ cup grated Parmesan cheese
½ tsp black pepper
¼ tsp salt
¼ tsp freshly grated nutmeg
9 lasagna noodles

SQUASH FILLING
1⅓ cups squash purée
1¼ cups 2% cottage cheese
2 eggs
3 tbsp whole-wheat bread crumbs
½ cup shredded light mozzarella cheese
¼ tsp each salt and black pepper

Heat oil in a large non-stick skillet set over medium heat. Add onion; cook, stirring often, until golden and very soft, about 30 minutes. Transfer to a bowl. In same skillet, in batches, cook spinach, with some water clinging to leaves, just until wilted. Squeeze out any excess moisture. Chop coarsely.

Meanwhile, in a saucepan, melt butter over medium heat. Whisk in flour; cook, stirring, for 2 minutes. Gradually whisk in milk; bring to a boil, whisking constantly. Reduce heat to medium-low; cook, whisking often, until thickened, about 8 minutes. Remove from heat; stir in Parmesan, pepper, salt and nutmeg. Stir in cooked spinach. Set aside 1 cup of mixture.

At the same time, in a large pot of boiling salted water, cook noodles until almost tender, 8 to 10 minutes. As noodles are done, arrange in a single layer on a damp kitchen towel.

Preheat oven to 375°F.

Squash filling: In a the bowl of a food processor, combine squash purée and cottage cheese; purée. Transfer to a large bowl; stir in eggs, bread crumbs, half of mozzarella plus salt and pepper.

Arrange 3 noodles in a single layer on bottom of a greased 13 x 9-inch baking dish. Spread with half the onions, half the squash filling and half the spinach mixture. Repeat layers once. Top with remaining 3 noodles and reserved 1 cup spinach mixture. Sprinkle with remaining mozzarella.

Bake in centre of preheated oven for 45 minutes or until golden and bubbly. Let stand for 10 minutes before serving.

NUTRITIONAL ANALYSIS PER EACH OF 8 SERVINGS: Calories 280; Protein 14g; Carbohydrate 30g (10%DV); Fat, total 11g (17%DV); Fat, saturated 5g (25%DV); Fat, trans 0g; Cholesterol 65mg (22%DV); Fibre 3g (12%DV); Sodium 370mg (15%DV).

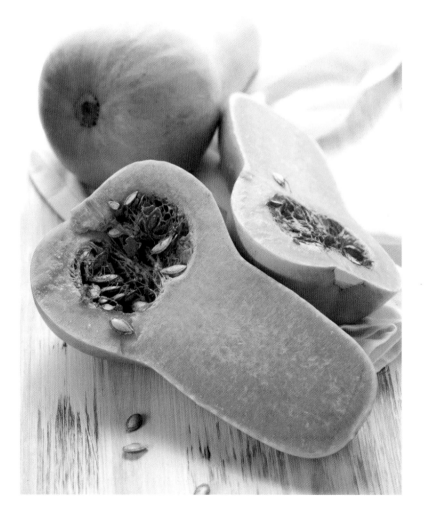

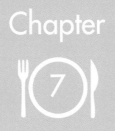
Delicious Desserts:

Sweet Endings, Sweet Dreams

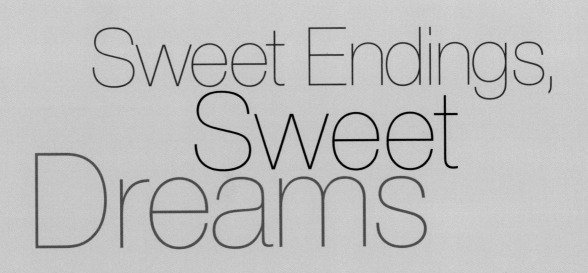

We now know that certain foods and nutrients can help with brain health and function in older adults.

But can food help improve our mood or ability to enjoy a good night's sleep, too?

The Mood-Altering Effects of Food

Researchers have looked at whether foods can affect mood by helping to promote the synthesis of a brain chemical called serotonin. Serotonin is a "neurotransmitter" that is disrupted in patients with depression. In fact, many antidepressant medications work to increase brain serotonin.

Serotonin is made in our bodies from tryptophan, an amino acid contained in most proteins that we eat. Surprisingly, the best way to increase brain serotonin is by eating carbohydrate, not protein. This is because the insulin released into your bloodstream after eating carbohydrate helps tryptophan gain entry to the brain by removing other amino acids from your blood and sending them to other tissues, like muscle. When you eat protein, the other amino acids in protein compete with tryptophan for entry into the brain.

Could increasing carbohydrates and therefore brain serotonin help elevate mood and be a more natural way to minimize reliance on the use of antidepressant medications?

Unfortunately, the vast majority of studies failed to show a change in mood, especially an improvement, following the ingestion of carbohydrate foods in either healthy adults or in those with depression. Further studies revealed why. Even small amounts of protein can impair carbohydrates' ability to increase brain tryptophan and consequently serotonin. Virtually all foods consumed by humans have sufficient protein in them to do this, although current research is attempting to identify specific proteins that may not do so.

Whether other food components can directly influence mood is largely unexplored. However, a recent study suggests that the bio-active components of green tea may actually play a direct role in improving calmness and reducing feelings of stress.

Researchers also looked at the opposite question: Can low levels of brain serotonin lead to carbohydrate cravings as a form of self-medication? It appears that some obese individuals and those with specific types of depression (e.g., seasonal affective disorder [SAD] or depression that occurs in the winter months when access to light is limited) may be susceptible to this. As a result, these people are more vulnerable to overeating in the face of the cravings.

We also know that women's appetites change throughout their menstrual cycle. Some women experience carbohydrate cravings in the premenstrual period. The data suggests that eating carbohydrates will not satisfy these cravings, so it is more important to recognize this as a vulnerable period. If you find yourself reaching for high-carb snacks and foods, check where you are in your menstrual cycle and put the craving into perspective. Acting on these carb cravings will not help you in the short term and could contribute to weight gain in the long run.

Sleep Effects of Food

The amount and quality of your sleep have enormous effects on your daily life and well-being. Increasingly, we hear about the negative effects of sleep deprivation on both physiological and psychological well-being.

Sleep deficits can lead to disordered eating, including overeating, and ultimately to obesity and its related disorders. So ensuring that you are getting enough sleep is one way to help maintain your body weight and avoid those disorders (high blood pressure, elevated blood cholesterol and type 2 diabetes) that increase your likelihood of cognitive decline and dementia.

Fortunately, following the principles needed for brain health—eating a diet rich in fruits, vegetables, whole grains and low-fat protein sources—can also improve your sleep. However, many ask if they can improve their sleep by eating the right food just before going to bed. Well, the answer remains unclear.

Research examining food and sleep focuses on brain serotonin, as it is also involved in sleep. Our brain serotonin levels naturally rise in the evening, and high levels of brain serotonin are thought to promote sleep. As mentioned, it is difficult to alter brain serotonin through food, as most foods do not have the right proportion of carbohydrate and protein to do so. Nevertheless, there is some evidence that drinking milk, especially milk that has been sweetened, may be able to alter brain serotonin—so there may be some wisdom in having a hot cup of milk before going to bed.

Important Caveats

There are two important caveats to these findings. One is that a poor diet, especially one that is low in vitamins (such as folate and vitamin B_{12}), can contribute to depression. So ensuring that you are eating an optimal diet and meeting your nutritional requirements is important for your mental health.

The other area under investigation is the relationship between poor intake of omega-3 fats and depression. Today, many Canadians have diets that are deficient in omega-3 fats. Again, we can overcome this deficiency by making wise choices when it comes to fats in our diet. Current research is also exploring whether omega-3 fats can be used alone or in combination with antidepressants to help the treatment of depression. While the results are preliminary, this area of research looks promising.

You won't feel the difference consuming foods that are high in omega-3 fats right away, but over time, you will enjoy the healthy benefits of these foods.

Nourishing the Soul to Benefit Mood and Sleep

Right now, evidence shows that there aren't any foods that alter our moods significantly in the short term. So why do people argue that foods have beneficial mood or sleep effects?

One answer is the psychological aspect of food. Certain foods remind us of nurturing moments in our lives: perhaps a loving mother preparing a nourishing meal for the family or a holiday meal with your entire extended family gathered around. Perhaps these psychological triggers inherent in food help improve our mood or relax us so we can sleep better.

In addition, the rituals we establish to help nurture ourselves, be it a cup of tea at the end of a long day or warm milk before bedtime, may provide important down time to help alleviate the negative effects of a stressful day.

While these benefits would be considered a placebo effect from a scientific perspective, they are an important part of nourishing ourselves.

How to Use This Information

While there is no scientific proof that foods can alter our moods or help us fall asleep faster, using food to nurture and comfort ourselves can help both mood and sleep, provided that food is not consumed in excess. The recipes in this section were developed to embrace this nurturing, rewarding and comforting quality of food. Yet, at the same time, the healthy ingredients, such as fruits, nuts and grains, are at the forefront of a brain-healthy diet. So make room for delicious, healthy eating and a few sweet treats, too. Enjoy!

Chapter 7
Delicious Desserts

Recipes

Mango and Fennel Granita   243

Roasted Cinnamon Plums   244
by Chef Chuck Hughes

The Most Delicious Nutritious Berry Crisp Ever   248

Crème Caramel   250

Sponge Cake with Peaches Macerated in White Wine   253

Warm Citrus Casserole   257

Warm Blueberry Brown Butter Cake Bites   258
by Chef Jeff McCourt

Almond Ginger Tart   261

Chocolate Avocado Cupcakes   263

Meringue Cups with Strawberry Rhubarb Topping   265

Vanilla Yogurt Cake with Marmalade Glaze   267

Mango and Fennel Granita

This is the ultimate adult snow cone! Scraping the mixture as it freezes gives this icy dessert a granular texture, which makes it an Italian favourite.

Prep time: 10 minutes
Freeze time: 3 hours
Serves 6 (¾ cup each)

4 ripe mangoes
1 fennel bulb
2 tbsp liquid honey

Peel and coarsely chop mangoes. Coarsely chop fennel; reserve fennel fronds for garnish.

Place mango and fennel pieces in the bowl of a food processor; purée until smooth. Stir in honey. Spread mixture evenly into a 13 x 9-inch baking tray or dish. Freeze, stirring and scraping with fork every 30 minutes, until it becomes shaved ice. Serve within 2 hours of forming.

NUTRITIONAL ANALYSIS PER SERVING: Calories 70; Protein 1g; Carbohydrate 19g (6%DV); Fat, total 0g; Fat, saturated 0g; Fat, trans 0g; Cholesterol 0mg; Fibre 2g (8%DV); Sodium 15mg (1%DV).

Roasted Cinnamon Plums

By Chef Chuck Hughes

The word "prune" comes from *prunum*, the Latin word for plum. A prune plum refers to any smaller-sized plum with a rich purple or bluish-black skin. Ripe plums can be stored in the refrigerator for up to 4 days.

Prep time: 5 minutes
Cook time: 30 minutes
Serves 8 (2 halves each)

8 ripe purple prune plums, halved and pitted
2 tbsp packed light brown sugar
1½ tsp ground cinnamon
Pinch salt
2 tsp finely grated lemon zest

Preheat oven to 350°F.

Place plum halves, cut-side up, in a large baking dish. Sprinkle with sugar, cinnamon, salt and lemon zest.

Bake in centre of preheated oven until soft, about 30 minutes.

NUTRITIONAL ANALYSIS PER SERVING: Calories 45; Protein 0.5g; Carbohydrate 11g (3.5%DV); Fat, total 0g; Fat, saturated 0g; Fat, trans 0g; Cholesterol 0mg; Fibre 1.5g (6%DV); Sodium 5mg (0%DV).

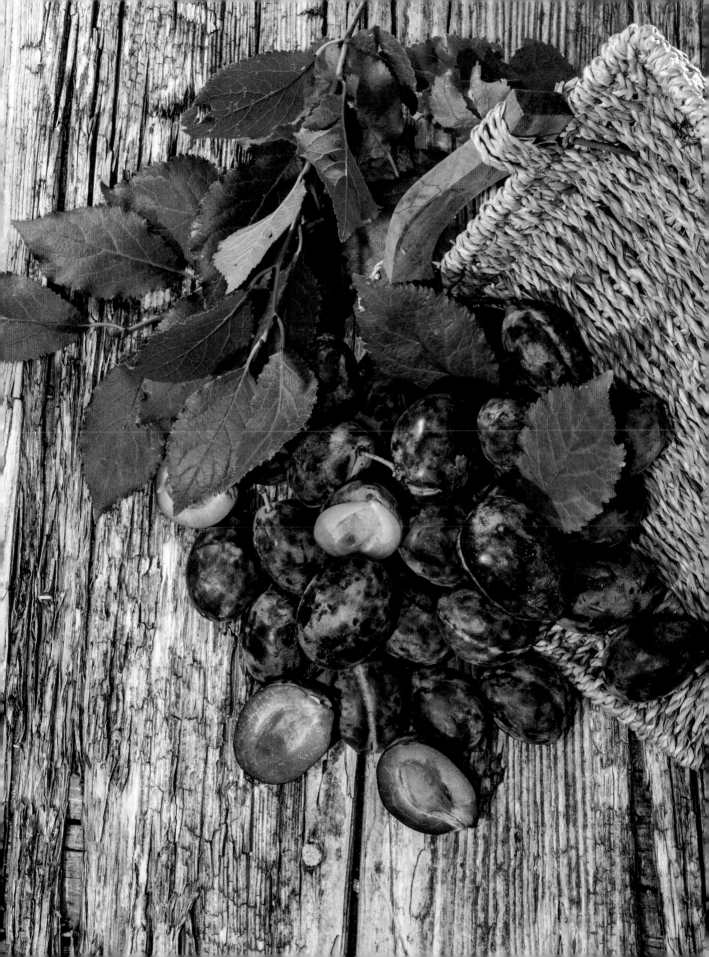

❧Health Savvy: Fresh Fruit Fundamentals

Although we're inundated with the message to paint our fruit crisper red and buy deeply coloured fruits, it's essential to consume a variety of fresh fruit: berries, apples, pears, bananas, melons, etc. But what to do when you overbuy and risk some of that fruit going to waste? Or, in the depths of winter, how do you ensure you're getting enough? Follow these buying and storage tips to maximize your grocery budget and guarantee your fruit cup runneth over. The best tip, of course, is to buy local as much as possible, buy in season as much as possible and buy only what you can consume in 3 to 5 days.

Berries Look for fairly firm, sweet-smelling berries with no signs of mould or mildew and no crushed berries in the box. Strawberries should be completely red with no white or green spots. Be wary of berries packed in juice-stained containers. Store berries loosely covered in the refrigerator. Blueberries will last for up to 2 weeks, strawberries from 3 to 6 days, and raspberries and blackberries from 2 to 3 days. Do not wash berries until ready to eat.

To freeze, place in a single layer (unwashed) on a large tray or cookie sheet. Freeze until firm (about one hour), pack in freezer bags (drawing off as much air as possible before sealing), and seal. Store for up to 12 months.

Apples and pears Look for firm apples, free of wrinkles and bruises. Do not purchase any overripe apples that have soft spots; they give off ethylene gas that will cause nearby apples to ripen too quickly and spoil. Apples will keep for up to 1 month.

Unlike most other fruits, pears don't ripen well on the tree. They are harvested just before they're mature and allowed to finish ripening under controlled conditions. Ripe pears spoil easily, so refrigerate them and use within a couple of days of purchase.

Peaches, plums and nectarines Choose fruit that's plump, relatively firm but not hard, with a smooth skin and a sweet and fruity scent. Fruit should give slightly to finger-tip pressure, especially along the seam. Avoid fruit that has wrinkled skin or a greenish tinge at the end, or excessively soft, bruised or blemished fruit. When still fairly firm to the touch, store peaches at room temperature out of direct sun until ripening begins and their skin yields slightly to gentle pressure. Once ripe, peaches should be refrigerated in a single layer for no longer than 5 days, plums for 4 days and nectarines for 7 days.

To freeze, first pit and slice fruit. Place in a single layer (unwashed) on a large tray or cookie sheet. Freeze until firm (about 1 hour), then pack in freezer bags (drawing off as much air as possible before sealing), and seal. Store for up to 12 months.

Mangoes, papayas, exotic fruits Choose mangoes that have unblemished yellow skin blushed with red, and a sweet, fruity scent. To measure for ripeness, squeeze gently. If it's ripe, it should give slightly but not be too soft. Unripe mangoes should be stored on a table or countertop at room temperature out of direct sun. Once ripe, refrigerate for up to 2 weeks. Papayas should ripen at room temperature and then be stored, loosely covered, for up to 1 week. Kiwis can be refrigerated for up to 2 weeks. Pineapples should not be stored in the fridge, unless you are trying to avoid ripening. They tend to take quite some time to ripen, then once ripened become overripe in 1 or 2 days.

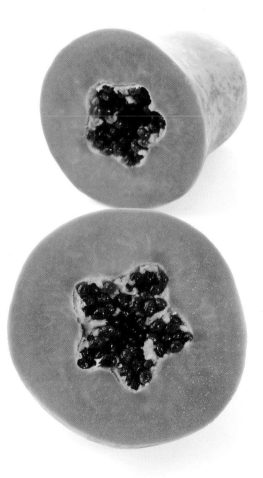

The Most Delicious Nutritious Berry Crisp Ever

This recipe, contributed by nutritionist Rena Mendelson, makes more topping than you'll need for just one crisp; leftovers can be stored in the freezer for up to 3 months.

Prep time: 25 minutes
Cook time: 45 minutes
Serves 8
(Makes enough topping for about 6 large crisps)

TOPPING
1½ cups cold unsalted butter, cut into small pieces
1½ cups whole-wheat flour
1½ cups packed light brown sugar
4 cups large-flake rolled oats
1 cup wheat or oat bran
½ cup wheat germ
½ cup ground flaxseed

FRUIT MIXTURE
6 cups chopped fruit (apples, pears, peaches, berries, plums, etc.)
¼ cup packed light brown sugar
2 tbsp all-purpose flour
1 tsp ground cinnamon
½ tsp ground ginger

Topping: In a large bowl, combine butter, flour, brown sugar, rolled oats, bran, wheat germ and flaxseed. Using fingertips, rub all ingredients together until crumbly mixture is formed. This will take quite a while because of the volume. (Mixture can be frozen for up to 3 months. Mixture will make about 6 large crisps, depending on the size of baking dish.)

Fruit mixture: In another large bowl, combine fruit, brown sugar, flour, cinnamon and ginger, mixing until fruit is well coated.

Preheat oven to 375°F.

Transfer fruit to an 8-inch square baking dish. Spread about 2 cups topping over entire surface of fruit. Bake in centre of preheated oven until thickened, bubbling and fruit is tender, 35 to 45 minutes. (Baked crisps can be frozen for up to 1 month. Thaw at room temperature; reheat in 200°F oven for 20 minutes.)

NUTRITIONAL ANALYSIS PER EACH OF 8 SERVINGS: Calories 190; Protein 3g; Carbohydrate 32g (11%DV); Fat, total 6g (9%DV); Fat, saturated 3.5g (18% DV); Fat, trans 0g; Cholesterol 15mg (5% DV); Fibre 3g (12%DV); Sodium 5mg (0%DV).

TIP—Pairing Fruit with Herbs and Spices

Up the flavour quotient of your crisp by pairing particular fruits with a variety of made-in-heaven spice and herb matches. Apples marry beautifully with cinnamon, of course, but they are also wonderful with aromatic cardamom, allspice or even five spice powder. The sweetness of pears is highlighted with crystallized and ground ginger or nutmeg. Don't be afraid to mingle herbs in with your sweet fruit. Berries get transported to another level of deliciousness when sprinkled with lemon juice and a hit of dried basil. Lavender and honey, rosemary and lime are perfect dates for apples, melons and berries.

Crème Caramel

Crème caramel, or flan, is a custard dessert common in Europe and South America. It differs from crème brûlée by having a liquid caramel sauce over the custard rather than a hard caramel top. The soft and creamy texture of this flan belies its reasonably low fat content (thanks to the use of 2% milk). Use a 6-cup flan or quiche-type mould for this dish.

Prep time: 15 minutes plus 2 hours to chill
Cook time: 1 hour
Serves 8

1½ cups granulated sugar
3 tbsp water
4 cups 2% milk
8 eggs, lightly beaten
1 tsp vanilla
Pinch salt

Preheat oven to 350°F.

Pour enough hot water into a 6-cup mould to fill: just before making the caramel, drain and set aside.

In a high-sided saucepan, combine ¾ cup sugar and 3 tbsp water; stir until a slurry the consistency of wet sand forms. Place saucepan over medium heat; without stirring, bring to a boil. Boil lightly, without stirring, until sugar melts and turns a medium dark brown (be careful not to overcook: the darker the sugar, the more bitter it will taste).

Immediately pour caramel into mould, turning it in all directions until caramel covers bottom and sides. As soon as the caramel stops running, turn mould upside down on a plate. At this stage, the caramel should have solidified against the sides and bottom of the mould.

Heat milk until a fine sheen appears on top (about 6 minutes in microwave). Remove from heat; cool.

In a bowl, whisk remaining ¾ cup sugar gradually into eggs; whisk in milk, vanilla and salt. Strain into caramel-lined mould. Place mould in a larger pan; fill pan with warm water to halfway up sides of mould.

Bake in centre of preheated oven for 1 hour or until a knife inserted in the custard comes out clean. Remove custard to a wire rack; cool to room temperature. Refrigerate until completely chilled, at least 2 hours.

To unmould, run a knife between custard and mould. Place a serving dish upside down over mould; invert quickly. Slice into 8 pie-shaped wedges and spoon 1 to 2 tbsp caramel over each wedge.

NUTRITIONAL ANALYSIS PER EACH OF 8 SERVINGS: Calories 320; Protein 10g; Carbohydrate 44g (15%DV); Fat, total 7g (11%DV); Fat, saturated 3g (15% DV); Fat, trans 0g; Cholesterol 196mg (65% DV); Fibre 0g; Sodium 148mg (6%DV).

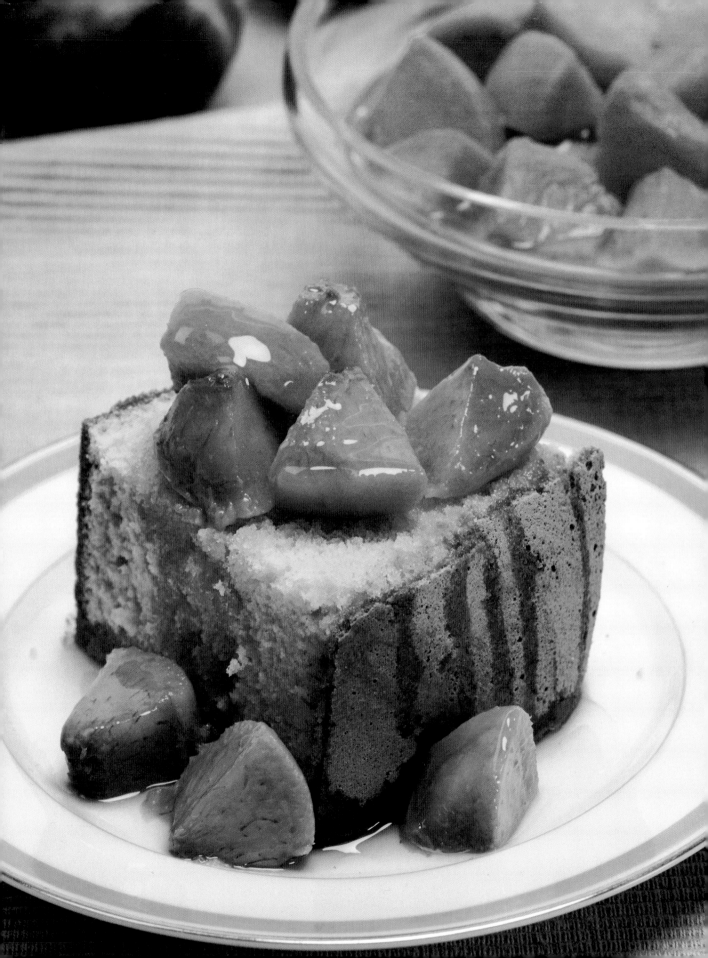

Sponge Cake with Peaches Macerated in White Wine

Macerated peaches are delicious on their own, but sponge cake is its heavenly made match! Simple and satisfying, this is the perfect end to any day of the week.

Prep time: 15 minutes
Cook time: 1 hour
Serves 12

1⅔ cups all-purpose flour
½ tsp salt
6 eggs
1½ cups granulated sugar
1 tsp vanilla
1 Peaches Macerated in White Wine (page 254)

Preheat oven to 350°F.

Line bottom of an 8-inch square baking pan with parchment paper; lightly grease bottom and sides of pan.

In a small bowl, combine flour and salt; set aside.

In a large bowl, beat eggs, adding ½ cup sugar at a time, until thickened and light in colour. Beat in vanilla. Slowly add flour, about ½ cup at a time, until lightly mixed. Continue until all flour has been added, being careful to not over-mix.

Pour batter into prepared baking pan. Bake in centre of preheated oven until tester inserted in centre comes out clean, 50 to 60 minutes. Cool in pan on wire rack.

Reserving juice, drain peaches. Transfer to a serving bowl; cover with plastic wrap and refrigerate until ready to serve. Transfer peach juice to a small pan set over medium heat. Cook until volume is reduced by approximately half. Remove from heat; let cool.

To serve, cut cake into 2 x 3-inch squares and place each square on a dessert plate. Cover each with 2 tbsp reduced peach juice; top with macerated peaches.

NUTRITIONAL ANALYSIS PER EACH OF 12 SERVINGS: Calories 170; Protein 4g; Carbohydrate 33g (11%DV); Fat, total 2.5g (4%DV); Fat, saturated 1g (5%DV); Fat, trans 0g; Cholesterol 105mg (35%DV); Fibre 0g; Sodium 170mg (7%DV).

TIP—Controlling the Colour of Your Cake

Use a light-coloured pan for the cake if you can, to ensure a nice golden-coloured cake.

Peaches Macerated in White Wine

Simple and exquisite, this dessert is best enjoyed in the late summer and early autumn, when fresh local peaches are available. The peaches do need the day to absorb the flavours from the cinnamon-flavoured wine, so be certain to make this ahead of time. Take note, peaches will begin to brown and lose their texture after a couple of days.

Prep time: 10 minutes plus 18 hours marinating time
Resting time: 24 hours
Serves 12 (2 peach halves each)

1 cup dry white wine
½ cup granulated sugar
6 peaches, preferably freestone
1 cinnamon stick (about 3 inches long)

Mix together white wine and sugar in an airtight container large enough to hold the peaches. Stir until sugar is almost dissolved. Peel peaches; halve and remove pits. Working over the container as much as possible to catch all the juices, cut peaches into large chunks; add to wine/sugar mixture. Add cinnamon stick. Cover and refrigerate for 18 to 24 hours. Serve as is or use as a topping for Sponge Cake (page 253).

NUTRITIONAL ANALYSIS PER SERVING: Calories 70; Protein 0g; Carbohydrate 13g (4%DV); Fat, total 0g; Fat, saturated 0g; Fat, trans 0g; Cholesterol 0mg; Fibre 1g (4%DV); Sodium 0mg.

❦Health Savvy: Stocking Your Sweet Pantry

Granulated sugar Granulated sugar is the most common form of sugar used today. It is the final product of the sugar-refining process, be it from beets or sugar cane. Stored in an airtight container in a cool dry place, granulated sugar will keep for up to 2 years. In baking, sugar plays multiple roles. It tenderizes, caramelizes, sweetens and enhances other flavours, enables fermentation (in yeast breads), and attracts and retains moisture. This multi-faceted role means that you cannot reduce sugar arbitrarily in a recipe. As a general rule, you can replace up to one-third of the sugar in a recipe with either fruit juice or another alternative without the texture, taste or look being affected.

Brown sugar Brown sugar is essentially granulated sugar with molasses added back in for colour and flavour. The added moisture from the molasses means that brown sugar makes chewier cookies and softer, more tender baked goods. Both light and dark brown sugars are almost as sweet as granulated sugar, and can be substituted in equal amounts for granulated sugar in most recipes (the exception being where aeration and creaming are vital to the foundation of the cake).

Honey Unlike granulated sugar, honey is not pure sweetener. It's made up of about 18% water, with dextrose, fructose and traces of vitamins and minerals making up the rest. It has fewer calories by weight than sugar, but is not quite as sweet as regular granulated sugar. By composition, it only has about 75% of the sweetening power of regular sugar. If you bake with honey, your baked goods will have a somewhat longer shelf life. It also caramelizes at a lower temperature than sugar, so recipes using a large amount of honey should be baked at slightly lower temperatures. If you simply substitute half of the sugar called for in a recipe with honey, your baked goods may be a touch heavier, denser and more moist.

Agave Sometimes called "nectar" and sometimes called "syrup," agave is a sweetener commercially produced in Mexico. It is used to replace granulated sugar in beverages and baked goods. Caution is required, however, when substituting agave, since it is 1.4 to 1.6 times sweeter than sugar. It consists primarily of glucose and fructose. Agave is generally available in light, amber, dark and raw varieties. Light agave nectar has a mild, almost neutral flavour and is most widely used in baking. The dark and raw varieties of agave have increasing amounts of caramel flavouring and are generally considered too strong for all-purpose baking.

Maple syrup Less viscous and more fluid than honey, maple syrup imparts a unique and distinctive flavour to baked goods. Like desserts made with honey or corn syrup, baked goods made with maple syrup tend to have a dense moist crumb and to be slightly heavier than those made with granulated sugar. Maple syrup is slightly less sweet than regular sugar. As a guide, 1½ cups maple syrup will sweeten to the same degree as 1 cup of granulated sugar. Do not substitute more than half the total sugar in a recipe with a liquid sweetener such as maple syrup. Also, you must reduce the amount of liquid in the recipe by ¼ cup for every 1 cup syrup used. Maple syrup comes in about five different grades of increasing intensity, reflecting the amount of water that has been evaporated.

Sugar substitutes It's easy to substitute a sugar replacement for granulated sugar in most conventional shortbread cookies. If using a product like Splenda, simply replace each cup of sugar with a cup of the substitute. If using a more specific baking product such as Splenda Sugar Blend for Baking®, use ½ cup for every cup of granulated sugar and increase the vanilla by ½ teaspoon.

Using a sugar substitute may yield slightly different results, however. Generally, cookies will not brown quite as much and they may take 3 to 5 minutes *less* time to bake, so watch your oven! Also, sugar substitutes will remain a bit grainy when creamed with the butter. Cookies made with a sugar substitute will not store for as long as those made with conventional granulated sugar.

Warm Citrus Casserole

Comforting on a cold winter's night, this fruit salad is packed full of the goodness of citrus fruits. Feel free to omit the brandy or to add it to the casserole but not flame it. This dish is wonderful by itself but also great over Sponge Cake (page 253) or waffles.

Prep time: 10 minutes
Cook time: 30 minutes
Serves 6

1 grapefruit, peeled and segmented
3 oranges, peeled and segmented
1 small tin (11 oz/284 mL) mandarin oranges, drained
3 tbsp packed light brown sugar
½ tsp ground nutmeg or mace
1 tbsp butter
3 tbsp brandy

Preheat oven to 350°F.

Combine grapefruit, oranges, mandarin oranges and their juices in an ovenproof 6-cup casserole dish. Sprinkle with brown sugar and nutmeg; dot with butter.

Bake in centre of preheated oven until liquid starts to simmer and small bubbles form at side of casserole dish, 25 to 30 minutes.

In a small pot set over medium heat, warm brandy; pour over casserole. Transfer casserole to kitchen counter or dinner table. Using a long match or a long barbecue lighter, and averting your face, light brandy until it flames. The flames will die down of their own accord within a few seconds (after many *oohs* and *aahs*, of course).

Serve casserole in small bowls or decorative glasses, such as martini glasses.

NUTRITIONAL ANALYSIS PER EACH OF 6 SERVINGS: Calories 100; Protein 1g; Carbohydrate 22g (7%DV); Fat, total 2g (3%DV); Fat, saturated 1.5g (8%DV); Fat, trans 0g; Cholesterol 5mg (2%DV); Fibre 2g (8%DV); Sodium 0mg.

Warm Blueberry Brown Butter Cake Bites

By Chef Jeff McCourt

Jeff McCourt is founder of Chefwise Consulting in Prince Edward Island and a respected teacher and board chair at the PEI Culinary Alliance. He also co-authored Flavours of Prince Edward Island.

I bake this dessert with almost any fruit—strawberries, raspberries, apples, pears. It follows seasonal availability where blueberries land right in the middle of these four ingredients; blueberries are my favourite, though. In this recipe, I have combined them with the nuttiness of the brown butter backed up by some toasted pecans as well as the heady aroma of freshly ground cardamom—a very exciting spice.

Prep time: 15 minutes
Cook time: 20 minutes
Makes 12 servings (2 bites each)

¼ lb unsalted butter
¾ cup granulated sugar
2 eggs
½ tsp vanilla
⅜ cup all-purpose flour (or scant ½ cup)
1 cup fresh blueberries, preferably small wild
½ tsp ground cardamom
¼ cup chopped pecans
Pinch salt

Preheat oven to 375°F. Generously coat two mini-muffin tins with cooking spray; set aside.

Melt butter in a small saucepan and heat until butter starts turning a light brown colour (see Tip on page 260). Pour browned butter into a medium-sized metal mixing bowl and cool for 3 to 4 minutes. Whisk together cooled browned butter and sugar. Mix in eggs, one at a time, beating well after each addition; stir in vanilla. Fold in flour, blueberries, cardamom, pecans and salt.

Place a scant 1 tbsp batter into each muffin cup, filling approximately three-quarters full. Bake in centre of preheated oven until tops are lightly browned and tester inserted in centre comes out clean, 18 to 20 minutes. Using a paring knife, quickly run knife around edges to ensure cakes will unmould. Cool in tins for 5 minutes and then unmould onto a wire rack. These bites are lovely served warm; however, they work equally well at room temperature.

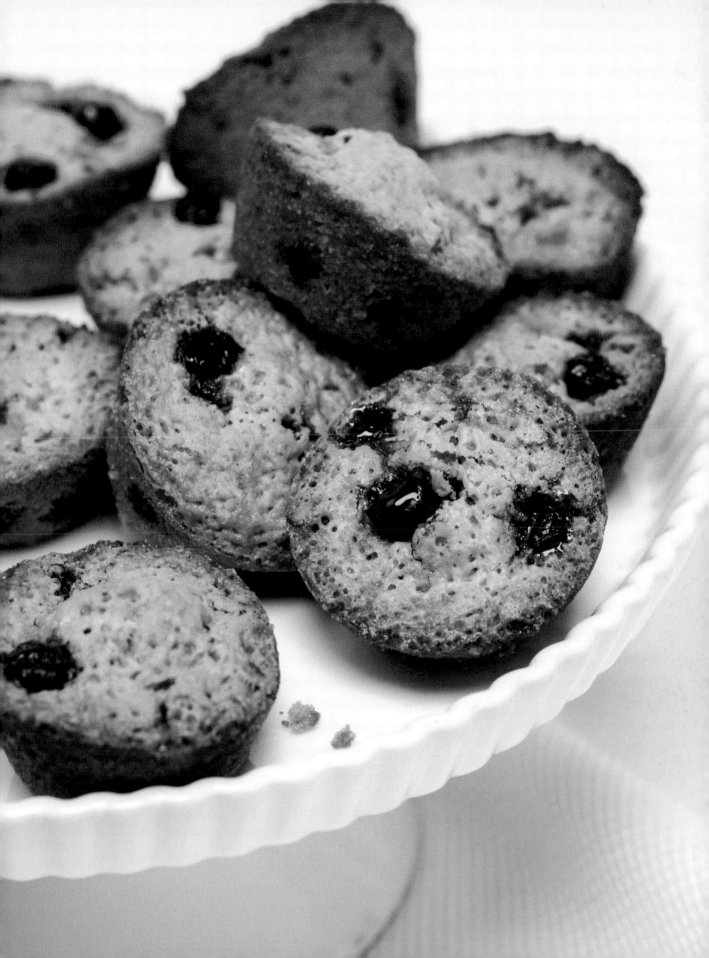

NUTRITIONAL ANALYSIS PER SERVING: Calories 160; Protein 2g; Carbohydrate 18g (6%DV); Fat, total 10g (15%DV); Fat, saturated 5g (25%DV); Fat, trans 0g; Cholesterol 55mg (18%DV); Fibre 1g (4%DV); Sodium 15mg (1%DV).

TIP—How to Brown Butter

Melt butter in a saucepan over medium heat. Once melted, it will begin to bubble—which means it is cooking out the water-based liquid in the butter. The final stage is the foaming stage; it is very obvious: the butter will start smelling very nutty. Also, the foam will start changing colour slightly; you may see small brown bits—caramelized milk solids—come up through the foam. When this happens, remove from heat and pour into a metal bowl to cool.

Almond Ginger Tart

Where possible, use nuts that have the skin on—while the nut itself is rich in healthy oils, the skin is rich in compounds that help reduce tissue damage and maintain heart health. These same compounds are believed to be culinary contributors to brain health.

Prep time: 25 minutes
Cook time: 1 hour
Serves 12

7 tbsp fine granulated sugar, plus extra for dusting cake pan
1 cup panko or very fine dry white bread crumbs
1 tbsp baking powder
1 cup roughly chopped natural (whole, skin-on) almonds
½ cup canola oil
½ tsp finely grated lemon zest
¼ cup finely chopped crystallized ginger
8 egg whites or 1 container (250 g) of "whites only" eggs
Icing sugar

Preheat oven to 350°F.

Line bottom of a 9-inch round springform pan with parchment paper; grease bottom and sides lightly. Dust bottom and sides with 1 tbsp sugar.

In the bowl of a food processor, pulse together remaining sugar plus bread crumbs, baking powder and almonds; add oil. Pulse until mixture is consistency of brown sugar. Add lemon zest and crystallized ginger; pulse 4 or 5 times, until distributed throughout batter. Transfer to a mixing bowl.

In a separate bowl, whip egg whites until stiff, but not glossy, peaks form. Mix 1 cup egg whites into batter to lighten. Using a spatula, gently fold half of remaining egg whites into batter by running a spatula down the side of the bowl to the bottom and lifting batter to the top. Continue until egg whites are distributed throughout the batter. Do not over-mix or the egg whites will collapse. Fold in second half of egg whites. Pour batter into prepared springform pan.

Bake in centre of preheated oven until toothpick inserted in centre comes out clean, 50 to 60 minutes. Cool in pan on rack for 10 minutes before removing from pan.

Sprinkle with icing sugar before serving. If you like, serve with fresh-cut fruit or berries.

NUTRITIONAL ANALYSIS PER SLICE: Calories 210; Protein 5g; Carbohydrate 21g (7%DV);
Fat, total 13g (20%DV); Fat, saturated 1g (5%DV); Fat, trans 0g; Cholesterol 0mg; Fibre 1g (4%DV);
Sodium 125mg (5%DV).

Kitchen Savvy: Chocolate Ravioli

For those post-dinner or evening cravings, arrange 12 unbaked wonton wrappers on a parchment paper–lined baking sheet. Place some chopped bittersweet chocolate (about 1 tbsp) on the left-hand side of each wrapper. Brush some water over the edges of each wrapper and fold the right side of the wonton over the chocolate; pinch edges together to seal. Brush surface with a tiny amount of canola oil. Bake in centre of preheated 350°F oven for about 7 minutes or until wontons are golden and chocolate has melted. Serve warm.

NUTRITIONAL ANALYSIS PER RAVIOLI: Calories 120; Protein 2g; Carbohydrate 13g (4%DV); Fat, total 6g (9%DV); Fat, saturated 2g (10%DV); Fat, trans 0g; Cholesterol 0mg; Fibre 1g (4%DV); Sodium 95mg (4%DV).

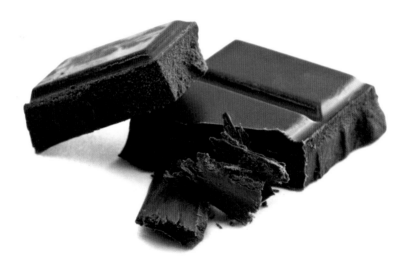

Chocolate Avocado Cupcakes

Avocado is a rich, creamy and surprisingly subtle replacement for eggs, binding the batter, keeping the muffins perfectly moist, and adding healthy fats to your dessert menu. Swap the milk for almond or coconut milk to make this a vegan-friendly treat.

Prep time: 10 minutes
Cook time: 25 minutes
Makes 12 cupcakes

1½ cups whole-wheat flour
4 tbsp (heaping) unsweetened cocoa powder, sifted
1 tsp baking powder
1 tsp baking soda
¼ tsp salt
1 ripe avocado
1 cup maple syrup
1/3 cup canola oil
1/3 cup milk
2 tsp vanilla

Preheat oven to 350°F. Grease a 12-cup muffin tin or line with muffin cups.

In a large bowl, whisk together flour, cocoa powder, baking powder, baking soda and salt.

In a separate bowl, mash avocado into smooth purée. Stir in maple syrup, oil, milk and vanilla. Transfer wet ingredients to flour mixture and stir until a smooth batter forms.

Divide batter evenly among prepared muffin cups. Bake in centre of preheated oven until toothpick inserted in centre of cupcake comes out clean, about 25 minutes.

Serve with fresh berries or balsamic-infused strawberries (see Tip, below).

NUTRITIONAL ANALYSIS PER SERVING: Calories 200; Protein 3g; Carbohydrate 32g (11%DV); Fat, total 8g (12%DV); Fat, saturated 1g (5%DV); Fat, trans 0g; Cholesterol 0mg; Fibre 3g (12%DV); Sodium 190mg (8%DV).

....

TIP—Up the Flavour Quotient of Your Strawberries with Balsamic Vinegar

A little bit of balsamic vinegar and black pepper is a great way to brighten the flavour of strawberries, especially during the winter months. Drizzle 1 tbsp balsamic vinegar over 2 cups sliced strawberries. Gently stir in 3 tbsp sugar and set aside, covered, for 1 hour at room temperature or for 3 to 4 hours in the refrigerator. Just before serving, add a pinch of freshly ground black pepper.

....

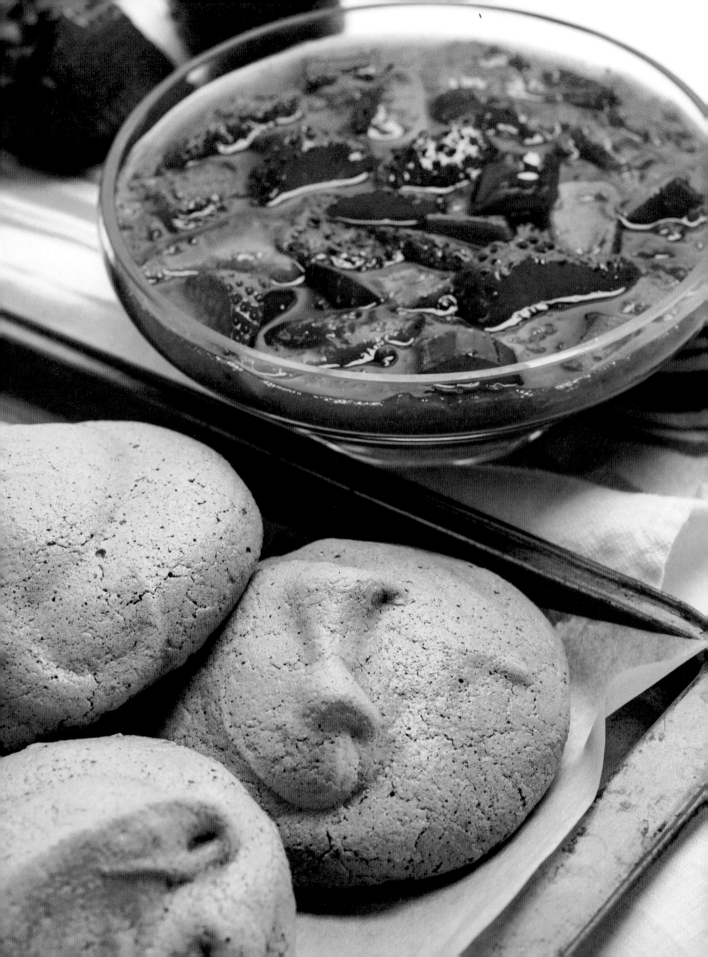

Meringue Cups with Strawberry Rhubarb Topping

The availability of high-quality, flash-frozen strawberries and rhubarb makes this a dessert you will enjoy all year round. Not too sweet, not too chocolatey, meringues will fare especially well in your kitchen during dry winter months. The topping is delicious served over pound cake, French toast, pancakes or waffles. You may even be tempted to eat it on its own!

Prep time: 15 minutes
Cook time: 1 hour
Serves 8 (¼ cup of topping each)

MERINGUE
4 egg whites
Pinch salt
1 cup granulated sugar
2 tbsp unsweetened cocoa powder, sifted
1 tbsp cornstarch
1 tsp vanilla

TOPPING
2 cups chopped fresh or frozen rhubarb
⅔ cup granulated sugar
⅓ cup water
1 tbsp cornstarch
1¾ cups sliced strawberries

Preheat oven to 250°F.

Meringue: Line a baking sheet with a piece of parchment paper. With a pencil, trace eight 3-inch circles onto parchment. Turn parchment over.

In a bowl, using an electric beater, beat egg whites with salt until soft peaks form. In a thin steady stream, beat in sugar until stiff glossy peaks form. Using a spatula, fold in cocoa powder, cornstarch and vanilla.

Mound a heaping ⅓ cup meringue onto outlined circles. Do not flatten.

Bake in centre of preheated oven until firm to the touch but still somewhat soft inside, about 1 hour. Transfer pan to a rack to cool. (Meringues can be stored in an airtight container at room temperature for up to 5 days.)

Topping: In a saucepan set over medium heat, combine rhubarb, sugar and water. Bring to a boil. Cook, stirring, until rhubarb has softened and broken down, about 5 minutes. Stir in cornstarch. Cook, stirring, for 2 minutes. Stir in strawberries; cook, stirring, for 2 minutes. Let cool. (Topping can be stored in an airtight container and refrigerated for up to 5 days. Bring to room temperature before serving.)

When ready to serve, place each meringue on a dessert plate. Lightly crush top of meringue to form a crater. Spoon topping into crater.

NUTRITIONAL ANALYSIS PER SERVING: Calories 190; Protein 2g; Carbohydrate 48g (16%DV); Fat, total 0g; Fat, saturated 0g; Fat, trans 0g; Cholesterol 0mg; Fibre 2g (8%DV); Sodium 35mg (1%DV).

TIP—Turning Greek Yogurt into Regular Yogurt

If all you have on hand is thick Greek yogurt, stir together ⅔ cup Greek yogurt with ⅓ cup milk to approximate 1 cup regular yogurt.

Vanilla Yogurt Cake with Marmalade Glaze

This is a perfect, simple cake to end any special occasion or weeknight repast. The acid in the yogurt ensures a tender crumb, as does the switch to cake and pastry flour—well worth the investment! The orange marmalade lends a polished finish, but the cake will work equally well with lemon marmalade.

Prep time: 10 minutes
Cook time: 30 minutes
Serves 12

CAKE
1 cup low-fat vanilla yogurt
3 tbsp canola oil
2 tbsp grated orange zest
3 tbsp orange juice
1 egg
2 tsp vanilla
2¼ cups sifted cake and pastry flour
½ cup granulated sugar
1 tbsp baking powder
½ tsp salt
¼ tsp baking soda

GLAZE
¾ cup orange marmalade
2 tbsp water

Preheat oven to 350°F. Lightly grease an 8-inch square baking pan.

Cake: In a bowl, stir together yogurt, oil, orange zest and juice, egg and vanilla.

In a separate bowl, combine flour, sugar, baking powder, salt and baking soda. Add flour mixture to yogurt mixture, stirring with a wooden spoon until just combined.

Transfer batter to prepared pan, smoothing top.

Bake in centre of preheated oven until cake tester inserted in centre of cake comes out clean, about 30 minutes. Let cool in pan on rack for 10 minutes.

Glaze: Meanwhile, heat marmalade and water in a small saucepan set over medium heat. Cook, stirring, until warmed through and liquefied, about 5 minutes. Pour over warm cake, spreading evenly.

NUTRITIONAL ANALYSIS PER SLICE: Calories 220; Protein 3g; Carbohydrate 41g (14%DV); Fat, total 4.5g (7%DV); Fat, saturated 0.5g (3%DV); Fat, trans 0g; Cholesterol 20mg (7%DV); Fibre 0g; Sodium 130mg (5%DV).

Acknowledgements

The great thing about writing a cookbook—aside from getting to test and taste all the fabulous recipes contained in it—are the amazing people who come together, not only to help put the food on the table (so to speak) and make it look beautiful, but to finesse our words, make sure that every single ingredient is reflected in a recipe's method and make the whole enterprise flourish and come together. We had the great fortune of working with such people. And because this book has had two incarnations—it first entered the world as an ebook, and now it is finding its place in printed book form—we had even more people rallying behind it.

That the photographs in this book look so utterly scrumptious and appealing, we owe thanks to food stylist extraordinaire Ettie Shuken and her extremely capable assistant, Gina St. Germain, a food stylist in her own right. David Shuken, our photographer, brought by sleight of hand and many a twist of light their visions of our recipes to the page, working umpteen hours to perfect the photographs, angles and the particular way an herb or a tomato slice looked.

Michael Nelson, our art director, is especially owed a keen sense of gratitude for his vision, his unfailing attention to detail and depth, and his unflagging sense of equanimity. Michael, we also owe you a kitchen full of thanks for the insight and perspective you brought to the design of the ebook (on which we based the design of the print book), the unique looking-glass through which you approach all things design and the time you spent propping and detailing every shot and every page.

Special thanks is due to Emily Richards and Heather Trim, as well as a bevy of Baycrest colleagues, who tested and retested our recipes until they were perfect enough to grace these pages. Ruth Hanley worked her magic to ensure that the recipes themselves were word perfect, spending many hours reviewing and correcting each little comma, semicolon and period. That we have such a fine index is due to Gillian Watts, who categorized not only each and every single recipe but also the mountain of information contained in this collection.

Barnaby Kalan, a wordsmith of the highest order, made our words resonate more deeply, clarified the science and in a profound way made what we wanted to tell you accessible. Thank you, Barnaby. We were so fortunate to have your input.

Without Marsha Rosen there simply would be no nutritional information. In her inimitable, friendly but decisive way, Marsha compiled the nutritionals for each recipe and then chided us until they were in the range she deemed acceptable. Thank you for your steadfastness, Marsha, for your good humour under an avalanche of work and for keeping us on the straight and narrow.

We also owe a pantry full of gratitude to Lillian Chan, whose whimsical and imaginative creativity is evident in the layout and colourful entries that bring each page to

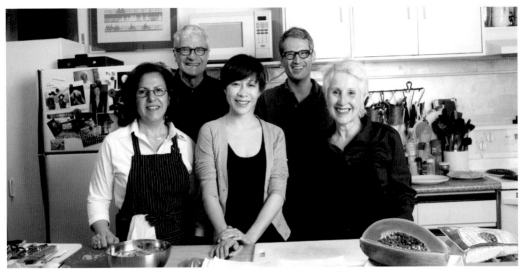

Our creative team extraordinaire. From left to right:
Gina St. Germain, Michael Nelson, Lillian Chan, David Shuken, Ettie Shuken.

life. Lillian knows everything there is to know about ereading and page layouts. She took us neophytes gently by the hand, instructing us on the intricacies and mazelike possibilities of edesign, never once intimidating us with the sheer vastness of her efforts and understanding.

In addition to talent, science and passion, this project, like all projects, needed funding to bring it to life. We were blessed by two organizations that took the leap of faith to provide the funds for all the groceries, development, writing and photography that went into this labour of love. To our supporters both in the Baycrest Foundation and in Cogniciti: thank you.

Thanks is also due to Lynn Posluns, without whose input and dedication this cookbook would not have been possible. She and Karen Baruch laid the foundation for us to proceed and were the initial shepherds who saw it take its fledgling steps. Margi Oksner was seminal in her tireless efforts to bring the book to life, gathering chefs' recipes and collating all the organizing that it entailed. Lori Radke and Corinne Rusch-Drutz were the ones who took the baton last, ensuring that the entire process was seamless, professional and utterly delightful. Without these Women of Baycrest, this book would still be languishing on some kitchen floor.

To our editor at HarperCollins, Brad Wilson, thank you for taking the leap of faith and making this recipe collection and the science that is at its foundation available to so many people. Thanks also to proofreader Tracy Bordian for her incredible eye for detail and to production editor Sarah Howden for guiding the project through to completion. Our cherished baby has grown up in your capable hands and is ready to meet the world.

About the Authors

Carol Greenwood, PhD

Born in Montreal, Carol attributes her love of food and cooking to having a mother who is both an excellent cook and a patient and skilled teacher. She proudly presented her first "homemade" cake to her family at about the age of 5, baked fresh from her new child's oven. This launched her lifelong passion for all things culinary. Her career in science has allowed her to travel worldwide and interact with individuals from many cultures. Through these experiences, she developed an enthusiasm for exploring foods and cuisines from around the globe.

Professionally, after completing her undergraduate studies at MacDonald College of McGill University, Carol received her MSc and PhD from the University of Toronto. It was during her PhD studies that she first started exploring the diet-brain-behaviour relationship. She then furthered this training for several years at MIT in Cambridge, Massachusetts, before returning to Canada.

Carol is currently a senior scientist at the Rotman Research Institute at Baycrest and a professor in the Department of Nutritional Sciences at the University of Toronto. As an expert on the relationship between diet, nutrition and brain health, she frequently lectures and serves on advisory boards both nationally and internationally.

She and her colleagues are working to understand what factors in our diet increase our risk of cognitive loss as we age, and what we can do proactively through our diet to help retain our brain function. Hers was the first research to show that the average North American diet, if consumed in middle age, can contribute to cognitive decline. Now, Carol and her colleagues are using brain-imaging technology to understand the biological factors that connect diet to dementia, and ultimately to identify food strategies that can help to set our brains up for healthy aging.

For her, the culmination of this cookbook fulfills a strong desire to translate current knowledge in nutrition and brain health sciences into accessible information and practical, yet delicious, recipes for all.

Joanna Gryfe

In awe of all things edible, Joanna has turned her passion for food and media into an exciting career.

After working in New York City for *The Rachel Ray Show*, Joanna revamped the show's web site as online food editor and had the amazing opportunity to edit and write for *Rachel Ray's Book of 10*. She returned to Canada, completing the food and media program at George Brown Chef School before her stint on the culinary production team of *Top Chef Canada*. Joanna currently works in Toronto, choosing and buying new television shows for Shaw Media's family of channels, including Food Network Canada.

Daphna Rabinovitch

Daphna Rabinovitch has, for as long as she can remember, been at her happiest in the kitchen. After earning an undergraduate degree from the University of Toronto and a graduate degree in Ottawa, Daphna completed her culinary training at the famed Tante Marie's Cooking School, where she studied both savoury cooking and baking for a year. While there, she trained under Brad Ogden, then-chef at The Campton Place Hotel, and under Jim Dodge at the illustrious Fairmount Hotel. Italy then beckoned, where Daphna worked with Lorenza de Medici at her ancestral home, Badia a Coltibuono, teaching classic Tuscan cooking to travelling groups of North Americans and cooking privately for the family and all social events.

Upon her return to Canada, Daphna became senior pastry chef for the David Wood Food Shops. From the world of pastry, Daphna was then hired by *Canadian Living* magazine as the Test Kitchen director, managing the Test Kitchen and supervising the testing of over 500 published recipes a year. Aside from contributing many recipes and stories herself, Daphna was the editor of *Canadian Living Cooks Step By Step*, a compendium of how-to recipes, which won the Cuisine Canada Culinary Book Award in 1999. A successful stint as co-host (along with Elizabeth Baird and Emily Richards) of the popular *Canadian Living Cooks* on the Food Network followed, where the show aired for four seasons.

After working as a freelance consultant for eight years, Daphna became director of product development and innovation for a local baking manufacturing company, sending cookies, tarts and brownies to all corners of the earth.

Daphna has now returned to her consulting practice, developing recipes for a variety of national and international food companies, consulting on cookbooks, writing about food, assisting food companies as an innovations specialist and food web specialist and teaching at local cooking schools.

References

Introduction

1. Novak, V. and I. Hajjar. The relationship between blood pressure and cognitive function. *Nature Reviews Cardiology.* 7:686–98, 2010.
2. Ledesma, M.D. and C.G. Dotti. Peripheral cholesterol, metabolic disorders and Alzheimer's disease. *Frontiers in Bioscience.* 4:181–94, 2012.
3. Meusel, L., et al. Vascular and metabolic contributors to cognitive decline and dementia risk in older adults with type 2 diabetes. *J Curr Clin Care.* Jan/Feb:6–16, 2012.
4. Larson, E. Prospects for delaying the rising tide of worldwide, late-life dementias. *International Psychogeriatrics.* 22:1196–202, 2010.
5. Alzheimer Society of Canada. About the Brain: Brain Health. http://www.alzheimer.ca/en/About-dementia/About-the-brain/Brain-health.
6. Shatenstein, B., et al. Diet quality and cognition among older adults from the NuAge study. *Exper Gerontol.* 47:353–360, 2012.
7. Parrott, M. and C. Greenwood. Dietary influences on cognitive function with aging: from high-fat diets to healthful eating. *Ann N Y Acad Sci.* 1114:389–97, 2007.
8. Solfrizzi, V., et al. Diet and Alzheimer's disease risk factors or prevention: the current evidence. *Expert Review of Neurotherapeutics.* 11(5):677–708, 2011.
9. Joseph, J., et al. Nutrition, Brain Aging, and Neurodegeneration. *The Journal of Neuroscience* 29:12795–12801, 2009. http://www.jneurosci.org/content/29/41/12795.full.pdf.
10. Morris, M.C., et al. Vitamin E and Cognitive Decline in Older Persons. *Archives of Neurology.* 59(7):1125–1132, 2002. http://archneur.jamanetwork.com/article.aspx?volume=59&issue=7&page=1125.
11. Kronenberg, G. et al. Folic acid, neurodegenerative and neuropsychiatric disease. *Current Molecular Medicine.* 9(3):315–23, 2009.
12. de Lau, L.M. Plasma vitamin B$_{12}$ status and cerebral white-matter lesions. *Journal of Neurology, Neurosurgery & Psychiatry.* 80(2):149–57, 2009.
13. Dangour, A.D. et al. B-vitamins and fatty acids in the prevention and treatment of Alzheimer's disease and dementia: a systematic review. *Journal of Alzheimer's Disease.* 22(1):205–24, 2010.
14. Sorgen, Carol. Eat Smart for a Healthier Brain. WebMD. http://www.webmd.com/diet/guide/eat-smart-healthier-brain.
15. Dietitians of Canada, at http://www.dietitians.ca/.
16. Perry, E. and M.J. Howes. Medicinal plants and dementia therapy: herbal hopes for brain aging? *CNS Neuroscience and Therapeutics.* 17(6):683–98, 2011.
17. Kalaria, R.N. et al. Alzheimer's disease and vascular dementia in developing countries: prevalence, management, and risk factors. *Lancet Neurology.* 7:812–826, 2008.
18. Frautschy, S.A. and G.M. Cole. Why pleiotropic interventions are needed for Alzheimer's disease. *Molecular Neurobiology.* 41(2–3):392–409, 2010.
19. Ng, T.P. et al. Curry consumption and cognitive function in the elderly. *American Journal of Epidemiology.* 164(9):898–906, 2006.
20. Williams, R.J. and J.P. Spencer. Flavonoids, cognition, and dementia: actions, mechanisms, and potential therapeutic utility for Alzheimer disease. *Free Radical Biology and Medicine.* 52(1):35–45, 2012.
21. Chonpathompikunlert, P. et al. Piperine, the main alkaloid of Thai black pepper, protects against neurodegeneration and cognitive impairment in animal model of cognitive deficit like condition of Alzheimer's disease. *Food and Chemical Toxicology.* 48(3):798–802, 2010.
22. Dahl, A. et al. Body mass index across midlife and cognitive change in late life. *Int J Obes* (Lond). 2012 Mar 27. doi: 10.1038/ijo.2012.37.
23. Barnes, D. and K. Yaffe. The projected effect of risk factor reduction on Alzheimer's disease prevalence. *Lancet Neurology.* 10:819–28, 2011.
24. Alzheimer Society of Canada. Alzheimer's Disease: Risk Factors. http://www.alzheimer.ca/en/About-dementia/Alzheimer-s-disease/Risk-factors.
25. Fiocco, A. et al. Sodium intake impacts cognitive function in older adults over 4 years depending on level of physical activity: The NuAge Study. *Neurobiol Aging.* 33(4):829.e21–8, 2012.

CHAPTER 1: Breaking the Fast

1. Bayer-Carter, J. et al. Diet intervention and cerebrospinal fluid biomarkers in amnestic mild cognitive impairment. *Arch Neurol.* 68:743–52, 2011.
2. Sacco, J.E. and V. Tarasuk. Health Canada's proposed discretionary fortification policy is misaligned with the nutritional needs of Canadians. *Journal of Nutrition.* 139(10):1980–1986, 2009.
3. Feart, C. et al. Adherence to a Mediterranean diet, cognitive decline, and risk of dementia. *JAMA.* 302:638–48, 2009.
4. Valls-Pedret, C. et al. Polyphenol-rich foods in the Mediterranean diet are associated with better cognitive function in elderly subjects at high cardiovascular risk. *Journal of Alzheimer's Disease.* 29:773–782, 2012.
5. Alhassan, S. et al. Dietary adherence and weight loss success among overweight women: results from the A TO Z weight loss study. *International Journal of Obesity.* 32(6):985–91, 2008.
6. ESHA. Food Processor. http://www.esha.com/foodprosql.
7. Health Canada. The Canadian Nutrient File. http://www.hc-sc.gc.ca/fn-an/nutrition/fiche-nutri-data/cnf_aboutus-aproposdenous_fcen-eng.php.
8. Ibid. Using the Nutrition Facts Table: % Daily

Value (Fact Sheet). http://www.hc-sc.gc.ca/fn-an/label-etiquet/nutrition/cons/fact-fiche-eng.php.

9. Ibid. Canada's Food Guide: Estimated Energy Requirements. http://www.hc-sc.gc.ca/fn-an/food-guide-aliment/basics-base/1_1_1-eng.php.

10. The National Academies Press. Protein and Amino Acids. Dietary reference intakes for energy, carbohydrate, fibre, fat, fatty acids, cholesterol, protein, and amino acids (macronutrients), p. 589–768. http://www.nap.edu/catalog.php?record_id=10490. Dietary Carbohydrates: Sugars and Starches (ibid., 265–338). Macronutrients and Healthful Diets (ibid., 769–879).

11. Dietitians of Canada. Dietary Fats. http://www.dietitians.ca/Dietitians-Views/Dietary-Fats.aspx.

12. Greenwood, C.E. and G. Winocur. High fat diets, insulin resistance and declining cognitive function. *Neurobiology of Aging.* 26S: S42–S45, 2005.

13. Dietitians of Canada. Food Sources of Fibre. http://www.dietitians.ca/Nutrition-Resources-A-Z/Factsheets/Fibre/Food-Sources-of-Fibre.aspx.

14. Health Canada. Dietary Reference Intakes. http://www.hc-sc.gc.ca/fn-an/nutrition/reference/table/ref_elements_tbl-eng.php.

15. Ibid. Sodium in Canada. http://www.hc-sc.gc.ca/fn-an/nutrition/sodium/index-eng.php.

16. Szajewska, H. and M. Ruszczynski. Systematic review demonstrating that breakfast consumption influences body weight outcomes in children and adolescents in Europe. *Critical Reviews in Food Science & Nutrition.* 50:113–119, 2011.

17. Bazzano, L., et al. Dietary intake of whole and refined grain breakfast cereals and weight gain in men. *Obesity Research.* 13:1952–60, 2005.

18. Wing, R. and S. Phelan. Long-term weight loss maintenance. *American Journal of Clinical Nutrition.* 82(1 Suppl):222S–225S, 2005.

19. Anderson, G. and S. Moore. Dietary proteins in the regulation of food intake and body weight in humans. *Journal of Nutrition.* 134:974S–9S, 2004.

20. Anderson, G. et al. Milk proteins in the regulation of body weight, satiety, food intake and glycemia. Nestle Nutrition Workshop Series. Pediatric Program 67:147–59, 2011.

21. Gilbert, J.-A. et al. Effect of proteins from different sources on body composition. *Nutrition Metabolism & Cardiovascular Diseases.* 21 Suppl 2:B16–31, 2011.

22. Wanders, A. et al. Effects of dietary fibre on subjective appetite, energy intake and body weight: a systematic review of randomized controlled trials. *Obesity Reviews.* 12:724–39, 2011.

23. Ford, H. and G. Frost. Glycaemic index, appetite and body weight. *Proceedings of the Nutrition Society.* 69(2):199–203, 2010.

24. Cline, Tami J. The Nutritional Benefits of Milk—PowerPoint presentation. http://www.docstoc.com/docs/122179264/Microsoft-PowerPoint---04---Cline---The-Nutritional-Benefits-of.

25. Tyler Herbst, S. Eggs. In: *Food Lover's Companion,* 4th edition, Barron's Educational Series. New York: Hauppauge; 2007: 237.

26. Centers for Disease Control and Prevention. Tips to Reduce Your Risk of Salmonella from Eggs. http://www.cdc.gov/Features/SalmonellaEggs/.

27. Harvard Health Publications and Harvard Medical School. Egg Nutrition and Heart Disease: Eggs aren't the dietary demons they're cracked up to be. http://www.health.harvard.edu/press_releases/egg-nutrition.

28. Heart and Stroke Foundation of Canada. Eggs 101. http://www.heartandstroke.com/site/apps/nlnet/content2.aspx?c=ikIQLcMWJtE&b=4869055&ct=7511425.

29. Kang, J., et al. Fruit and vegetable consumption and cognitive decline in aging women. *Annals of Neurology.* 57:713–720, 2005.

30. Joseph, J., et al. Nutrition, Brain Aging, and Neurodegeneration. *The Journal of Neuroscience* 29:12795–12801, 2009. http://www.jneurosci.org/content/29/41/12795.full.pdf.

31. Daviglus, M. et al. National Institutes of Health State-of-the-Science Conference Statement: Preventing Alzheimer's Disease and Cognitive Decline. *NIH Consens State Sci Statements.* 2010 Apr 26–28;27(4):1–30. http://consensus.nih.gov/2010/alzstatement.htm.

32. Barclay, A. et al. Glycemic index, glycemic load, and chronic disease risk: a meta-analysis of observational studies. *American Journal of Clinical Nutrition.* 87:627–37, 2008. http://konopka-dr.de/pdf/Barclay08LowGl.pdf.

33. Wikipedia contributors. Glycemic Index. *Wikipedia, the Free Encyclopedia.* http://en.wikipedia.org/wiki/Glycemic_index.

CHAPTER 2: Morning Brain Boosters

1. Kaplan, R.J. et al. Cognitive performance is associated with glucose regulation in healthy elderly persons and can be enhanced with glucose and dietary carbohydrates. *American Journal of Clinical Nutrition.* 72:825–36, 2000.

2. Owen, L. and S.I. Sunram-Lea. Metabolic Agents That Enhance ATP Can Improve Cognitive Functioning: A Review of the Evidence for Glucose, Oxygen, Pyruvate, Creatine, and L-Carnitine. *Nutrients.* 3:735–755, 2011. http://www.ncbi.nlm.nih.gov/pmc/articles/PMC3257700/?tool=pubmed.

3. Papanikolaou, Y. et al. Better cognitive performance following a low-glycaemic-index compared with a high-glycaemic-index carbohydrate meal in adults with type 2 diabetes. *Diabetologia.* 49:855–62, 2006.

4. Barclay, A. et al. Glycemic index, glycemic load, and chronic disease risk: a meta-analysis of observational studies. *American Journal of Clinical Nutrition.* 87:627–37, 2008. http://konopka-dr.de/pdf/Barclay08LowGl.pdf.

5. Kaplan, R.J. et al. Dietary protein, carbohydrate, and fat enhance memory performance in the healthy elderly. *American Journal of Clinical Nutrition.* 74:687–93, 2001.

6. Smith, A. Effects of caffeine on human behavior.

Food and Chemical Toxicology. 40:1243–55, 2002.

7. Snel, J. and M. Lorist. Effects of caffeine on sleep and cognition. *Progress in Brain Research.* 190:105–17, 2011.

8. Health Canada. Caffeine: It's Your Health. http://www.hc-sc.gc.ca/hl-vs/iyh-vsv/food-aliment/caffeine-eng.php.

9. Tim Hortons. Canadian Nutrition Calculator. http://www.timhortons.com/ca/en/menu/nutrition-calculator.html.

10. Starbucks. Nutritional information for Double Chocolaty Chip Frappucino Blended Crème. http://www.starbucks.com/menu/drinks/frappuccino-blended-beverages/double-chocolaty-chip-frappuccino-blended-creme.

11. Second Cup. Chillatte nutritional information. http://www.secondcup.com/other-drinks/?nutcat=7&productid=36.

12. Oude Griep, L. et al. Colors of fruit and vegetables and 10-year incidence of stroke. *Stroke.* 42:3190–3195, 2011.

13. Parrott, M. and C. Greenwood. Dietary influences on cognitive function with aging: from high-fat diets to healthful eating. *Ann N Y Acad Sci.* 1114:389–97, 2007.

CHAPTER 3: Lunch for All

1. National Institute of General Medical Sciences. Circadian Rhythms Fact Sheet. http://www.nigms.nih.gov/Education/Factsheet_CircadianRhythms.htm.

2. Esquirol, Y. et al. Shift work and cardiovascular risk factors: new knowledge from the past decade. *Archives of Cardiovascular Diseases.* 104(12):636–68, 2011.

3. Pan, A. et al. Rotating night shift work and risk of type 2 diabetes: two prospective cohort studies in women. *PLoS Med.* 2011 Dec;8(12):e1001141.

4. Young, K.W.H. and C.E. Greenwood. Shift in diurnal feeding patterns in nursing home residents with Alzheimer's disease. *Journal of Gerontology Series A: Biological Sciences and Medical Sciences.* 56:M700–M706, 2001.

5. Kang, J. et al. Fruit and vegetable consumption and cognitive decline in aging women. *Annals of Neurology.* 57:713–720, 2005.

CHAPTER 4: Afternoon Brain Boosters

1. Yoon, C. et al. Aging, circadian arousal patterns and cognition. In Park D. & Schwarz N., editors: *Cognitive Aging: A Primer, 2nd Edition.* Philadelphia, PA: Psychology Press, Taylor & Francis; 2008: 353–363.

2. Greenwood, C.E. and G. Winocur. High fat diets, insulin resistance and declining cognitive function. *Neurobiology of Aging.* 26S: S42–S45, 2005.

3. Fiocco, A. et al. Sodium intake impacts cognitive function in older adults over 4 years depending on level of physical activity: The NuAge Study. *Neurobiol Aging.* 33(4):829.e21–8, 2012.

4. Heart and Stroke Foundation. Healthy Eating: Salt. http://www.heartandstroke.com/site/c.ikIQLcM-WJtE/b.3484241/k.6D9D/Healthy_living__Salt.htm.

5. Hitti, Miranda. Pistachios May Lower LDL Cholesterol. *WebMD Health News.* http://www.webmd.com/cholesterol-management/news/20080911/pistachios-may-lower-ldl-cholesterol.

CHAPTER 5: Appetizing Appetizers

1. Rolls, B.J. Sensory-specific satiety. *Nutrition Reviews.* 44(3): 93–101, 1986.

2. Cunnane, S.C. et al. Fish, docosahexaenoic acid and Alzheimer's disease. *Progress in Lipid Research.* 48(5):239–56, 2009.

3. Health Canada. Mercury in Fish—Consumption Advice: Making Informed Choices about Fish. http://www.hc-sc.gc.ca/fn-an/securit/chem-chim/environ/mercur/cons-adv-etud-eng.php.

4. Health Canada. Fish and Seafood Fact Sheets: Farmed Salmon. http://www.ats.agr.gc.ca/seamer/4801-eng.htm.

CHAPTER 6: The Dinner Plate

1. Ibid. Canada's Food Guide: Estimated Energy Requirements. http://www.hc-sc.gc.ca/fn-an/food-guide-aliment/basics-base/1_1_1-eng.php.

2. United States Department of Agriculture. MyPlate. http://www.choosemyplate.gov/.

3. Soni, M. et al. Vitamin D and cognitive function. *Scandinavian Journal of Clinical & Laboratory Investigation.* 72(S243) 70–82, 2012.

4. Annweiler, C., et al. Low serum vitamin D concentrations in Alzheimer's disease: A systematic review and meta-analysis. *Journal of Alzheimer's Disease.* 33(3):659–674, 2013.

5. Self Nutrition Data. Nutrition Facts: Nuts, coconut milk, raw (liquid expressed from grated meat and water). http://nutritiondata.self.com/facts/nut-and-seed-products/3113/2.

6. Hogervorst, E. et al. High tofu intake is associated with worse memory in elderly Indonesian men and women. *Dementia and Geriatric Cognitive Disorders.* 26 (1): 50–7, 2008.

7. White, L.R. et al. Brain aging and midlife tofu consumption. *Journal of the American College of Nutrition.* 19 (2): 242–55, 2000.

8. Clarkson, T.B., et al. The role of soy isoflavones in menopausal health: report of The North American Menopause Society/Wulf H. Utian Translational Science Symposium in Chicago, IL (October 2010). *Menopause.* 18(7):732–753, 2011.

9. United States Department of Agriculture, A.R.S., USDA–Iowa State University Database on the Isoflavone Content of Foods. Release 1.3 - 2002. Nutrient Data Laboratory website. http://www.nal.usda.gov/fnic/foodcomp/Data/isoflav/isoflav.html.

10. Mayo Clinic. Red wine and resveratrol: Good for

your heart? http://www.mayoclinic.com/health/red-wine/hb00089.

11. Tyas, S.L. Alcohol use and the risk of developing Alzheimer's disease. http://pubs.niaaa.nih.gov/publications/arh25-4/299-306.htm.

12. Sun, Q. et al. Alcohol consumption at midlife and successful ageing in women: a prospective cohort analysis in the Nurses' Health Study. *PLoS Medicine.* September; 8(9): e1001090, 2011.

13. Samieri, C., et al. Long-term adherence to the Mediterranean diet is associated with overall cognitive status, but not cognitive decline, in women. *Journal of Nutrition.* 143(4): 493–499, 2013.

14. Hong, J., et al. Alcohol consumption promotes mammary tumor growth and insulin sensitivity. *Cancer Letters.* 294(2): 229–235, 2010.

15. Heart and Stroke Foundation. Excessive Alcohol Consumption. http://www.heartandstroke.com/site/c.ikIQLcMWJtE/b.3484033/k.380A/Excessive_alcohol_consumption.htm.

CHAPTER 7: Delicious Desserts

1. Lemmens, S.G. et al. Influence of consumption of a high-protein vs. high-carbohydrate meal on the physiological cortisol and psychological mood response in men and women. *PLoS One.* 6(2):e16826, 2011, at http://www.ncbi.nlm.nih.gov/pubmed/21304815.

2. Choi, S. et al. Meal ingestion, amino acids and brain neurotransmitters: effects of dietary protein source on serotonin and catecholamine synthesis rates. *Physiology & Behavior.* 98(1–2):156–62, 2009.

3. Scholey, A. et al. Acute neurocognitive effects of epigallocatechin gallate (EGCG). *Appetite.* 58(2):767–70, 2012.

4. Wurtman, R.J. and J.J. Wurtman. Brain serotonin, carbohydrate-craving, obesity and depression. *Obesity Research.* 3(Suppl 4):477S–480S, 1995.

5. Trout, K.K. et al. Insulin sensitivity, food intake, and cravings with premenstrual syndrome: a pilot study. *Journal of Women's Health.* 17(4):657–65, 2008.

6. Peuhkuri, K. et al. Diet promotes sleep duration and quality. *Nutrition Research.* 32(5):309–19, 2012.

7. Miller, A.L. The methylation, neurotransmitter, and antioxidant connections between folate and depression. *Alternative Medicine Review.* 13(3):216–26, 2008.

8. Appleton, K.M. et al. Updated systematic review and meta-analysis of the effects of n-3 long-chain polyunsaturated fatty acids on depressed mood. *American Journal of Clinical Nutrition.* 91(3):757–70, 2010.

Glossary of Cooking Terms

Al dente In Italian, this means "to the tooth"; it describes how pasta should be cooked only until a slight resistance is felt when the cooked pasta is eaten.

Asian chili paste Many different varieties are available, but they are all hot, so use sparingly. Store well-sealed in the refrigerator, where it will keep for several months.

Asian chili sauce Different from Asian chili paste, this is a blend of chilies, vinegar, salt and sugar that may or may not include tomato, dried shrimp, garlic and fresh ginger. Sauces vary from mild and thin to very thick and hot. As a guideline, Southeast Asian chili sauces are sweeter and more garlicky than those from Korea or China. If you want a good all-purpose one, buy sriracha, named for the town in southern Thailand where these sauces were first produced.

Au gratin A dish, either sweet or savoury, topped with cheese or moistened bread crumbs, most often browned in the oven or under the broiler.

Bain marie Basically a double boiler (can be as makeshift as placing a stainless steel bowl over a pot on top of an element, or a pan in a larger roasting pan inside the oven) that provides a stable cooking temperature.

Bake To cook by dry heat in an oven. Best results transpire from not overcrowding your oven to allow for the full circulation of heat. (This is also true when frying in a skillet.)

Batter An uncooked pourable mixture, usually containing eggs and flour, used for coating foods or to make pancakes or cakes. It can be thick or thin.

Blanch To boil food—often vegetables—briefly in boiling water, then immerse them immediately in cold water to stop the cooking process. Blanching can loosen the skin of a tomato, heighten the colour of a green bean and remove the bitterness from an eggplant or the saltiness of other foods.

Blend The mixing together of two or more ingredients until smooth; usually done with a wooden spoon, whisk, mixer or blender.

Boil To heat liquid of any kind until bubbles aggressively break the surface.

Braise A time-honoured slow-cooking method used to tenderize tough cuts of meat. The food is first generally browned over a hot stove and then immersed in liquid and cooked over low heat (either stovetop or in the oven) for an extended amount of time.

Broil Whereby a food is cooked or browned directly under the broiler element in the oven.

Chiffonade To cut leafy-type vegetables into thin, uniformly sized strips.

Chop A method of cutting food into approximately ½-inch pieces.

Cube This generally results in a more uniform size than chopping, which is considered to be coarse. Pieces should be a uniform ½ inch.

Dice The cutting of food into small—generally about ¼ inch in size—equal-sized cubes.

Edamame Young, tender, green soybeans that are boiled and often eaten straight from the pod after being generously salted.

Flake To break off small pieces of fish with a fork to test for doneness or to use in a dish.

Fold A baking technique used to combine a light mixture, such as beaten egg whites, into a heavier mixture, such as whipped cream, to minimize deflation. To fold, use a spatula to cut vertically through the two mixtures right to the bottom of the bowl, then bring some of the heavier mixture up from the bottom to the top; constantly repeat this motion while rotating the bowl.

Fry: Pan-fry The cooking of food in a skillet with just enough oil to coat the bottom of the skillet and to prevent the food from sticking to the pan. **Deep-fry** The cooking of food by submerging it in hot oil. **Stir-fry** The cooking of food in a little oil, usually over high heat, with constant stirring.

Grease The coating of a dish with a fat (e.g., cooking spray, butter or oil) to prevent food from sticking.

Harissa A hot chili sauce common to North Africa; used both in cooking and as a condiment.

Jicama A large bulbous root vegetable with a thin paper-like skin and a sweet, crunchy interior. Usually available from November through May.

Julienne A method of cutting food, most often vegetables, into matchstick-size strips.

Knead The method by which bread is pushed and turned to develop the gluten inside the flour.

Lemongrass A tropical grass with long leaves shaped like blades with a clean lemon aroma and flavour. Generally, only the lower 6 inches of the interior stalk are used. Most ideally used fresh, sliced extremely thinly or chopped very finely.

Lukewarm Refers to a temperature similar to body temperature.

Macerate A method of tenderizing or flavouring fruit by immersing in liquid.

Marinate A method of tenderizing or flavouring meats, poultry or vegetables by soaking in a highly seasoned liquid that tends to include an acid to aid in the tenderization or flavouring.

Mince To chop into very fine pieces.

Miso A fermented soybean paste used in soups, sauces, dressings and marinades. Usually available in a variety of colours (white, yellow and very dark, almost chocolatey) and strengths. For a rounded all-purpose miso, it's best to purchase a yellow miso, which will keep for several weeks in the refrigerator.

Mix To combine two or more ingredients either by stirring, beating or whisking.

Mousse An airy savoury or sweet mixture, lightened by beaten egg whites or whipped cream. Sometimes set with gelatin.

Pinch Generally, about $1/8$ teaspoon, or anything less than $1/4$ teaspoon.

Poach The cooking of foods, generally fish or eggs, by submerging or partially submerging in a simmering liquid.

Purée To mash into a very fine textured mixture, either in a blender, food processor or food mill.

Reduce The process of evaporating liquid in an uncovered pan over high heat to concentrate both flavour and texture.

Refresh Submerging of cooked food in ice water to stop the cooking process and to set colour and flavour.

Roast Cooking foods uncovered in a dry oven.

Sauté Cooking in a skillet, over high heat, while stirring.

Score Whereby shallow incisions are made in the skin, flesh or fat of a food before cooking to help flavours penetrate or to help maintain a food's shape or to tenderize a food. Can also refer to the cutting of sweet dessert bars into uniform portions.

Sear Browning meat or poultry quickly in a skillet or in the oven over high heat.

Simmer Heating a liquid so that it just barely reaches a bubble.

Steam Cooking food in a covered container over a small amount of liquid.

Stew Slow-cooking a food submerged in a flavourful liquid either on the stovetop or in an oven at low heat.

Thai chilies The most common available in North America are the small hot bird pepper chilies. Red pepper chilies are milder than the green or unripe variety.

Tofu Iron rich, tofu is made from liquid extracted from ground, cooked soybeans. The resulting curds are drained and pressed. The firmness of the consequent tofu is determined by how much whey has been pressed out. Tofu is available in soft, semi-firm, firm and extra firm.

Wasabi A pungent green rhizome, akin to horseradish.

Whip Beating to soft or stiff peaks using a whisk or electric mixer.

INDEX

A

agave, 255
alcohol, 223
almonds, 129–30
    Almond Ginger Tart, 261
    Fresh Fried and Roasted Almonds with Spicy
        Marinated Olives, 168
    Golden Quinoa with Raisins and Almonds, 109
    Thai-Inspired Almond and Peanut Dipping
        Sauce, 140
appetizers
    Coconut Shrimp, 161
    Cinnamon-Skewered Lamb Kebabs, 164
    Figs with Walnuts, Gorgonzola and Balsamic
        Drizzle, 162
    Fresh Fried and Roasted Almonds with Spicy
        Marinated Olives, 168
    Malaysian Fish Cakes with Easy Dipping
        Sauce, 155–56
    Persian Platter, 160
    Roasted Squash Soup with Roasted Pumpkin
        Seeds, 166
    Salmon Tartare with Wasabi-Spiked Avocado
        "Mousse," 147
    Summer Rolls with Thai Dipping Sauce, 150
    Sushi Stacks, 153
    Thai Shrimp on Lemongrass Skewers, 148
    Whitefish "Tartare," 159
appetizers, skewered, 148, 164
apples
    buying and storing, 246
    varieties, 48
    Autumn Fruit Turnovers, 46
    Chicken with Rhubarb Chutney over Dark
        Greens, 83
    Farfalle with Walnuts, Goat Cheese, Arugula
        and Caramelized Apples, 230–32
    On-the-Go Fruit Salad, 49
    Winter Fruit Compote, 34
apricots, 60
    dried, 60
    Bet-You-Can't-Eat-Just-One Cereal Cookies, 61
    Winter Fruit Compote, 34
Argentinean Steak Sandwich, 73
arugula, 84
    Chickpea and Herb Salad with Warm Lemon
        Dressing, 93
    Farfalle with Walnuts, Goat Cheese, Arugula
        and Caramelized Apples, 230–32
    Grilled Salmon with Green Salad and Apple
        Vinaigrette, 95
    Scallop Niçoise Salad, 88
Asian Greens and Rice Noodle Salad, 87
Asian Salmon Burgers, 187
asparagus
    Basa and Asparagus Steamed in White Wine, 183

    Four-Season Frittata, 77
    Pesto Orzo with Roasted Trout and Peas, 80–81
Autumn Fruit Turnovers, 46
avocado
    Chocolate Avocado Cupcakes, 263
    Corn, Black Bean and Tomato Salad, 97
    Haddock Wraps with Crunchy Southwestern
        Salad, 179
    Halibut with Two Tomato and Avocado Salsa, 184
    Salmon Tartare with Wasabi-Spiked Avocado
        "Mousse," 147
    Sushi Stacks, 153

B

Banana Bread with Flaxseed and Wheat Germ, 58
bananas
    Banana Bread with Flaxseed and Wheat Germ,
        58
    Parliament Hill Smoothie, 36
bánh mì, 75
baozi, 75
barley, 106
    Sweet Pepper and Barley Risotto Tart with
        Spinach and Pine Nuts, 111–12
bars/squares
    Date–Pecan Oatmeal Squares, 54
    Granola Bites with Figs and Dates, 57
    Squash Squares with a Whole-Wheat Crust,
        53
Basa and Asparagus Steamed in White Wine, 183
beans, 182. *See also* beans, green; chickpeas
    Black Bean Soup, 198
    Breakfast Burritos, 31
    Corn, Black Bean and Tomato Salad, 97
    Herbed Fish Stew, 181
    Mediterranean Stuffed Peppers, 102
    Ribollita, 197
    Scallop Niçoise Salad, 88
    Spicy Smoky Succotash, 202
beans, green
    Four-Season Frittata, 77
    Grilled Salmon with Green Salad and Apple
        Vinaigrette, 95
    Malaysian Fish Cakes with Easy Dipping
        Sauce, 155–56
    Provençal-Style Rabbit with Polenta, 214–17
    Scallop Niçoise Salad, 88
    Toasted Sesame Green Beans, 189
bean sprouts
    Peanut Coleslaw, 219
beef
    Argentinean Steak Sandwich, 73
    Cinnamon-Skewered Lamb Kebabs, 164
    Flank Steak with Pine Nut, Herb and Currant
        Stuffing, 224
    Thyme-Roasted Beef Tenderloin with Three-
        Mushroom Ragout, 221–22

berries. *See also* blueberries; cranberries
    The Most Delicious Nutritious Berry Crisp
      Ever, 248–49
    Parliament Hill Smoothie, 36
Bet-You-Can't-Eat-Just-One Cereal Cookies, 61
Bite-Size Nut Scones, 141
Black Bean Soup, 198
blueberries
    Blintz Envelopes with Blueberries, 9–10
    Cranberry Pumpkin Seed Crunchy Snack, 124
    Delicious Low-Fat, High-Fibre Blueberry
      Muffins, 44
    Warm Blueberry Brown Butter Cake Bites,
      258–60
    Whole-Wheat Oatmeal Blueberry Pancakes
      with Ricotta Topping, 6
bok choy, 84
    Asian Greens and Rice Noodle Salad, 87
bran
    The Most Delicious Nutritious Berry Crisp
      Ever, 248–49
bread
    Breakfast Crostini with Ricotta, Honey and
      Figs, 27
    Fruit Bruschetta, 28
    Overnight Swiss Chard, Sun-Dried Tomato and
      Mushroom Strata, 21
    Whitefish "Tartare," 159
    biscuits and scones:
      Bite-Size Nut Scones, 141
      Cheese and Herb Biscuits, 64
    flatbreads:
      Breakfast Pizza with Potatoes and Tomato,
        62
      Pear, Spinach and Blue Cheese Flatbread
        with Onion Jam, 115
    pitas:
      Argentinean Steak Sandwich, 73
      Persian Platter, 160
      Saag Paneer Sandwich, 74
      Shakshuka with Warmed Zaatar Pita, 13–14
    quick breads:
      Banana Bread with Flaxseed and Wheat
        Germ, 58
    tortillas:
      Breakfast Burritos, 31
      Haddock Wraps with Crunchy Southwestern
        Salad, 179
Breakfast Burritos, 31
Breakfast Crostini with Ricotta, Honey and Figs,
    27
Breakfast Pizza with Potatoes and Tomato, 62
breakfast
    and body weight, 3
broccoli, 84
    Cream of Broccoli Soup, 100
    Four-Season Frittata, 77
Brussels sprouts, 84
    Scallop Niçoise Salad, 88
bulgur, 106

Cracked Wheat and Chayote or Zucchini Pilaf,
    213
burgers
    Asian Salmon Burgers, 187
butter, 50
    how to brown, 260
buttermilk, 11
    Bite-Size Nut Scones, 141
    Cheese and Herb Biscuits, 64
    Delicious Low-Fat, High-Fibre Blueberry
      Muffins, 44
    Fennel-Spiced Asiago Biscotti, 123

C

cabbage, 84
    Hot and Sour Soup, 195
    Marinated Tofu over Wilted Napa Cabbage and
      Vegetables, 193–94
    Peanut Coleslaw, 219
    Ribollita, 197
caffeine, 41–42
cakes
    Sponge Cake with Peaches Macerated in White
      Wine, 253–54
    Warm Blueberry Brown Butter Cake Bites,
      258–60
    Vanilla Yogurt Cake with Marmalade Glaze,
      267
calories, 17–18
Canada's Food Guide, 173
canola oil, 51
Caramelized Onion and Tomato Phyllo Tart, 78
carbohydrates, xviii
    and cognitive function, 41
    in diet, xviii
carrots
    Asian Greens and Rice Noodle Salad, 87
    Bet-You-Can't-Eat-Just-One Cereal Cookies, 61
    Crunchy Southwestern Salad, 180
    Hot and Sour Soup, 195
    Marinated Tofu over Wilted Napa Cabbage and
      Vegetables, 193–94
    Moroccan Chicken Stew with Couscous and
      Homemade Harissa, 203–4
    Peanut Coleslaw, 219
    Ribollita, 197
cashews, 131
cauliflower, 84
    Tandoori-Spiced Lamb with Roasted
      Cauliflower Purée, 225–26
celery
    Crunchy Southwestern Salad, 180
    Grilled Salmon with Green Salad and Apple
      Vinaigrette, 95
    Shaved Green Salad with Spicy Grilled Shrimp,
      86
cereal
    Easy Maple Granola, 29
cereal (as ingredient)
    Bet-You-Can't-Eat-Just-One Cereal Cookies, 61
    Granola Bites with Figs and Dates, 57

Granola Parfait, 29
Ceviche Lettuce Wraps, 98
cheese
    Cheese and Herb Biscuits, 64
    Fennel-Spiced Asiago Biscotti, 123
    Figs with Walnuts, Gorgonzola and Balsamic
      Drizzle, 162
    Four-Season Frittata, 77
    Overnight Swiss Chard, Sun-Dried Tomato and
      Mushroom Strata, 21
    Pear, Spinach and Blue Cheese Flatbread with
      Onion Jam, 115
    Roasted Fruit and Vegetable Stuffed Chicken,
      206
cheese, cheddar
    Breakfast Burritos, 31
    Breakfast Pizza with Potatoes and Tomato, 62
    Cheese and Herb Biscuits, 64
    Four-Season Frittata, 77
cheese, cottage, 11
    Blintz Envelopes with Blueberries, 9–10
    Squash, Spinach and Onion Lasagna, 234–35
cheese, feta
    Greek-Style Vinaigrette, 92
    Persian Platter, 160
    Shakshuka with Warmed Zaatar Pita, 13–14
cheese, goat
    Farfalle with Walnuts, Goat Cheese, Arugula
      and Caramelized Apples, 230–32
    Thin-Crust Pizza with Balsamic-Glazed
      Tomatoes and Pesto, 113–14
cheese, mozzarella
    Saag Paneer Sandwich, 74
    Squash, Spinach and Onion Lasagna, 234–35
cheese, Parmesan
    Chickpea and Herb Salad with Warm Lemon
      Dressing, 93
    Parmesan and Pepper Wonton Crackers, 134
    Pesto Orzo with Roasted Trout and Peas, 80–81
    Polenta, 217
    Ribollita, 197
    Sweet Pepper and Barley Risotto Tart with
      Spinach and Pine Nuts, 111–12
cheese, ricotta
    Breakfast Crostini with Ricotta, Honey and
      Figs, 27
    Persian Platter, 160
    Whole-Wheat Oatmeal Blueberry Pancakes
      with Ricotta Topping, 6
cherries
    Chili Chocolate Bark with Cherries and
      Pistachios, 125
    Persian Platter, 160
chicken. See also turkey
    Chicken with Rhubarb Chutney over Dark
      Greens, 83
    Four-Season Frittata, 77
    Grilled Chicken with Pomegranate Vinaigrette,
      207
    Provençal-Style Rabbit with Polenta, 214–17

    Moroccan Chicken Stew with Couscous and
      Homemade Harissa, 203–4
    Peruvian-Spiced Grilled Chicken with Cracked
      Wheat and Chayote or Zucchini Pilaf, 212
    Roasted Fruit and Vegetable Stuffed Chicken,
      206
    Spicy Honeyed Chicken Thighs with Peanut
      Coleslaw, 218–19
    Thin-Crust Pizza with Balsamic-Glazed
      Tomatoes, Goat Cheese and Pesto, 113–14
chickpeas
    Chickpea and Herb Salad with Warm Lemon
      Dressing, 93
    Iberian Chickpea Soup, 199
    Indian-Spiced Chickpeas, 127
    Moroccan Chicken Stew with Couscous and
      Homemade Harissa, 203–4
chocolate
    Chili Chocolate Bark with Cherries and
      Pistachios, 125
    Chocolate Avocado Cupcakes, 263
    Chocolate Ravioli, 262
cholesterol, xviii–xix
    in eggs, 17
Cinnamon-Skewered Lamb Kebabs, 164
circadian rhythms, 69
    in cognitive function, 119
citrus fruits, 152, 257. See also grapefruit, lemons;
  limes; oranges
    Citrus Vinaigrette, 92
    Warm Citrus Casserole, 257
cocoa
    Meringue Cups with Strawberry Rhubarb
      Topping, 265–66
coconut
    Coconut Shrimp, 161
    Malaysian Fish Cakes with Easy Dipping
      Sauce, 155–56
coconut milk
    Poached Coconut Fish, 186
    Thai Shrimp on Lemongrass Skewers, 148
coffee, 41–42
collard greens, 85
cookies
    Bet-You-Can't-Eat-Just-One Cereal Cookies,
      61
    Fennel-Spiced Asiago Biscotti, 123
coriander (fresh)
    Argentinean Steak Sandwich, 73
    Asian Salmon Burgers, 187
    Crunchy Southwestern Salad, 180
    Haddock Wraps with Crunchy Southwestern
      Salad, 179–80
    Poached Coconut Fish, 186
    Thai Shrimp on Lemongrass Skewers, 148
corn
    Corn, Black Bean and Tomato Salad, 97
    Crunchy Southwestern Salad, 180
    Four-Season Frittata, 77
    Spicy Smoky Succotash, 202

cornmeal, 106
    Polenta, 217
couscous, 106
    Cracked Wheat and Chayote or Zucchini Pilaf, 213
    Moroccan Chicken Stew with Couscous and Homemade Harissa, 203–4
crackers
    Parmesan and Pepper Wonton Crackers, 134
    Seaweed and Sesame Wonton Crackers, 133
cranberries
    dried, 55
    Bet-You-Can't-Eat-Just-One Cereal Cookies, 61
    Cranberry Pumpkin Seed Crunchy Snack, 124
    Turkey Shepherd's Pie with Mushrooms, Spinach, Cranberries and Sweet Potatoes, 209–10
    Wild Rice Salad, 108
    Winter Fruit Compote, 34
Cream of Broccoli Soup, 100
Crème Caramel, 250
cruciferous vegetables, 23, 84–85
Crunchy Southwestern Salad, 180
cucumber
    Shaved Green Salad with Spicy Grilled Shrimp, 86
    Summer Rolls with Thai Dipping Sauce, 150
    Sushi Stacks, 153
currants, 60
    Curried Lentil and Wheatberry Salad with Mango, 105
    Flank Steak with Pine Nut, Herb and Currant Stuffing, 224
Curried Lentil and Wheatberry Salad with Mango, 105

D

daikon, 85
dairy products, 3, 11–12, 14–15, 19. *See also* cheese; milk
    including in diet, 174–75
dates, 59
    Date–Pecan Oatmeal Squares, 54
    Granola Bites with Figs and Dates, 57
Delicious Low-Fat, High-Fibre Blueberry Muffins, 44
depression, 239–40
    omega-3 fats and, 240
desserts
    Almond Ginger Tart, 261
    Autumn Fruit Turnovers, 46
    Banana Bread with Flaxseed and Wheat Germ, 58
    Chili Chocolate Bark with Cherries and Pistachios, 125
    Chocolate Avocado Cupcakes, 263
    Chocolate Ravioli, 262
    Crème Caramel, 250
    Date–Pecan Oatmeal Squares, 54
    Granola Bites with Figs and Dates, 57
    Mango and Fennel Granita, 243

    Meringue Cups with Strawberry Rhubarb Topping, 265–66
    The Most Delicious Nutritious Berry Crisp Ever, 248–49
    Roasted Cinnamon Plums, 244
    Sponge Cake with Peaches Macerated in White Wine, 253–54
    Squash Squares with a Whole-Wheat Crust, 53
    Vanilla Yogurt Cake with Marmalade Glaze, 267
    Warm Blueberry Brown Butter Cake Bites, 258–60
    Warm Citrus Casserole, 257
dips/dipping sauces
    Easy Dipping Sauce, 156
    Roasted Edamame Bean Dip, 138
    Thai-Inspired Almond and Peanut Dipping Sauce, 140
dressings/vinaigrettes (salad)
    Apple Vinaigrette, 95
    Citrus Vinaigrette, 92
    Greek-Style Vinaigrette, 92
    Peanut Coleslaw, 218
    Pesto Sauce, 80
    Pomegranate Vinaigrette, 207
    Sun-dried Tomato Vinaigrette, 92
    Tarragon Vinaigrette, 86

E

Easy Dipping Sauce, 156
Easy Maple Granola, 29
edamame
    Asian Greens and Rice Noodle Salad, 87
    Roasted Edamame Bean Dip, 138
eggplant
    Argentinean Steak Sandwich, 73
    Mediterranean Stuffed Peppers, 102
eggs, 16–17
    Almond Ginger Tart, 261
    Crème Caramel, 250
    Four-Season Frittata, 77
    Meringue Cups with Strawberry Rhubarb Topping, 265–66
    Morning Hash with Faux Poached Eggs, 19
    Overnight Swiss Chard, Sun-Dried Tomato and Mushroom Strata, 21
    Shakshuka with Warmed Zaatar Pita, 13–14
    Sponge Cake with Peaches Macerated in White Wine, 253–54
    Squash Squares with a Whole-Wheat Crust, 53
egg substitutes, 17
estrogen, 190

F

falafel, 75
Farfalle with Walnuts, Goat Cheese, Arugula and Caramelized Apples, 230–32
farro, 106
fats, cooking, 50–51
fats, dietary
    and brain health, 157–58
    and cholesterol, xviii–ix

flavour without fat, 152
monounsaturated, 50
omega-3, 50
and overeating, 145
fennel (bulb)
Basa and Asparagus Steamed in White Wine, 183
Crunchy Southwestern Salad, 180
Fennel-Spiced Asiago Biscotti, 123
Herbed Fish Stew, 181
Mango and Fennel Granita, 243
Shaved Green Salad with Spicy Grilled Shrimp, 86
fibre, xiii, xix
health benefits, xiii
figs
dried, 60
Breakfast Crostini with Ricotta, Honey and Figs, 27
Figs with Walnuts, Gorgonzola and Balsamic Drizzle, 162
Granola Bites with Figs and Dates, 57
Winter Fruit Compote, 34
fish, 158. *See also* salmon; seafood
Basa and Asparagus Steamed in White Wine, 183
Ceviche Lettuce Wraps, 98
Haddock Wraps with Crunchy Southwestern Salad, 179
Halibut with Two Tomato and Avocado Salsa, 184
Herbed Fish Stew, 181
Malaysian Fish Cakes with Easy Dipping Sauce, 155–56
Pesto Orzo with Roasted Trout and Peas, 80–81
Poached Coconut Fish, 186
Sushi Stacks, 153
Whitefish "Tartare," 159
Flank Steak with Pine Nut, Herb and Currant Stuffing, 224
flaxseeds, 135
Banana Bread with Flaxseed and Wheat Germ, 58
The Most Delicious Nutritious Berry Crisp Ever, 248–49
flours, 55
folate, xiii
Four-Season Frittata, 77
Fresh Fried and Roasted Almonds with Spicy Marinated Olives, 168
fruit. *See also* berries; fruit, dried; fruit juices; specific fruits
fresh, 246–47
frozen, 211
Fruit Bruschetta, 28
Meringue Cups with Strawberry Rhubarb Topping, 265–66
The Most Delicious Nutritious Berry Crisp Ever, 248–49
Warm Citrus Casserole, 257

fruit, dried
Autumn Fruit Turnovers, 46
Breakfast Burritos, 31
Granola Bites with Figs and Dates, 57
Winter Fruit Compote, 34
fruit juices
Flank Steak with Pine Nut, Herb and Currant Stuffing, 224
Grilled Salmon with Green Salad and Apple Vinaigrette, 95

G
garlic
Argentinean Steak Sandwich, 73
Basa and Asparagus Steamed in White Wine, 183
Harissa, 204
Peruvian-Spiced Grilled Chicken with Cracked Wheat and Chayote or Zucchini Pilaf, 212
Pesto Orzo with Roasted Trout and Peas, 80–81
Roasted Tomato and Garlic Soup with Rice, 101
Shakshuka with Warmed Zaatar Pita, 13–14
Thai Dipping Sauce, 151
Thai-Inspired Almond and Peanut Dipping Sauce, 140
Turkey Shepherd's Pie with Mushrooms, Spinach, Cranberries and Sweet Potatoes, 209–10
ginger
Almond Ginger Tart, 261
Asian Greens and Rice Noodle Salad, 87
Asian Salmon Burgers, 187
Hot and Sour Soup, 195
Peanut Coleslaw, 219
Poached Coconut Fish, 186
Roasted Edamame Bean Dip, 138
Tandoori-Spiced Lamb with Roasted Cauliflower Purée, 225–26
Thai-Inspired Almond and Peanut Dipping Sauce, 140
Thai Shrimp on Lemongrass Skewers, 148
glucose
and cognitive function, 32
glycemic index, 32–33
Golden Quinoa with Raisins and Almonds, 109
grains. *See also* oats; rice
and hunger, 3–4
including in diet, 106–7
Cracked Wheat and Chayote or Zucchini Pilaf, 213
Curried Lentil and Wheatberry Salad with Mango, 105
Easy Maple Granola, 29
Golden Quinoa with Raisins and Almonds, 109
Moroccan Chicken Stew with Couscous and Homemade Harissa, 203–4
Polenta, 217
Sweet Pepper and Barley Risotto Tart with Spinach and Pine Nuts, 111–12

granola
    Easy Maple Granola, 29
    Granola Bites with Figs and Dates, 57
    Granola Parfait, 29
Granola Bites with Figs and Dates, 57
Granola Parfait, 29
grapefruit
    Warm Citrus Casserole, 257
Greek-Style Vinaigrette, 92
greens. *See also* arugula; lettuce; Swiss chard
    cruciferous vegetables, 23, 84–85
    Asian Greens and Rice Noodle Salad, 87
    Easy Kale Chips, 137
Grilled Chicken with Pomegranate Vinaigrette, 207
Grilled Salmon with Green Salad and Apple
    Vinaigrette, 95

H

Haddock Wraps with Crunchy Southwestern Salad,
    179
Halibut with Two Tomato and Avocado Salsa, 184
Harissa, 204
hazelnuts, 130
healthy eating
    and brain health, ix–x
herbs. *See also* coriander
    Argentinean Steak Sandwich, 73
    Cheese and Herb Biscuits, 64
    Chickpea and Herb Salad with Warm Lemon
        Dressing, 93
    Flank Steak with Pine Nut, Herb and Currant
        Stuffing, 224
    Herbed Fish Stew, 181
    Persian Platter, 160
    Pesto Orzo with Roasted Trout and Peas, 80–81
    Summer Rolls with Thai Dipping Sauce, 150
honey, 255
    Breakfast Crostini with Ricotta, Honey and
        Figs, 27
    Granola Bites with Figs and Dates, 57
    Spicy Honeyed Chicken Thighs with Peanut
        Coleslaw, 218–19
    Squash Squares with a Whole-Wheat Crust, 53
hormone replacement therapy (HRT), 190–91
hors d'oeuvres, 145
Hot and Sour Soup, 195

I

Iberian Chickpea Soup, 199
Indian-Spiced Chickpeas, 127
isoflavones, 190–92

J

jicama, 277
    Corn, Black Bean and Tomato Salad, 97
    Crunchy Southwestern Salad, 180

K

kale, 85
    Easy Kale Chips, 137
kiwi, 247

L

lamb
    Cinnamon-Skewered Lamb Kebabs, 164
    Lamb Stew with Root Vegetables, 229
    Tandoori-Spiced Lamb with Roasted
        Cauliflower Purée, 225–26
leeks
    Basa and Asparagus Steamed in White Wine,
        183
    Herbed Fish Stew, 181
    Lamb Stew with Root Vegetables, 229
    Thyme-Roasted Beef Tenderloin with Three-
        Mushroom Ragout, 221–22
legumes. *See also* beans; chickpeas
    Curried Lentil and Wheatberry Salad with
        Mango, 105
lemongrass
    how to bruise, 186
    Poached Coconut Fish, 186
    Thai Shrimp on Lemongrass Skewers, 148
lemons
    Chickpea and Herb Salad with Warm Lemon
        Dressing, 93
    Fresh Fried and Roasted Almonds with Spicy
        Marinated Olives, 168
    Gremolata, 214–16
    Lemon Thyme Turkey with Spicy Smoky
        Succotash, 200
lentils
    Curried Lentil and Wheatberry Salad with
        Mango, 105
lettuce
    Ceviche Lettuce Wraps, 98
    Crunchy Southwestern Salad, 180
    Grilled Salmon with Green Salad and Apple
        Vinaigrette, 95
    Haddock Wraps with Crunchy Southwestern
        Salad, 179
    Malaysian Fish Cakes with Easy Dipping
        Sauce, 155–56
limes
    Ceviche Lettuce Wraps, 98
    Easy Dipping Sauce, 156
    Haddock Wraps with Crunchy Southwestern
        Salad, 179
    Poached Coconut Fish, 186
    Thai Shrimp on Lemongrass Skewers, 148

M

macadamia nuts, 131
Malaysian Fish Cakes with Easy Dipping Sauce,
    155–56
mango, 151, 247
    Curried Lentil and Wheatberry Salad with
        Mango, 105
    Mango and Fennel Granita, 243
    On-the-Go Fruit Salad, 49
    Summer Rolls with Thai Dipping Sauce, 150
maple syrup, 255–56
    Cranberry Pumpkin Seed Crunchy Snack, 124

Easy Maple Granola, 29
Granola Bites with Figs and Dates, 57
margarine, 50
Marinated Tofu over Wilted Napa Cabbage and
Vegetables, 193–94
mayonnaise alternatives, 76
Mediterranean diet, xv, 223
Mediterranean ingredients, xv
Mediterranean Stuffed Peppers, 102
Provençal-Style Rabbit with Polenta, 214–17
menopause, 190–92
Meringue Cups with Strawberry Rhubarb Topping,
265–66
milk, 11. *See also* buttermilk
Crème Caramel, 250
Overnight Swiss Chard, Sun-Dried Tomato and
Mushroom Strata, 21
Parliament Hill Smoothie, 36
Squash, Spinach and Onion Lasagna, 234–35
Whole-Wheat Oatmeal Blueberry Pancakes
with Ricotta Topping, 6
minerals
Miso-Glazed Tofu with Toasted Sesame Green
Beans, 188
mood-altering effects of food, 239–41
Morning Hash with Faux Poached Eggs, 19
Moroccan Chicken Stew with Couscous and
Homemade Harissa, 203–4
The Most Delicious Nutritious Berry Crisp Ever,
248–49
muffins
Delicious Low-Fat, High-Fibre Blueberry
Muffins, 44
mushrooms
Hot and Sour Soup, 195
Overnight Swiss Chard, Sun-Dried Tomato and
Mushroom Strata, 21
Poached Coconut Fish, 186
Ribollita, 197
Thyme-Roasted Beef Tenderloin with Three-
Mushroom Ragout, 221–22
Turkey Shepherd's Pie with Mushrooms,
Spinach, Cranberries and Sweet Potatoes,
209–10
mustard greens, 85

N

nectarines, 246
noodles. *See also* pasta
Asian Greens and Rice Noodle Salad, 87
Ceviche Lettuce Wraps, 98
nori
Seaweed and Sesame Wonton Crackers, 133
Sushi Stacks, 153
nuts. *See also* specific nuts
Easy Maple Granola, 29
Homemade Nut Butter in Minutes, 37
Southwestern-Spiced Nuts, 128

O

oats, 55
Bet-You-Can't-Eat-Just-One Cereal Cookies, 61
Cranberry Pumpkin Seed Crunchy Snack, 124
Date–Pecan Oatmeal Squares, 54
Delicious Low-Fat, High-Fibre Blueberry
Muffins, 44
Easy Maple Granola, 29
The Most Delicious Nutritious Berry Crisp
Ever, 248–49
Whole-Wheat Oatmeal Blueberry Pancakes
with Ricotta Topping, 6
oils, 50–51
okra
South African Peanut Stew, 233
olive oil, 51
olives
pitting, 114
Fresh Fried and Roasted Almonds with Spicy
Marinated Olives, 168
Provençal-Style Rabbit with Polenta, 214–17
Thin-Crust Pizza with Balsamic-Glazed
Tomatoes, Goat Cheese and Pesto, 113–14
omega-3 fatty acids, xii, 157–58
and depression, 240
including in diet, 157–58
omega-6 fatty acids, 157
onions
Caramelized Onion and Tomato Phyllo Tart, 78
Chicken Stew with Couscous and Homemade
Harissa, 203–4
Pear, Spinach and Blue Cheese Flatbread with
Onion Jam, 115
Squash, Spinach and Onion Lasagna, 234–35
On-the-Go Fruit Salad, 49
oranges
Autumn Fruit Turnovers, 46
Date–Pecan Oatmeal Squares, 54
Vanilla Yogurt Cake with Marmalade Glaze, 267
Warm Citrus Casserole, 257
Wild Rice Salad, 108
Winter Fruit Compote, 34
Overnight Swiss Chard, Sun-Dried Tomato and
Mushroom Strata, 21

P

pancakes
Whole-Wheat Oatmeal Blueberry Pancakes
with Ricotta Topping, 6
panini, 75
papaya, 247
Ceviche Lettuce Wraps, 98
Parliament Hill Smoothie, 36
Parmesan and Pepper Wonton Crackers, 134
parsnip
Lamb Stew with Root Vegetables, 229
pasta. *See also* noodles
Curried Lentil and Wheatberry Salad with
Mango, 105
Farfalle with Walnuts, Goat Cheese, Arugula
and Caramelized Apples, 230–32

Four-Season Frittata, 77
Pesto Orzo with Roasted Trout and Peas,
  80–81
Squash, Spinach and Onion Lasagna, 234–35
pastry
  Autumn Fruit Turnovers, 46
  Caramelized Onion and Tomato Phyllo Tart, 78
  Squash Squares with a Whole-Wheat Crust, 53
peaches, 246
  Fruit Bruschetta, 28
  Peaches Macerated in White Wine, 254
  Roasted Fruit and Vegetable Stuffed Chicken,
    206
  Sponge Cake with Peaches Macerated in White
    Wine, 253–54
  Peanut Coleslaw, 219
peanuts, 131
  Peanut Coleslaw, 219
  South African Peanut Stew, 233
  Summer Rolls with Thai Dipping Sauce, 150
  Thai-Inspired Almond and Peanut Dipping
    Sauce, 140
pears, 246
  Autumn Fruit Turnovers, 46
  Pear, Spinach and Blue Cheese Flatbread with
    Onion Jam, 115
  Winter Fruit Compote, 34
peas (green)
  Asian Greens and Rice Noodle Salad, 87
  Four-Season Frittata, 77
  Hot and Sour Soup, 195
  Marinated Tofu over Wilted Napa Cabbage and
    Vegetables, 193–94
  Pesto Orzo with Roasted Trout and Peas, 80–81
  Poached Coconut Fish, 186
pecans, 130
  Cracked Wheat and Chayote or Zucchini Pilaf,
    213
  Cranberry Pumpkin Seed Crunchy Snack, 124
  Date–Pecan Oatmeal Squares, 54
  Granola Bites with Figs and Dates, 57
  Warm Blueberry Brown Butter Cake Bites,
    258–60
  Wild Rice Salad, 108
peppers, hot
  Black Bean Soup, 198
  Ceviche Lettuce Wraps, 98
  Haddock Wraps with Crunchy Southwestern
    Salad, 179
  Harissa, 204
  Malaysian Fish Cakes with Easy Dipping
    Sauce, 155–56
  Poached Coconut Fish, 186
  Roasted Tomato and Garlic Soup with Rice, 101
  Saag Paneer Sandwich, 74
  Spicy Smoky Succotash, 202
  Thai-Inspired Almond and Peanut Dipping
    Sauce, 140
  Thai Shrimp on Lemongrass Skewers,
    148

peppers, sweet
  roasting, 114
  Argentinean Steak Sandwich, 73
  Curried Lentil and Wheatberry Salad with
    Mango, 105
  Four-Season Frittata, 77
  Marinated Tofu over Wilted Napa Cabbage and
    Vegetables, 193–94
  Mediterranean Stuffed Peppers, 102
  Peanut Coleslaw, 219
  Roasted Fruit and Vegetable Stuffed Chicken,
    206
  Shakshuka with Warmed Zaatar Pita, 13–14
  Spicy Smoky Succotash, 202
  Sweet Pepper and Barley Risotto Tart with
    Spinach and Pine Nuts, 111–12
  Thin-Crust Pizza with Balsamic-Glazed
    Tomatoes, Goat Cheese and Pesto, 113–14
Persian Platter, 160
Peruvian-Spiced Grilled Chicken with Cracked
  Wheat and Chayote or Zucchini Pilaf, 212
pesto
  Pesto Orzo with Roasted Trout and Peas, 80–81
  Thin-Crust Pizza with Balsamic-Glazed
    Tomatoes, Goat Cheese and Pesto, 113–14
phyllo dough
  Autumn Fruit Turnovers, 46
  Caramelized Onion and Tomato Phyllo Tart, 78
phytochemicals
  and brain health, xi–xii, xiii–xiv
pineapple, 247
pine nuts, 130
  Fennel-Spiced Asiago Biscotti, 123
  Flank Steak with Pine Nut, Herb and Currant
    Stuffing, 224
  Sweet Pepper and Barley Risotto Tart with
    Spinach and Pine Nuts, 111–12
pistachios, 130–31
  Chili Chocolate Bark with Cherries and
    Pistachios, 125
pitas
  Argentinean Steak Sandwich, 73
  Persian Platter, 160
  Saag Paneer Sandwich, 74
  Shakshuka with Warmed Zaatar Pita, 13–14
Pizza Dough, 63
pizza dough (as ingredient)
  Breakfast Pizza with Potatoes and Tomato, 62
  Pear, Spinach and Blue Cheese Flatbread with
    Onion Jam, 115
  Thin-Crust Pizza with Balsamic-Glazed
    Tomatoes, Goat Cheese and Pesto, 113–14
plums, 246
  Roasted Cinnamon Plums, 244
Poached Coconut Fish, 186
Polenta, 217
pomegranate
  removing seeds, 49
  Grilled Chicken with Pomegranate Vinaigrette,
    207

Haddock Wraps with Crunchy Southwestern
 Salad, 179
On-the-Go Fruit Salad, 49
poppy seeds, 135
potatoes
 Breakfast Pizza with Potatoes and Tomato, 62
 Cream of Broccoli Soup, 100
 Morning Hash with Faux Poached Eggs, 19
 Scallop Niçoise Salad, 88
potatoes, sweet
 Breakfast Pizza with Potatoes and Tomato, 62
 Lamb Stew with Root Vegetables, 229
 Morning Hash with Faux Poached Eggs, 19
 South African Peanut Stew, 233
 Sweet Potato Waffles, 8
 Turkey Shepherd's Pie with Mushrooms,
  Spinach, Cranberries and Sweet Potatoes,
  209–10
prosciutto
 Breakfast Pizza with Potatoes and Tomato, 62
protein,
 and brain health, xviii
 healthy sources, xviii
 and hunger, 3
prunes, 60
pumpkin seeds (pepitas), 135
 Bet-You-Can't-Eat-Just-One Cereal Cookies, 61
 Cranberry Pumpkin Seed Crunchy Snack, 124
 Roasted Squash Soup with Roasted Pumpkin
  Seeds, 166

Q

quesadilla, 75
quinoa, 107
 Golden Quinoa with Raisins and Almonds, 109
 Warm Quinoa Salad over Bitter Greens, 277

R

rabbit
 Provençal-Style Rabbit with Polenta, 214–17
radishes
 Corn, Black Bean and Tomato Salad, 97
 Crunchy Southwestern Salad, 180
 Grilled Salmon with Green Salad and Apple
  Vinaigrette, 95
 Summer Rolls with Thai Dipping Sauce, 150
raisins, 59
 Bet-You-Can't-Eat-Just-One Cereal Cookies, 61
 Chicken with Rhubarb Chutney over Dark
  Greens, 83
 Cracked Wheat and Chayote or Zucchini Pilaf,
  213
 Golden Quinoa with Raisins and Almonds, 109
 Granola Bites with Figs and Dates, 57
rhubarb
 Chicken with Rhubarb Chutney over Dark
  Greens, 83
 Meringue Cups with Strawberry Rhubarb
  Topping, 265–66
Ribollita, 197
rice, 107

Roasted Tomato and Garlic Soup with Rice, 101
 Sushi Stacks, 153
 Wild Rice Salad, 108
Roasted Cinnamon Plums, 244
Roasted Edamame Bean Dip, 138
Roasted Fruit and Vegetable Stuffed Chicken, 206
Roasted Squash Soup with Roasted Pumpkin
 Seeds, 166
Roasted Tomato and Garlic Soup with Rice, 101
rutabaga, 85
 Lamb Stew with Root Vegetables, 229

S

Saag Paneer Sandwich, 74
salads
 Asian Greens and Rice Noodle Salad, 87
 Chickpea and Herb Salad with Warm Lemon
  Dressing, 93
 Corn, Black Bean and Tomato Salad, 97
 Curried Lentil and Wheatberry Salad with
  Mango, 105
 Grilled Salmon with Green Salad and Apple
  Vinaigrette, 95
 Peanut Coleslaw, 219
 Scallop Niçoise Salad, 88
 Shaved Green Salad with Spicy Grilled Shrimp,
  86
 Warm Quinoa Salad over Bitter Greens, 277
 Wild Rice Salad, 108
salmon, 158
 smoking, 96
 Asian Salmon Burgers, 187
 Grilled Salmon with Green Salad and Apple
  Vinaigrette, 95
 Poached Coconut Fish, 186
 Salmon Tartare with Wasabi-Spiked Avocado
  "Mousse," 147
 Sushi Stacks, 153
salmonella, 17
sandwiches
 Argentinian Steak Sandwich, 73
 Breakfast Burritos, 31
 Ceviche Lettuce Wraps, 98
 Saag Paneer Sandwich, 74
sauces/salsas
 Balsamic Drizzle, 162
 Blueberry Sauce, 9
 Chimichurri Sauce, 73
 Gremolata, 214–16
 Harissa, 204
 Pesto, 80
 Strawberry Rhubarb Topping, 265–66
 Two Tomato and Avocado Salsa, 184
seafood
 Coconut Shrimp, 161
 Scallop Niçoise Salad, 88
 Shaved Green Salad with Spicy Grilled Shrimp,
  86
 Thai Shrimp on Lemongrass Skewers, 148
Seaweed and Sesame Wonton Crackers, 133

seeds. *See* specific seeds

serotonin, 239–40

sesame seeds, 136

    Salmon Tartare with Wasabi-Spiked Avocado "Mousse," 147

    Seaweed and Sesame Wonton Crackers, 133

    Sushi Stacks, 153

    Toasted Sesame Green Beans, 189

Shakshuka with Warmed Zaatar Pita, 13–14

Shaved Green Salad with Spicy Grilled Shrimp, 86

shortening, 50

sleep effects of food, 69, 240–41

small plates, 165

snacks

    snack-time healthy swaps, 137

sodium, xix

    and brain health, xix

soups

    Black Bean Soup, 198

    Cream of Broccoli Soup, 100

    Hot and Sour Soup, 195

    Iberian Chickpea Soup, 199

    Ribollita, 197

    Roasted Squash Soup with Roasted Pumpkin Seeds, 166

    Roasted Tomato and Garlic Soup with Rice, 101

snow peas

    Asian Greens and Rice Noodle Salad, 87

    Marinated Tofu over Wilted Napa Cabbage and Vegetables, 193–94

sour cream, 12

South African Peanut Stew, 233

Southwestern-Spiced Nuts, 128

soy foods and menopause, 190–92

spices, 126

    and brain health, xiii–xiv

Spicy Honeyed Chicken Thighs with Peanut Coleslaw, 218–19

Spicy Smoky Succotash, 202

spinach

    Argentinean Steak Sandwich, 73

    Pear, Spinach and Blue Cheese Flatbread with Onion Jam, 115

    Ribollita, 197

    Saag Paneer Sandwich, 74

    South African Peanut Stew, 233

    Squash, Spinach and Onion Lasagna, 234–35

    Sweet Pepper and Barley Risotto Tart with Spinach and Pine Nuts, 111–12

    Turkey Shepherd's Pie with Mushrooms, Spinach, Cranberries and Sweet Potatoes, 209–10

Sponge Cake with Peaches Macerated in White Wine, 253–54

squash

    Cracked Wheat and Chayote or Zucchini Pilaf, 213

    Roasted Squash Soup with Roasted Pumpkin Seeds, 166

    Squash, Spinach and Onion Lasagna, 234–35

    Squash Squares with a Whole-Wheat Crust, 53

strawberries, 246

    Fruit Bruschetta, 28

    Meringue Cups with Strawberry Rhubarb Topping, 265–66

sugar, 255

sugar substitutes, 256

Summer Rolls with Thai Dipping Sauce, 150

Sun-Dried Tomato Vinaigrette, 92

sunflower seeds, 136

super foods, 23

supplements, 23–24

Sushi Stacks, 153

sweeteners, 255–56

Sweet Pepper and Barley Risotto Tart with Spinach and Pine Nuts, 111–12

Swiss chard

    Chicken with Rhubarb Chutney over Dark Greens, 83

    Morning Hash with Faux Poached Eggs, 19

    Overnight Swiss Chard, Sun-Dried Tomato and Mushroom Strata, 21

    Thyme-Roasted Beef Tenderloin with Three-Mushroom Ragout, 221–22

T

Tandoori-Spiced Lamb with Roasted Cauliflower Purée, 225–26

tapas, 165

tartine, 75

tea, 152

Thai Dipping Sauce, 151

Thai-Inspired Almond and Peanut Dipping Sauce, 120, 121, 140

Thai Shrimp on Lemongrass Skewers, 148

Thin-Crust Pizza with Balsamic-Glazed Tomatoes, Goat Cheese and Pesto, 113–14

Thyme-Roasted Beef Tenderloin with Three-Mushroom Ragout, 221–22

Toasted Sesame Green Beans, 189

tofu

    Hot and Sour Soup, 195

    Marinated Tofu over Wilted Napa Cabbage and Vegetables, 193–94

    Miso-Glazed Tofu with Toasted Sesame Green Beans, 188

    Roasted Edamame Bean Dip, 138

tomatoes

    Black Bean Soup, 198

    Breakfast Pizza with Potatoes and Tomato, 62

    Caramelized Onion and Tomato Phyllo Tart, 78

    Corn, Black Bean and Tomato Salad, 97

    Cracked Wheat and Chayote or Zucchini Pilaf, 213

    Four-Season Frittata, 77

    Halibut with Two Tomato and Avocado Salsa, 184

    Herbed Fish Stew, 181

    Mediterranean Stuffed Peppers, 102

Moroccan Chicken Stew with Couscous and
  Homemade Harissa, 203–4
Provençal-Style Rabbit with Polenta, 214–17
Ribollita, 197
Roasted Tomato and Garlic Soup with Rice, 101
Saag Paneer Sandwich, 74
Shakshuka with Warmed Zaatar Pita, 13–14
Spicy Smoky Succotash, 202
Thin-Crust Pizza with Balsamic-Glazed
  Tomatoes, Goat Cheese and Pesto, 113–14
tomatoes, sun-dried
  Flank Steak with Pine Nut, Herb and Currant
    Stuffing, 224
  Halibut with Two Tomato and Avocado Salsa,
    184
  Overnight Swiss Chard, Sun-Dried Tomato and
    Mushroom Strata, 21
  Sun-Dried Tomato Vinaigrette, 92
tortillas
  Breakfast Burritos, 31
  Haddock Wraps with Crunchy Southwestern
    Salad, 179
turkey. *See also* chicken
  Lemon Thyme Turkey with Spicy Smoky
    Succotash, 200
  Turkey Shepherd's Pie with Mushrooms,
    Spinach, Cranberries and Sweet Potatoes,
    209–10
turnips, 85

V

Vanilla Yogurt Cake with Marmalade Glaze, 267
vegetables. *See also* specific vegetables
  fresh vs. frozen, 271
  Grilled Salmon with Green Salad and Apple
    Vinaigrette, 95
  Lamb Stew with Root Vegetables, 229
  Marinated Tofu over Wilted Napa Cabbage and
    Vegetables, 193–94
vinaigrettes. *See* dress ings
vinegars, 152
vitamins, xv
  vitamin B$_{12}$, xiii, 240
  vitamin E, xii

W

waffles
  Sweet Potato Waffles, 8
walnuts, 130
  Banana Bread with Flaxseed and Wheat Germ,
    58
  Bet-You-Can't-Eat-Just-One Cereal Cookies, 61
  Bite-Size Nut Scones, 141

Farfalle with Walnuts, Goat Cheese, Arugula
    and Caramelized Apples, 230–32
  Figs with Walnuts, Gorgonzola and Balsamic
    Drizzle, 162
  Persian Platter, 160
  Pesto Orzo with Roasted Trout and Peas, 80–81
Warm Blueberry Brown Butter Cake Bites, 258–60
Warm Citrus Casserole, 257
Warm Quinoa Salad over Bitter Greens, 227
wheatberries, 107
  Curried Lentil and Wheatberry Salad with
    Mango, 105
wheat bran, 55
wheat germ, 55
  Banana Bread with Flaxseed and Wheat Germ,
    58
  The Most Delicious Nutritious Berry Crisp
    Ever, 248–49
Whitefish "Tartare," 159
Whole-Wheat Oatmeal Blueberry Pancakes with
  Ricotta Topping, 6
Wild Rice Salad, 108
Winter Fruit Compote, 34
wonton wrappers
  Chocolate Ravioli, 262
  Parmesan and Pepper Wonton Crackers, 134
  Salmon Tartare with Wasabi-Spiked Avocado
    "Mousse," 147
  Seaweed and Sesame Wonton Crackers, 133

Y

yogurt, 11–12
  how to thicken, 226
  turning Greek yogurt into regular yogurt, 266
  Crunchy Southwestern Salad, 180
  Granola Parfait, 29
  Haddock Wraps with Crunchy Southwestern
    Salad, 179
  Parliament Hill Smoothie, 36
  Vanilla Yogurt Cake with Marmalade Glaze,
    267

Z

zaatar, 14
  Shakshuka with Warmed Zaatar Pita, 13–14
zucchini
  Cracked Wheat and Chayote or Zucchini Pilaf,
    213
  Four-Season Frittata, 77
  Moroccan Chicken Stew with Couscous and
    Homemade Harissa, 203–4
  Roasted Fruit and Vegetable Stuffed Chicken,
    206